Trends and Variations in Fertility in the United States

Clyde V. Kiser / Wilson H. Grabill /

Arthur A. Campbell

1968 / HARVARD UNIVERSITY PRESS

Cambridge, Massachusetts

American Public Health Association
VITAL AND HEALTH STATISTICS MONOGRAPHS

Trends and Variations in
Fertility in the United States

PREFACE

Probably no subject is more relevant to the status of our future human resources than that of levels, trends, and differentials in the fertility[1] of women in the United States.

As one of the monographs in a series on vital and health statistics in the 1960 census period, this volume is concerned mainly with census and registration data on fertility for this period. However, both census and vital statistics for previous periods are used to analyze trends, a task facilitated by the existence of a monograph on fertility for the 1950 census period which two of the current authors helped to prepare.[2]

Like its predecessor, this monograph is based largely upon official data. Also like its predecessor, it traces trends and differentials in fertility by geographic area, color, nativity, rural-urban residence, and by several indices of socioeconomic status. However, the present monograph contains important materials not covered in the previous monograph, as the following brief content analysis indicates.

The first three chapters are innovations. Chapter 1 contains a brief description of current fertility levels and expected future trends in the world setting. Rates estimated by the United Nations are given for the more developed and the less developed areas as a whole and for regions within each area. Chapter 2 describes some of the medical and biological aspects of fertility. It includes materials from various sources on matters such as maternal and fetal mortality. The materials in Chapter 3 on fecundity and family planning, taken largely from private surveys and particularly from the Growth of American Families Study,[3] are especially valuable in that the differentials in family planning are impressively complementary to differentials in fertility by color, geographic region, urban-rural residence, and the various indices of socioeconomic status.

Chapter 4, which concerns color, nativity, and ethnic groups, was represented in the previous monograph. However, the present volume

[1]Following the definitions adopted by the Population Association of America shortly after its founding in 1931, the present authors use the term "fertility" to mean *actual birth performance*. They use the term "fecundity" to mean physiological *capacity* to participate in reproduction.

[2]Wilson H. Grabill, Clyde V. Kiser, and Pascal K. Whelpton, *The Fertility of American Women* (New York: John Wiley and Sons, 1958).

[3]Pascal K. Whelpton, Arthur A. Campbell, and John E. Patterson, *Fertility and Family Planning in the United States* (Princeton: Princeton University Press, 1966).

in this and other chapters gives special emphasis to fertility trends among nonwhite persons; it also provides some new data on the fertility of persons of Puerto Rican origin. Similarly, although Chapter 5, on residence, presents the trends for the conventional urban, rural nonfarm, and rural farm areas, it reflects the declining importance of the rural population and the increasing importance of the metropolitan area.

Chapter 6 analyzes fertility rates by migration status and also by region of birth in relation to region of residence. Some of these rates are used to explore hypotheses regarding the relative importance of origins and destinations in affecting fertility.

Chapter 7, dealing with marital characteristics, points up the differences by color in marital stability and presents an estimate of the fertility lost among white and nonwhite groups because of marital instability. It notes the greater sensitivity of nonwhite fertility to change in age at marriage than that of white fertility. The following and closely related Chapter 8, on illegitimacy, is another innovation. It discusses the nature and limitations of existing data, measures, and results.

Chapters 9 to 11 discuss trends and differentials in fertility in relation to education of the wife, occupation of the husband, and income and other indices of socioeconomic status. The first two indices are considered singly, and trends in the fertility differentials by each since 1940 or earlier are considered. Also presented for the first time is the analysis of data from the 1960 census on fertility of women classified on the basis of the multiple indices of occupation, education, and income of the husband. Another important innovation is the inclusion of data on fertility in relation to religion of the wife or couple. These data come partly from special surveys and partly from the data collected by the 1957 Current Population Survey.

Chapter 12, concerning fertility in relation to economic trends, is also new; it reviews some of the recent work on this subject and presents some data that were prepared at the Scripps Foundation for Research in Population Problems.

Chapter 13 gives data for birth and marriage cohorts. The cohort approach is also utilized in various other chapters; for instance, the tracing of fertility of given birth cohorts in 1940, 1950, and 1960 by color and educational attainments of the wife.

Appendix A describes the concepts and measures used in the cohort fertility analyses based on vital statistics, and Appendix B provides an analysis of the quality of data on children ever born in the 1960 census and in the Current Population Surveys.

Substantively, the monograph shows that among white persons the fertility differentials by region, urban-rural residence, and socioeconomic status have continued to decline. However, the differentials in fertility by color, and possibly also those by religion, have widened in recent years. The enhancement of the white-nonwhite differential in fertility is well documented by census data. The increase in the differential in fertility by religion is strongly suggested by several unofficial surveys, but it cannot be definitively documented because of the absence of official data on the subject for this country for dates other than 1957.

The 1970 census results concerning trends and differentials in fertility will be awaited with interest. The 1960 census probably marked the end of the postwar increases in the fertility of young women. These increases were marked by a narrowing of the fertility differentials among white women but not among the nonwhite. The average number of children ever born among women under 25 years old will probably be lower in 1970 than in 1960, at least for the white group. The oral pill became available to the public in 1960 and the intrauterine device somewhat later. It will be of interest to learn the impact of these new methods on the trends and differentials in fertility developing during the current decennial period.

Although the three authors of the present volume worked together a great deal, each had major responsibility for certain chapters. Grabill and Campbell shared responsibility for the chapters on medical and biological characteristics of births and on cohort fertility. Campbell was the chief author of the chapters on the control of fertility, illegitimacy, and economic trends. Grabill was mainly responsible for the chapters on residence and marital characteristics. Kiser undertook the chapters on color and ethnic groups, migration, education, occupation, and income. All participated in the preparation of the summary.

The authors wish first of all to pay their respects to the late Pascal K. Whelpton. His indirect contribution to the present volume was made not only by virtue of his co-authorship of the preceding volume, which was repeatedly used as a basis for comparison with 1960 results, but also by his role in the Growth of American Families Study, on which Chapter 3 of the present volume is based, and by his development of the cohort approach to the study of fertility, on which Chapter 13 is based. In a broader sense, his influence extends to all aspects of this volume—an influence arising from his long professional association and personal friendship with each of the three authors of this volume.

The authors are indebted to many organizations and individuals. They are indebted to Mr. Mortimer Spiegelman and to the Committee on Vital and Health Statistics Monographs of the Statistics Section of the American Public Health Association for the invitation to prepare the monograph. They wish to thank the Rockefeller Foundation and the Milbank Memorial Fund for supporting the preparatory work of the Committee and the United States Public Health Service for bearing the major costs of the monograph program. It should also be noted that the report on *Women by Number of Children Ever Born,* published by the Bureau of the Census from the 1960 census enumeration, was prepared largely with funds for the present monograph. Without that report, this monograph would not have been attempted. The authors are grateful to the Bureau of the Census and the National Center for Health Statistics for their heavy contributions toward collection, processing, and tabulation of data required in this and other monographs. The monograph benefited from the critical comments of Mr. Sam Shapiro on a draft of Chapter 2.

Clyde V. Kiser is grateful to Dr. Frank G. Boudreau for his interest in the project at its early stages and to Dr. Alexander Robertson for his interest at later stages. He wishes to thank Miss Myrna E. Frank for her invaluable assistance in processing the statistical materials and drafting the tables and charts in his chapters. He acknowledges with gratitude the work of Miss Betty Vorwald and Mrs. Sally F. Klepper in typing successive drafts of the manuscript.

Wilson H. Grabill is grateful to Dr. Paul C. Glick for especially helpful suggestions for the chapter on marital status, and to Dr. Conrad Taeuber and Dr. Maria Davidson, who reviewed several of the chapters. He wishes to thank Mrs. Joyce Phipps for her work on processing the statistical materials in his chapters. He acknowledges with thanks the work of Mrs. Lydia Walters, Miss Evelyn Hoffman, and Mrs. Leona Luck in clerical operations, typing of drafts of the manuscript for his parts, and typing of final tables for the whole monograph for photo-offset reproduction.

Arthur A. Campbell wishes to thank Mrs. Alice Clague for her help in assembling data on illegitimacy and for her suggestions concerning the analysis of these data. He also wishes to thank Mrs. Dorothy Herrell for typing drafts of the chapters for which he was primarily responsible.

It is hoped that this monograph will be useful to the growing number of research and civic groups concerned with problems of population dynamics in the United States and other countries, as well as for teaching and reference.

Clyde V. Kiser
Wilson H. Grabill
Arthur A. Campbell

January 1968

CONTENTS

TABLES

FIGURES

FOREWORD

Rapid advances in medical and allied sciences, changing patterns in medical care and public health programs, an increasingly health-conscious public, and the rising concern of voluntary agencies and government at all levels in meeting the health needs of the people necessitate constant evaluation of the country's health status. Such an evaluation, which is required not only for an appraisal of the current situation, but also to refine present goals and to gauge our progress toward them, depends largely upon a study of vital and health statistics records.

Opportunity to study mortality in depth emerges when a national census furnishes the requisite population data for the computation of death rates in demographic and geographic detail. Prior to the 1960 census of population there had been no comprehensive analysis of this kind. It seemed appropriate, therefore, to develop for intensive study a substantial body of death statistics for a three-year period centered around that census year.

A detailed examination of the country's health status must go beyond an examination of mortality statistics. Many conditions such as arthritis, rheumatism, and mental diseases are much more important as causes of morbidity than of mortality. Also, an examination of health status should not be based solely upon current findings, but should take into account trends and whatever pertinent evidence has been assembled through local surveys and from clinical experience.

The proposal for such an evaluation, to consist of a series of monographs, was made to the Statistics Section of the American Public Health Association in October 1958, and a Committee on Vital and Health Statistics Monographs was authorized. The members of this Committee and of the Editorial Advisory Subcommittee created later are:

Committee on Vital and Health Statistics Monographs

Mortimer Spiegelman, Chairman
Paul M. Densen, D. Sc.
Robert D. Grove, Ph.D.
Clyde V. Kiser, Ph.D.
Felix Moore
George Rosen, M.D., Ph.D.

William H. Stewart, M.D. (withdrew June 1964)
Conrad Taeuber, Ph.D.
Paul Webbink
Donald Young, Ph.D.

Editorial Advisory Subcommittee

Mortimer Spiegelman, Chairman
Duncan Clark, M.D.
E. Gurney Clark, M.D.
Jack Elinson, Ph.D.

Eliot Freidson, Ph.D. (withdrew
   February 1964)
Brian MacMahon, M.D., Ph.D.
Colin White, Ph.D.

The early history of this undertaking is described in a paper that was presented at the 1962 Annual Conference of the Milbank Memorial Fund.[1] The Committee on Vital and Health Statistics Monographs selected the topics to be included in the series and also suggested candidates for authorship. The frame of reference was extended by the Committee to include other topics in vital and health statistics than mortality and morbidity, namely fertility, marriage, and divorce. Conferences were held with authors to establish general guidelines for the preparation of the manuscripts.

Support for this undertaking in its preliminary stages was received from the Rockefeller Foundation, the Milbank Memorial Fund, and the Health Information Foundation. Major support for the required tabulations, for writing and editorial work, and for the related research of the monograph authors was provided by the United States Public Health Service (Research Grant CH 00075, formerly GM 08262). Acknowledgment should also be made to the Metropolitan Life Insurance Company for the facilities and time that were made available to Mr. Spiegelman, now retired from its service, who proposed and administered the undertaking and served as general editor. The National Center for Health Statistics, under the supervision of Dr. Grove and Miss Alice M. Hetzel, undertook the sizable tasks of planning and carrying out the extensive mortality tabulations for the period 1959-1961. Dr. Taeuber arranged for the cooperation of the Bureau of the Census at all stages of the project in many ways, principally by furnishing the required population data used in computing death rates and by undertaking a large number of varied special tabulations. As the sponsor of the project, the American Public Health Association furnished assistance through Dr. Thomas R. Hood, its Deputy Executive Director.

---

[1]Mortimer Spiegelman, "The Organization of the Vital and Health Statistics Monograph Program," *Emerging Techniques in Population Research (Proceedings of the 1962 Annual Conference of the Milbank Memorial Fund;* New York: Milbank Memorial Fund, 1963), p. 230. See also Mortimer Spiegelman, "The Demographic Viewpoint in the Vital and Health Statistics Monographs Project of the American Public Health Association," *Demography,* vol. 3, No. 2 (1966), p. 574.

Because of the great variety of topics selected for monograph treatment, authors were given an essentially free hand to develop their manuscripts as they desired. Accordingly, the authors of the individual monographs bear the full responsibility for their manuscripts, and their opinions and statements do not necessarily represent the viewpoints of the American Public Health Association or of the agencies with which they are affiliated.

Berwyn F. Mattison, M.D.
Executive Director
American Public Health Association

NOTES ON TABLES

1. Regarding 1959-61 mortality data:
   a. Deaths relate to those occurring in the United States (including Alaska and Hawaii);
   b. Deaths are classified by place of residence (if pertinent);
   c. Fetal deaths are excluded;
   d. Deaths of unknown age, marital status, nativity, or other characteristics have not been distributed into the known categories, but are included in their totals;
   e. Deaths were classified by cause according to the *Seventh Revision of the International Statistical Classification of Diseases, Injuries, and Causes of Death* (Geneva: World Health Organization, 1957);
   f. All death rates are average annual rates per 100,000 population in the category specified, as recorded in the United States census of April 1, 1960;
   g. Age-adjusted rates were computed by the direct method using the age distribution of the total United States population in the census of April 1, 1940 as a standard.[1]
2. Symbols used in tables of data:
   - - - Data not available;
   . . . Category not applicable;
   - Quantity zero;
   0.0 Quantity more than zero but less than 0.05;
   * Figure does not meet the standard of reliability of precision:
       a) Rate or ratio based on less than 20 deaths;
       b) Percentage or median based on less than 100 deaths;
       c) Age-adjusted rate computed from age-specific rates where more than half of the rates were based on frequencies of less than 20 deaths.
3. Geographic classification:[2]
   a. Standard Metropolitan Statistical Areas (SMSA's): except in the New England States, "an SMSA is a county or a group of contiguous counties which contains at least one city of 50,000 inhabitants or more or 'twin cities' with a combined population of at least 50,000 in the 1960 census. In addition, contiguous counties are included in an SMSA if, according to specified criteria, they are (a) essentially metropolitan in character and (b) socially and economically integrated with the central city or cities."

---

[1] Mortimer Spiegelman and H.H. Marks, "Empirical Testing of Standards for the Age Adjustment of Death Rates by the Direct Method," *Human Biology*, 38:280 (September 1966).

[2] National Center for Health Statistics, *Vital Statistics of the United States, 1960*, vol. II, *Mortality*, Part A, sec. 7, p. 8.

In New England, the Division of Vital Statistics of the National Center for Health Statistics uses, instead of the definition just cited, Metropolitan State Economic Areas (MSEA's) established by the Bureau of the Census, which are made up of county units.

b. Metropolitan and nonmetropolitan: "Counties which are included in SMSA's or, in New England, MSEA's are called metropolitan counties; all other counties are classified as nonmetropolitan."

c. Metropolitan counties may be separated into those containing at least one central city of 50,000 inhabitants or more or twin cities as specified previously, and into metropolitan counties without a central city.

4. Sources:

In addition to any sources specified in the figures, text tables, and appendix tables, the deaths and death rates for the period 1959-61 are derived from special tabulations made at the National Center for Health Statistics, Public Health Service, U. S. Department of Health, Education, and Welfare, for the American Public Health Association.

Trends and Variations in Fertility in the United States

1 / The World Setting

Although this volume is concerned with fertility trends and differentials in the United States, it may be well here to describe briefly the world setting of this subject. The countries of the world are frequently dichotomized as those of low fertility and those of high fertility. There are exceptions, but the countries of low fertility tend to be the more developed countries, and the countries of high fertility tend to be the less developed countries. Again with certain important exceptions, the modernized countries of low fertility are those of Europe, North America, and Oceania and the less developed countries of high fertility are those of Asia, Africa, and Latin America.[1]

Prior to World War II population growth in the less developed countries was much slower than today because the high birth rates were offset by high death rates. Population growth in the modernized countries was also much slower than today because both birth and death rates were low. Indeed, there was much concern about the "small family" system that prevailed among the urban white-collar workers in the modern Western nations.

Since World War II there has been rapid population growth throughout the world. This has resulted from the dramatic decline in death rates in the less developed areas and from a postwar increase in birth rates over a decade or more in the modernized countries.

The population growth in the underdeveloped areas has become a matter of increasing concern to thoughtful persons of all religions and ideologies. The decline in death rates in underdeveloped areas has been the result of the application of medical discoveries to large populations through intensive public health programs, of a wave of humanitarian interest in the underprivileged nations of the world, and of international development programs of the United Nations and its specialized agencies and other organizations. The decline gave evidence that reductions in mortality, particularly the saving of infant lives, may now be attained easily, at relatively small expense, but without substantial improvement in levels of living of the population.

The great growth of population and the gloomy predictions for future growth have stimulated research in the physiology of reproduction and in simple methods of fertility control. The oral pill and the intrauterine device are believed by some to provide grounds for optimism that population growth will be controlled within two or three decades. The first Pan American Assembly on Population, held in Cali, Colombia, August 11-14, 1965,[2] and the International Conference on Family Planning Projects, held in Geneva, Switzerland, August 23-27, 1965,[3] were impressive for their indication of indigenous interest in Latin America and Asia in both research and action programs in human reproduction. Furthermore, both types of programs are frequently carried out under medical auspices in these areas. For instance, medical and public health groups in Santiago, Chile, have sponsored clinical and community research on abortion, reproductive processes, and the prevalence and effectiveness of various types of contraceptives. The opposition of the Catholic Church to the use of certain techniques of contraception may be strong in most of Latin America, but the Church has manifested a great concern over the health hazards of provoked abortion.

In Asia, Japan has recently demonstrated the possibility of cutting a birth rate in half within a decade, largely by means of making abortion freely available. In this case abortions are legal, and for the most part, medically attended. However, even where abortions are not legal—as in Latin America—their incidence is high. This fact, and the frequent resort to sterilization in countries like Puerto Rico, indicate the lengths to which families are willing to go to avoid excessive childbearing.

To put the United States in the setting of the modernized world, one might say that the postwar level of fertility in the United States was among the highest. Virtually all modernized countries experienced increases in marriage and fertility rates after the war. The increases were more sustained in the United States and Canada than in Europe. Birth rates have been reduced drastically in Hungary, Greece, and Italy. They have been declining in the United States from 1957 to the time of this writing. There are at least suggestive indications that this will eventually involve some decline in completed fertility for cohorts.[4]

The United States has experienced, as have other modern countries, a contraction of differences in fertility by urban-rural residence and by socioeconomic status.[5] It shares with others a sharp and persistent difference in fertility according to labor force status of women, and also the difficulty of ascertaining how much of this is selective and how much is determinative. Fertility rates tend to be relatively low among married women in the labor force. Some women may work because they have no young children. Others may refrain from having children, or more children, because they want to work.

A striking enhancement of the fertility differentials by color in the United States may have its counterpart in other countries with bi-racial populations, but the data for other countries are not adequate for definitive documentation.

Special studies have suggested that fertility differentials by religion within the United States have also widened; and at least a "persist-ence" of important fertility differentials by religion has been found in the Netherlands.[6]

A fairly optimistic prediction for relatively low crude birth rates was made in 1963 and published in 1966 by the United Nations.[7] Projections were prepared on the basis of several assumptions; those presented in Table 1.1, adapted from the report, are "medium" estimates.

For the world as a whole, the medium estimate was 32.9 for the period 1965-70. This estimate declines continuously for the remainder of the century, reaching 25.7 for the period 1995-2000.

The postulation of a decline in the crude birth rate for the world as a whole is based upon the assumption that a decline in the high birth rates of the less developed countries will occur. The relatively low rates estimated for the more developed areas as a whole remain on the average at the 18-19 level from 1965 to 2000. For the less developed areas as a whole, the medium estimates are 39.4 for the period 1965-70 and 28.0 for the period 1995-2000.

With respect to specific regions, the rates are conspicuously low for Japan and Europe for the years 1965-70 and conspicuously high for South Asia, Africa, Tropical South America, Middle America (mainland), and Melanesia. However, the projected decline for South Asia is well marked, from about 42 in 1965-70 to about 27 in 1995-2000. The medium estimate for 1995-2000 is only 13.2 for Japan and 15.9 for Europe. The 1965-70 rates are 15.6 for Japan and 16.6 for Europe.

In making the medium estimates for Northern America, "the crude birth and death rates in the original population projection for the United States were taken as calculated by the United States Bureau of the Census, an adjustment being made to allow for somewhat different birth and death rates in Canada."[8] Apparently, these cal-culations are the "Series C" projections prepared by the Bureau of the Census,[9] which are given for single years 1963-86. Five-year averages yield medium estimates for the United States alone of 20.1

Table 1.1   "Medium" estimates of crude birth rates per 1,000
population for the world, more and less developed
areas, and major regions: 1965-2000

Area	1965-70	1975-80	1985-90	1995-2000
World total[a]	32.9	31.6	28.5	25.7
More developed	18.5	19.4	19.0	18.3
Less developed[a]	39.4	36.5	31.8	28.0
East Asia[b]	30.7	27.3	22.9	19.9
Mainland region[c]	32.3	28.2	23.8	20.4
Japan	15.6	16.8	13.6	13.2
Other East Asia[d]	37.5	31.8	26.5	23.3
South Asia[e]	42.1	38.6	32.3	26.9
Europe	16.6	16.4	16.4	15.9
U.S.S.R.	19.4	19.9	20.7	19.3
Africa	45.4	44.6	42.2	40.0
North America[f]	21.3	23.6	23.0	22.2
Latin America	39.0	37.2	33.6	30.3
Tropical South America	41.2	38.8	35.2	31.0
Middle America (mainland)	42.8	40.8	36.9	32.6
Temperate South America	25.5	23.5	21.2	21.0
Caribbean	38.2	36.1	32.4	28.4
Oceania[g]	24.4	25.5	25.4	25.3
Australia and New Zealand	21.5	22.8	22.6	22.1
Melanesia[h]	40.7	41.4	40.9	41.1

Source: Adapted from United Nations, "World Population
Prospects as Assessed in 1963," Population Studies, No. 41, 1966,
Table 7.1, p. 34.

[a]Not including areas listed in footnotes b, e, and g.

[b]Not including Hong Kong, Mongolia, Macao, and Ryukyu Islands.

[c]Mainland China only.

[d]Not including Ryukyu Islands.

[e]Not including Israel and Cyprus.

[f]Corresponding to immigration assumption made in original
projections.

[g]Not including Polynesia and Micronesia.

[h]Assumed same as Middle Africa.

for the years 1965-70 and 22.4 for 1975-80. These are 1.2 points below the estimates for North America as a whole, and presumably a difference of this magnitude would apply to the later periods considered.

The estimates of relative stability of birth rates for most of the more developed regions and of decline of the rates for the less developed areas, of course, are open to question. Whether there will be an increase or a decrease in the crude birth rate of the more developed countries depends a great deal on the nature of economic and political conditions.

The projected decline of 11.4 points in the crude birth rate of the less developed areas may give comfort to those who are concerned about the population explosion. It should be noted, however, that the medium estimates of death rates for these areas are 17.3 for 1965-70 and 9.2 for 1995-2000, showing a decline in the death rates of 8.1 points over this period. Hence the projected decline in the crude rate of natural increase is only 3 points, i.e. from 22.1 in 1965-70 to 18.8 in 1995-2000.

Other recent publications of the United Nations have pointed out that fertility levels distinguish the more developed countries from the less developed countries more sharply than any other available and readily measurable criterion.[10]

It is therefore clear that the primary differential in fertility in the world setting is that between the more developed and the less developed areas. The two groups of countries may also differ with respect to which stage of the trend in fertility differentials they occupy. Stated briefly, within the more developed areas there appears now to be a narrowing of previously wide fertility differentials by urban-rural residence, educational attainment, and socioeconomic status. Presumably, the differentials are now diminishing in these areas because family planning is practiced rather widely in all elements of the population.

In many of the less developed areas, in contrast, fertility differentials by socioeconomic status have scarcely emerged, partly because of the virtual absence of family planning at any level of society and partly because of the lack of economic differentiation of the population. Appreciable differentials in fertility in the less developed areas are frequently found by religion and sometimes by urban-rural residence and socioeconomic status. The avidity of the search for the emergence of differentials in fertility in the less developed countries is due to the common belief that such an emergence precedes a decline in fertility.

It is hoped that the analysis in this volume of trends and differentials in fertility in the United States may be of some use to demographers throughout the world.

This chapter presents statistical data on certain medical and biological aspects of fertility. Chapter 3 also includes material of this kind, but the data in that chapter relate primarily to factors influencing the probability of conception. The present chapter is about the risks of maternal and fetal death, the relation of fertility to longevity, the extent to which deliveries are attended by physicians, and the fertility of certain groups characterized by special medical problems.

Maternal Mortality

A shining chapter in the history of public health is the reduction in maternal mortality made in the present century, especially since 1930-34.[1] Between the years 1930-34 and 1963, the maternal mortality rate per 100,000 live births was reduced by 94 percent, from 636 to 36 (Table 2.1). The foundation for this reduction was laid down over a period of many years; significant developments include the first general use of obstetric forceps in the seventeenth century (this invention was held as a trade secret for over a century by the

Table 2.1   Maternal mortality rates by color: United States, selected years, 1915-63

(Rates per 100,000 live births. Deaths are classified according to the International Lists used at the time)

Year	Total	White	Nonwhite
1963	35.8	24.0	96.9
1962	35.2	23.8	95.9
1961	36.9	24.9	101.3
1960	37.1	26.0	97.9
1955	47.0	32.8	130.3
1950	83.3	61.1	221.6
1945	207.2	172.1	454.8
1940	376.0	319.8	773.5
1935-39[a]	493.9	439.9	875.5
1930-34[a]	636.0	575.4	1,080.7
1915-19[a]	727.9	700.3	1,253.5

Source: National Center for Health Statistics, Vital Statistics of the United States: 1963, Vol. II, Mortality, Part A, Table 1-14.

[a]Birth-Registration States.

inventor's heirs) and the use of antiseptics and attention to general asepsis in the nineteenth century, following discoveries by Semmelweis, Holmes, Lemaire, and Lister. In the early part of the present century hospital standards of sanitation were much improved; medical research into pregnancy and its complications was under way; advances were made in nutrition, obstetrical surgery, and anesthesia; postgraduate training and certification of specialists in obstetrics was begun; and medical schools began to teach general practitioners the need for prenatal care. However, as of 1915, about 40 percent of confinements were still being attended by midwives.[2] As the public became better informed about childbirth, prenatal care became more and more common and the proportion of confinements attended by physicians (especially in hospitals) increased. Still later, the improvement accelerated with the introduction of sulfas, penicillin, and the broad-spectrum antibiotics. In contrast to the rapid improvement up to the late 1950's, there was little improvement between that time and 1963 (the latest year for which published data were available). The recent leveling off in the rate of maternal mortality, as shown by the data in Table 2.1, does not mean that an irreducible minimum has been reached. It is noteworthy that several states had rates in the period 1961-63 that were far below those shown for the nation as a whole.

In 1963 only 1,466 maternal deaths were reported, as compared with 4,098,020 live births. That number does not include all deaths of women before, during, or after childbirth but only those whose death certificates designated maternal causes for the deaths.

Ideally, the maternal death rate should be related to the number of pregnancies rather than to the number of live births. If it is assumed, for purposes of illustration, that 15 percent of pregnancies do not result in a live birth, and that 2 percent of live births reflect plural deliveries, then for every 100,000 live births there are roughly 116,500 pregnancies. On that basis, a maternal death rate of 36 per 100,000 live births would equal about 31 maternal deaths per 100,000 pregnancies, which in turn would imply that 99,969 out of 100,000 women either survive the hazards of pregnancy or else die from some other reported cause than maternal mortality. Pregnancy may lower the death rate for nonmaternal causes in the case of some women insofar as they receive better medical care during pregnancy than at other times, and it may increase the death rate in the case of others insofar as it creates or aggravates an underlying health condition.

Of the 1,466 maternal deaths reported in 1963, 797 were of white women and 619 of nonwhite women. There were 280 reported deaths from toxemias of pregnancy and the postpartum period, 280 from abortions (both spontaneous and induced), 248 from hemorrhage (bleeding), 164 from sepsis (infection), 96 from ectopic pregnancies, and 398 from other complications of pregnancy, childbirth, and the puerperium, such as birth injuries.[3] Many of these conditions could be reduced with proper care before, during, and after birth, but not all women receive such care. It should also be noted that maternal deaths are few as compared with the much larger number of women who have one complication or another during pregnancy but do not die. Estimates of the annual number of spontaneous and induced abortions run into the high hundreds of thousands, but reliable figures are not available.

Maternal mortality is lowest at age 20-24 and increases with age. The rates decrease with order of birth up to the third and then rise, being very high for women who have had eight or more pregnancies. To some extent, the high maternal mortality among women who have had many children reflects a lack of prenatal care among the poor.[4]

Most women receive medical care at the time of live birth, and many also receive such care at other times during pregnancies. In 1963, 99.1 percent of white (live) births occurred in hospitals, 0.5 percent were attended by a physician not in a hospital, and 0.4 percent were attended by a midwife, other person, or person not specified. For nonwhite births, the corresponding figures were 87.9 percent, 2.4 percent, and 9.7 percent, respectively.

Women consult obstetricians and gynecologists for reasons other than pregnancy, as for female disorders and for prescription of contraceptives. It may be of interest to note that according to health survey interviews made between July and September 1963, for a nationwide probability sample of the civilian noninstitutional population, 8 million women aged 15 and over consulted specialists in obstetrics and gynecology in the preceding 12-month period.[5] For every live birth, there were at least two women who consulted a specialist. These comprised 17.1 percent of women 15 and over with family income of $7,000 or more, 14.4 percent of those with a family income of $4,000-$6,999, 8.1 percent with a family income of $2,000-$3,999, and 3.5 percent with a family income under $2,000. Women with low income may see a physician who is not a specialist more often than other women, but these data do indicate that people with money obtain more specialized care. The average number of visits per person consulting an obstetrician or gynecologist was 3.9 per year; this is well below the average that would arise from pregnancy considerations per se. According to health interview survey data for the period from July 1963 to June 1964, women made 35,403,000 physician visits (including those to general practitioners) for purposes of prenatal and postnatal care.[6] The ratio of the 35,403,000 physician visits reported in the health survey to 4,100,000 live births reported by vital statistics yields an understated average of 8.6 visits per mother. The average is understated for pregnant women who are under medical care because not all mothers receive prenatal and postnatal care.

The Relation Between Fertility and Longevity

It is known that death rates are somewhat higher, age for age, among single, widowed, and divorced persons than among married persons. The differences by marital status are much greater for men than for women. Marriages probably are somewhat selective of healthy lives. Also, married persons more often than single, widowed, and divorced persons may have someone to look after them when they are sick or may be more apt to have a sensible diet, regular hours, and so forth. Given favorable conditions, single persons do not necessarily have higher death rates than married persons. For example, there is evidence that Roman Catholic monks and nuns have lower age-specific death rates than prevail in the general population.[7] On a priori grounds it could be argued that death rates should tend to be higher among women who have borne many children than among women who have borne few children, because the women with many children tend to be in the lower socioeconomic groups, which are less able to afford adequate diet and medical care than the upper socioeconomic groups. That argument, although seemingly plausible, may be incorrect, as is noted below.

Using data for Australia for about 195,000 women dying between 1909 and 1928, with some but perhaps insufficient control on age at marriage, Dorn and McDowell found a strong positive correlation between the average number of children ever born and age at death after the end of the childbearing ages.[8] Using genealogical records for 2,614 women born before 1824, Freeman concluded that there was at best only a small positive correlation between length of life after age 45 and the number of offspring the women had produced.[9] Which of these two somewhat conflicting findings is correct? Perhaps census data can be used to throw new light on the issue of whether or not fertility is strongly related to longevity, although the data are for surviving women rather than for women who have died, and the data for successive censuses are affected by sampling variability, migration, and occasional errors of reporting. (Differences in reporting of race, for example, may arise when the enumerator determines race by observation, as in the 1940 census, and where the person himself reports race in self-enumeration procedures, as in the 1960 census; also, age is approximated for a small percentage of people.)

Table 2.2 presents data for white and nonwhite women in specified age cohorts of completed fertility. Most of the data are from the censuses of 1940 and 1960, because data on children ever born were not tabulated from the 1950 census for women over age 59 (for reasons of economy). Perhaps some readers would prefer comparisons for native white and Negro women instead of white and nonwhite women, but 1960 census data for the former are available only by broad groupings of advanced ages: 55-64 and 65 and over. The fertility rates shown for 1940 are those originally published in the 1940 census reports and are not strictly comparable with those from later censuses, in which estimates were made for women with no report on children ever born; similar adjustments are not available for women of older age.

It may be determined from the table (by computation, not shown) that among white women there is little difference between the proportions of single women and of women ever married surviving from age 45-49 in 1940 to age 65-69 in 1960 and from age 60-64 in 1940 to age 80-84 in 1960. There is also little change in the fertility of the women. Among nonwhite women, however, there is evidence that relatively fewer single women than women ever married survive to advanced ages. Also, there is a marked tendency for nonwhite women surviving to advanced ages to be more fertile than those enumerated earlier at a younger age. For nonwhite persons, then, there appears to be some relation between fertility and longevity. Could this perhaps be because of healthier living conditions on farms than in nonfarm areas?

Further, but more limited, evidence of the relationship between fertility and longevity appears in data for native white women, shown in Table 2.3. Here, women with five or more children ever born appear to survive in larger proportion than those with fewer than

Table 2.2 Women in specified birth cohorts of completed fertility, 1940, and survivors to 1960, by marital status and number of children ever born per 1,000 women: United States

Color, age, and census	Women (thousands)			Children ever born per 1,000 women		
	Total	Single	Ever married	Total women	Women ever married	Mothers ever married
WHITE						
45-49, 1940	3,651	326	3,325	2,719[a]	3,020[a]	3,544[a]
55-59, 1950	3,307	264	3,043	2,689	2,922	3,517
65-69, 1960	3,025	253	2,772	2,684	2,929	3,544
60-64, 1940	2,165	207	1,958	3,047	3,413	4,015
80-84, 1960	824	83	742	3,090	3,435	4,057
NONWHITE						
45-49, 1940	350	18	332	3,185[a]	3,385[a]	4,308[a]
55-59, 1950	260	10	250	3,214	3,344	4,403
65-69, 1960	270	11	259	3,292	3,432	4,475
60-64, 1940	143	7	136	3,954	4,199	4,906
80-84, 1960	53	2	52	4,224	4,374	5,161

Source: U.S. Bureau of the Census, 1940 Census of Population, Differential Fertility, 1940 and 1910—Fertility for States and Large Cities, Table 3; 1950 Census of Population, Fertility, P-E, No. 5C, Table 1; and 1960 Census of Population, Women by Number of Children Ever Born, PC(2)-3A, Tables 4 and 5.

[a]Rates shown for 1940 are those originally published; adjusted rates which include estimates of children for women with no report on children ever born are available for women 45-49 but not for those 60-64 in 1940. The following adjusted rates are from 1940 data presented in Tables 4 and 5 of the 1950 census report on Fertility.

Color of woman	Children ever born per 1,000 women 45-49 years old, 1940 (adjusted)		
	Total women	Women ever married	Mothers ever married
White	2,704	2,969	3,539
Nonwhite	3,120	3,288	4,291

Table 2.3   Proportion of native white women 45–54 years old in 1950
surviving to 1960, by number of children ever born: United
States

Children ever born	Number (thousands)		Percent surviving, 1950–60
	45–54, 1950	55–64, 1960	
Total women	6,648	6,346	95.5
Single	573	548	95.6
Ever married	6,076	5,798	95.4
Childless ever married	1,173	1,155	98.5
1 child ever born	1,188	1,093	92.0
2 children	1,314	1,243	94.6
3 children	863	825	95.6
4 children	556	523	94.0
5 and 6 children	546	534	97.7
7 or more	436	425	97.6
Children ever born per 1,000 total women	2,323	2,324	...

Source: U.S. Bureau of the Census, 1950 Census of Population,
Fertility, P-E, No. 5C, Table 12, and 1960 Census of Population, Women
By Number of Children Ever Born, PC(2)-3A, Table 8.

five children. Again, farm-nonfarm background may possibly be involved to some degree. An exception appears for childless women
ever married, but this may be more apparent than real. It is quite
possible that some of the women reported in 1950 as having one
child ever born were misreported as childless in the 1960 census;
the percentages surviving to 1960 for childless women and for one-
child women, if averaged, would match those for other categories
instead of being respectively higher and lower.

Fetal Mortality

Definition and Measurement. The definition of a fetal death recom-
mended by the World Health Organization is "death prior to the
complete expulsion or extraction from its mother of a product of
conception, irrespective of the duration of pregnancy."[10] This definition includes all fetal losses that might otherwise be classified as
abortions (induced or spontaneous), miscarriages, or stillbirths.

The basic problem in measuring the level of fetal mortality is the difficulty in recognizing a fetal death during the early months of gestation. It is believed that many early fetal deaths are undetected. Research by Hertig and Rock suggests that fetal mortality is very high in the first month of pregnancy and that it gradually decreases as gestation proceeds.[11]

However, there is an alternative view—that the risk of fetal death rises to a peak at about ten weeks of gestation and then declines. On the basis of information derived from medical records for patients, a large majority of whom began prenatal care early in pregnancy, Shapiro, Jones, and Densen have presented evidence on the level of fetal mortality at various gestational ages for 6,844 pregnancies, including 970 fetal deaths, observed in 1958 and 1959 by doctors participating in the Health Insurance Plan of Greater New York.[12] The authors calculated that the risk of fetal death reached a major peak at 10 weeks of gestation, then declined to very low levels, and rose slightly around 40 weeks of gestation. Although they acknowledged that the observed risks of fetal death in the early weeks of gestation are understatements, they note that "there are some circumstances that suggest that they may not be gross understatements. Potter points out that the 'embryonic sac develops normally only where it contains an embryo, but it may actually grow for about three months with a very abnormal embryo or none at all,' and then concludes that 'more abortions occur at 10 to 14 weeks than at any other time.' The last is, of course, a speculation since there are no data free of the problems discussed."[13]

Our idea of how high the level of fetal mortality actually is, then, depends to a major extent on our view of the shape of the curve of mortality risks in the early months of gestation. If this curve starts at a very high point shortly after conception and gradually descends, then the risk of fetal loss is very high. On the basis of a hypothetical curve of this kind, for example, Erhardt has estimated a fetal death rate of 295 deaths per 1,000 pregnancies."[14] If, however, the curve starts at a relatively low point shortly after conception, rises to a peak at about 10 weeks, and then descends, the risk of fetal loss is much lower. We do not yet have the evidence needed to choose either of these alternatives with confidence, so we must limit the present discussion to observed levels of fetal mortality.

The study by Shapiro, Jones, and Densen showed a fetal death rate of 142 fetal deaths per 1,000 pregnancies.[15] A series of 2,713 pregnancy histories collected in the Growth of American Families

Study in 1955 from white married women 18-39 years old yielded a fetal death rate of 129.[16] Interviews with similar women in 1960 indicated a fetal death rate of 131.[17] This is about the same as the rate observed in the Indianapolis Fertility Study of 1941.[18] A number of studies reviewed by the investigators in the Princeton Fertility Study suggested that a rate of about 120 would be a reasonable order of magnitude for the contemporary white metropolitan population of the United States.[19]

Data from the registration of fetal deaths generally yield much lower estimates. In the United States only ten registration areas (nine states and one city) require the registration of all fetal deaths, regardless of the gestational age at which the death occurs.[20] Other registration areas require the reporting of only those fetal deaths occurring after varying periods of gestation, most commonly 20 weeks. In the ten areas requiring complete reporting, the fetal death rate was 67 fetal deaths per 1,000 pregnancies in 1963, or about half the value of estimates based on data from interview surveys. The ten areas showed great variation in fetal death rates; the lowest was for Maine (17 per 1,000), and the highest was for New York City (117 per 1,000). These differences do not reflect actual differences in fetal mortality, but differences in the degree of completeness of reporting fetal deaths.

Although the level of fetal mortality in the United States has not been accurately determined, it is at least 12 to 14 percent of all pregnancies. This means that many women will have had a fetal death by the end of the reproductive period. In the 1955 Growth of American Families Study 21 percent of the wives 18-39 years old reported one or more fetal deaths. Among those who had ever been pregnant, the proportion was 25 percent. Among those who had been pregnant four times, almost half reported a fetal death; among those who had been pregnant six or more times, slightly over 60 percent reported a fetal death.[21] It is apparent from these figures that fetal loss is a fairly common experience among women in the reproductive years of life.

Trends in Fetal Mortality. The downward trend in fetal mortality shown in Fig. 2.1 represents an understatement of the actual reduction of fetal loss in the United States since the 1920's. All of the changes that have occurred in the registration of fetal deaths have widened the coverage of gestational ages included and improved the registration of recognized fetal deaths. In spite of these changes, observed fetal mortality rates have declined greatly, which means that actual fetal mortality has fallen by a very considerable amount. Just how great the decline has been, however, is unknown.

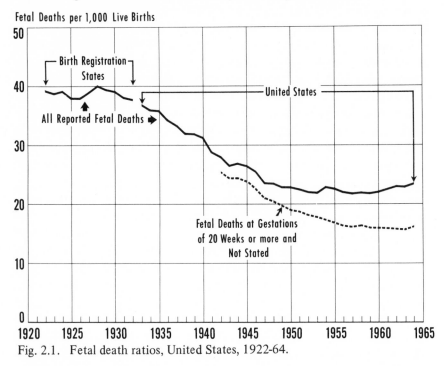

Fig. 2.1. Fetal death ratios, United States, 1922-64.

The measures presented in Fig. 2.1 are ratios of fetal deaths to live births. These measures are used because the under-registration of fetal deaths makes it impossible to estimate accurately the total number of pregnancies to use as a basis for a fetal death rate (fetal deaths per 1,000 pregnancies).

Of particular interest is the trend from 1942 to 1964 in the fetal death ratios for fetal deaths occurring after 20 weeks of gestation. These are more completely registered than earlier fetal deaths because they are more easily recognized. As Fig. 2.1 shows, the decline in fetal death ratios for gestational ages of 20 weeks or more has been faster than for earlier fetal deaths. The widening gap between the two curves is evidently due to the improved registration of earlier fetal deaths.

The fetal death ratio for gestational ages of 20 weeks or more was 16.4 in 1964. This represents an understatement of the actual situation, but the degree of understatement is difficult to determine. The data studied by Shapiro, Jones, and Densen showed a fetal mortality rate for gestational ages of 20 weeks or more of 19.4 fetal deaths per 1,000 pregnancies.[22] This corresponds to a fetal death ratio of 22.6 fetal deaths per 1,000 live births. The 1964 ratio for the United States is 27 percent below this level. Assuming that the actual ratio for the United States is higher than for the enrollees in the Health Insurance Plan of Greater New York (H.I.P.), the group studied by Shapiro and his associates, we may say with some assurance that fetal deaths at gestational ages of 20 weeks or more are under-registered by at least one-third in the United States.

The ten registration areas that require the registration of all fetal deaths, regardless of gestational age, show a higher fetal death ratio for deaths after 20 weeks of gestation than do those areas requiring the registration of only those fetal deaths occurring at the later gestational ages. The ten areas as a group showed a ratio of 19.6 fetal deaths per 1,000 live births in 1963, which was well above the ratio of 15.8 for the entire United States in that year. The highest ratio was observed for New York City—25.8 fetal deaths at gestational ages 20 weeks or more per 1,000 live births.

Correlates of Fetal Mortality. The risk of fetal death is not uniform. As we have seen in the preceding discussion, fetal mortality varies with time; it also varies with certain characteristics of the mother and the fetus. In spite of the many measurement problems involved in estimating fetal mortality, certain relations stand out clearly. A few of these are described below.

1. Color. Fetal mortality rates for the nonwhite population of the United States are more than twice as high as for the white population. In 1963 the ratio of all registered fetal deaths to live births was 19.9 per 1,000 for the white group and 40.2 for the nonwhite. The ratios for gestational ages 20 weeks or more were 13.7 and 26.7 for the white and nonwhite categories, respectively. Assuming that under-registration of nonwhite fetal deaths is greater than for white fetal deaths, these comparisons suggest that the risk of a fetal death is much greater for a nonwhite than for a white pregnant woman.

2. Age of Mother. Data from several sources indicate that the risk of fetal death is somewhat greater when the mother is under 20 than when she is 20-24, but that after the low-risk ages 20-24 are passed, the risk of fetal death rises sharply. The H.I.P. data investigated by

Shapiro, Jones, and Densen showed a fetal death rate of 97 for women aged 20-24 and 219 for those aged 35 or over.[23] Vital statistics data, though at a much lower level, show the same kind of relation to age of mother.

3. Order of Pregnancy. The risk of fetal death rises with order of pregnancy. The H.I.P. data referred to above show 97 fetal deaths per 1,000 pregnancies for first pregnancies and a rate of 186 for fourth and higher-order pregnancies.[24]

4. Previous Fetal Loss. The H.I.P. data also show that the risk of fetal death is twice as high for women whose preceding pregnancy ended in fetal death as for those whose preceding pregnancy ended in live birth. The fetal mortality rates for the two groups are 222 and 110, respectively.[25]

5. Plurality. The risk of fetal death is considerably greater when more than one fetus is present. Vital statistics data for 1963 show that the ratios of fetal deaths at gestational ages of 20 weeks or more to live births are 15.0 per 1,000 for single deliveries, 41.6 for twin deliveries, and 60.7 for other deliveries.

6. Sex. The risk of fetal death is apparently slightly greater for male than for female fetuses. In 1963 there were 16.2 fetal deaths at gestational ages of 20 weeks or more per 1,000 live births for males, and 14.9 for females.

7. Legitimacy. The risk of having a fetal death is apparently greater for unmarried women than for married women. The following table shows the ratio of fetal deaths per 1,000 live births for fetal deaths at gestational ages of 20 weeks or more in 1963:

	White	Nonwhite
Legitimate	12.9	25.0
Illegitimate	20.4	30.3

Regardless of color, the risk of fetal death is greater for the unmarried woman. It is doubtful that very much of this difference is due to the greater likelihood that an unmarried woman will have an induced abortion, since the great majority of illegally induced abortions are never registered. The difference is probably due to the poorer medical care that a pregnant unmarried woman receives.

Attendant at Birth and Place of Delivery

A large majority of births in the United States occur in hospitals and are attended by physicians. Although this suggests that mothers and newborn infants generally receive excellent care, it does not necessarily follow that births outside hospitals are inadequately attended. In the Netherlands, for example, most births occur in the home and about one-third of all deliveries are attended by midwives. Yet, the infant mortality rate in the Netherlands is lower than in the United States. This observation is made simply to serve as an indication that there are many factors affecting the health of the mother and new-born infant in addition to the place of delivery and the person in attendance. Nevertheless, in the United States, deliveries outside hospitals generally receive less adequate attention than those occurring in hospitals.

In the vital statistics of the United States, the category "physician in hospital" has been used for many years to describe the place of birth and attendant at delivery. This includes all births in hospitals, regardless of the type of attendant shown on the birth certificate, and all births in "clinics" that were reported as having been attended by physicians. A special tabulation of 1964 births indicated that a few births in hospitals were attended by a person other than a physician. A very few (0.1 percent of all births) were attended by nurse-midwives in hospitals, and a larger proportion (2.4 percent) were attended by "other and not specified" persons.

Altogether, 97.5 percent of the births in 1964 are classified as having been attended by "physician in hospital"; 0.7 percent were attended by a physician elsewhere; 1.5 percent were attended by midwives outside of hospitals; and 0.3 percent were classified as "other and not specified."

The present situation represents a substantial change from earlier years. In 1940 only 55.8 percent of births were attended by a physician in a hospital. Great progress in the hospitalization of deliveries was made during the 1940's, so that by 1951, 90.0 percent of births were delivered by physicians in hospitals. The 95 percent mark was reached in 1956, and further progress has since been made.

Even now, however, there is considerable variation by color and geographic area. Deliveries are least adequately attended among non-white women in the South. In Mississippi only 54.8 percent of the nonwhite births were delivered by physicians in hospitals in 1964; an additional 4.6 percent were delivered by physicians in other places (presumably, the mother's home in most cases), and 39.5 percent were delivered by midwives.

There is very little variation in the proportion of white births delivered by physicians in hospitals. In many states the proportion is above 99.0 percent, and in no state is it below 96.0 percent.

Inmates of Institutions

Fertility data from the 1960 census for women inmates of institutions are presented in Table 2.4. According to the definitions used in the decennial census, inmates of institutions are persons for whom care or custody is provided in such types of places as mental hospitals; home and schools for the mentally or physically handicapped; places providing specialized medical care for persons with tuberculosis or other chronic disease; nursing and domiciliary homes for the aged and dependent; and prisons and jails. Excluded are persons in general service wards of hospitals, persons receiving out-patient care from institutions, and persons receiving care in places not classified as institutions.

Table 2.4   Institutional status of women 35-44 years old, by children ever born, color of woman, and type of institution: United States, 1960

Color of woman and type of institution	All women		Percent single	Women ever married		Children ever born per woman ever married reporting
	Number	Prevalence rate[a]		Total	Reporting on children ever born	
White	11,007,175	...	6	10,351,697	b	2.6
Inmates of institutions	55,663	506	55	25,277	15,567	2.1
Mental hospitals	36,753	334	46	19,757	11,691	2.1
Homes and schools for mentally handicapped	10,814	98	98	232	114	1.9
Chronic disease hospitals	767	7	46	418	220	1.6
Tuberculosis hospitals	1,877	17	15	1,603	1,257	2.8
Homes for aged and dependent	3,197	29	53	1,505	931	2.1
Correctional institutions	1,745	16	11	1,561	1,227	2.4
All other institutions	510	5	61	201	127	1.3
Nonwhite	1,329,166	...	7	1,235,878	b	3.1
Inmates of institutions	11,443	861	33	7,641	4,161	2.3
Mental hospitals	7,126	536	34	4,719	2,142	2.3
Homes and schools for mentally handicapped	580	44	96	25	8	c
Chronic disease hospitals	147	11	30	103	38	c
Tuberculosis hospitals	1,238	93	29	880	592	3.1
Homes for aged and dependent	394	30	26	291	126	1.9
Correctional institutions	1,865	140	16	1,565	1,230	2.0
All other institutions	93	7	c	58	25	c

Source: U.S. Bureau of the Census, 1960 Census of Population, Vol. I., Characteristics of the Population, Part 1, U.S. Summary, Table 190; and Women by Number of Children Ever Born, PC(2)-3A, Table 46.

[a]Inmates per 100,000 total women of given age and color.

[b]Nonreports allocated, except for special tabulation of institutional inmates. Because most data for inmates come from office records of institutions, which do not always show children ever born, the proportion of nonreports is often high.

[c]Percent or rate not shown where base is less than 100.

It may be noted from the table that only 55,663 white women 35-44 years old were classified as inmates of institutions out of a total of 11,007,175 white women of this age in the total population of the United States. Only 506 per 100,000 white women 35-44 years old and 861 per 100,000 nonwhite women of this age were classified as inmates of institutions. Thus, most women of nearly completed childbearing age were "at large" in the general population and few were in institutions. The proportions in institutions were considerably greater for women of successively older ages (not shown). As a group, women inmates of institutions have borne fewer children on the average than women in the general population, even if comparisons are limited to women who have ever married. (Inmates of institutions are more generally single than women not in institutions.)

The majority of women inmates of institutions are in mental hospitals and institutions for the mentally handicapped. Mental illness is known to be a serious problem in modern societies. According to Plunkett, over one million Americans were hospitalized in 1959 for mental illness in federal, state, and private institutions, and in psychiatric units of general hospitals, of whom many had been hospitalized at least once previously for mental illness.[26] With present-day methods of treatment in a first-rate hospital, about seven out of ten may expect sufficient improvement for discharge, often in a fairly short interval of time.[27] Of course, some persons do not have mental disorders sufficiently serious to require hospitalization, so the rate of hospitalization for mental illness is an index of severe problems rather than mild disorders. The prevalence of mental illness increases with age and is greater for single and divorced persons than married persons. In the census data for inmates of mental hospitals (Table 2.4) the women are noticeably less fertile than women in the general population. In contrast, using data collected in the middle 1950's by Hollingshead and Redlich, Bean found no difference between the fertility of women who were former patients of mental hospitals and a group of women matched with reference to major characteristics who had never been hospitalized for mental illness.[28]

The fertility of certain types of mental patients has been studied, most notably by Franz Kallmann, Charles Goldfarb, L. Erlenmeyer-Kimling, and Erik Essen-Moller. The most comprehensive work has been done with schizophrenics. In a study conducted by the State of New York in its mental hospitals a sample of inmates admitted in the two three-year periods 1934-36 and 1954-56 were compared: first, with each other, and second, with the general population.[29] That study, like previous studies, found that most marriages occur before the onset of the disease, but the proportion married among inmates in the 1954-56 sample was higher than the earlier sample.

Changes occurred in the family size among married schizophrenics which almost paralleled those occurring among the general population. Fewer women were childless, and more were having two- or three-child families. The proportion of women with only one child in the 1954-56 sample was not markedly different from the 1934-36 sample but was higher than that of the general population. Because of the high proportion unmarried, schizophrenics as a whole produce fewer children than the general population.[30]

Essen-Moller, in explanation of the high proportion of single women in institutions, suggested that perhaps the close bond of marriage tended to keep many married women out of mental hospitals. Widows and divorcees, often with the benefit of close relatives, tend to be committed at an earlier stage of schizophrenia.[31]

It may be noted that many more white than nonwhite women were in homes and schools for mentally handicapped. For the most part, these are places for mental defectives, who enter them in early childhood and spend most of their lives there. Such facilities are apparently more generally available for white than nonwhite persons, but some or many of the nonwhite persons may be in mental hospitals rather than in homes or school for mental defectives.

Tuberculosis has plagued societies for many centuries. The death rate for tuberculosis in the United States has sharply declined with improved levels of living and the introduction of modern drugs. The mortality rate for all forms of tuberculosis was 194 per 100,000 population in 1900, 6.1 in 1960, and 4.3 in 1964.[32] There is no cure for tuberculosis at the present time, but in the majority of instances the disease can be arrested and persons suffering from it can lead a normal life. Severe cases are hospitalized, and after improvement, sent home.

The prevalence rate for inmates of tuberculosis hospitals at ages 35-44 years old was 17 per 100,000 white females and 93 per 100,000 nonwhite females. The higher rate of tuberculosis hospitalization for nonwhite than white females can be explained by the larger proportions of the former with little education and with congested living conditions. Female inmates of tuberculosis hospitals have had more children, on the average, than females of corresponding age in the general population, a circumstance that probably reflects their lower socioeconomic status.

The fertility of women in correctional institutions is below that of the general population. Not only are women with children less likely to be in trouble with the law, but those who do get into difficulties are more apt to be placed on probation than single or married women without children.

Deafness

An overall view of hearing impairments in the national population is presented below, followed by fertility data for "the deaf community" of the Washington, D.C., Metropolitan Area. Hearing impairments in the population in relation to fertility are of interest from several points of view. Some hearing impairments are of hereditary or genetic origin, as noted below. Regardless of the cause, there are occasional problems of adjustment to society when either the parents or the children have hearing impairments.

Prevalence. Hearing impairments differ in kind and degree. According to audiometer tests made in medical examinations between 1960 and 1962 by the National Health Survey for a nationwide probability sample of 6,672 persons 18-79 years of age in the civilian noninstitutional population, 97.3 percent had hearing ability in at least the better ear that would cause no significant difficulty with faint speech or difficulty only with faint speech, 1.6 percent had frequent difficulty with normal speech, and the remaining 1.1 percent required loud speech, shouted or amplified speech, or did not understand even amplified speech.[33] The speech-reception thresholds were not measured directly but were estimated on the basis of results of the audiometer tests. Rates for hearing impairments increase greatly with age, especially after age 45. Among adults 18-44 years old, for example, the audiometer tests indicated that only 0.3 percent needed loud speech, shouted or amplified speech, or were not able to understand even amplified speech, as compared with the figure just given of 1.1 percent for all ages, 18-79.

Another type of information on the prevalence of hearing impairments in the population comes from interview surveys in which respondents are expected to report impaired hearing when there is "deafness or serious trouble with hearing." In interview surveys thus far made, the determination of what is "serious" is left to the respondent to decide. The rates of persons with hearing impairments are lower in interview surveys than rates from audiometric examinations. Interview surveys made from July 1959 to June 1961 indicated that there were about 6,231,000 persons in the civilian noninstitutional population of the United States who had impaired hearing, or 35.3 per 1,000 population.[34] Recently, a "hearing ability scale" was developed for use with interview surveys, based on a series of questions indicative of ability to hear and interpret loud noises, speech, and so forth.[35] Applied to a portion of persons who reported impaired hearing in the health interview surveys, preliminary findings are that *without the use of a hearing aid,* 75 percent of the persons with impaired hearing were able to hear and understand most of the words spoken; only 3 percent were unable to hear even loud noises.

Genetics. Genetic aspects are thought to be relatively far more common in the small minority of deaf persons who have early total deafness (born deaf or became deaf early in childhood) than in the case of deafness at more advanced ages. A population study of early total deafness in the State of New York, covering a sample of 8,200 deaf residents over 12 years old with early total deafness, indicated that about one-half of the deafness was genetically determined.[36] Autosomal dominant genes accounted for approximately 10 percent of the cases, with the remainder of the inherited deafness being mainly of autosomal recessive origin. An average penetrance of only 50 percent was observed for the dominant genes, while the importance of the recessive component was emphasized by a finding that at least 45 different recessive genes may produce early total deafness when homozygous. (It may be of some interest to note that in 176 cases of fertile deaf by deaf matings studied, 147 matings produced only hearing children [294 such children], 15 matings produced some hearing children [23] and some deaf children [18], and 14 matings produced only deaf children [34].) According to McCabe, prenatal influences such as rubella, and complications such as hypoxia, inmaturity, and trauma are considerably more important as causes of early total deafness than heredity. Also, viral infections, drug toxicities, head injuries, and inflammatory ear conditions are common causes of early total deafness.[37]

Deaf Community Study. The Deaf Community Study, conducted by Jerome D. Schein, was an investigation of the social and vocational activities of residents of the Washington, D.C., Metropolitan Area who were 18-64 years old, not living in an institution, and deaf.[38] Deafness was defined as inability to hear and understand conversation even with electronic amplification. A relatively small group of persons with a hearing loss who indicated that they considered themselves deaf by joining an organization of deaf persons was also included. The study was based on interviews with 1,132 deaf persons, who were estimated (by two independent validation studies) to comprise 90.5 percent of all the adult noninstitutionalized deaf adults 18 and over living in the Washington area on July 1, 1962. Excluded were students attending Gallaudet College, the world's only college for the deaf. It is possible that the deaf persons in the Washington, D.C., Metropolitan Area have a higher socioeconomic status than deaf persons nationally. About half of the deaf adults interviewed had completed more than 12 years of school, whereas it is known that nationally less than 7 percent of young deaf persons ever go to college. The average annual earnings for white male deaf persons in the study was $6,473, compared to the SMSA average of $5,514 for all white males in the 1960 census; white deaf females compared just as favorably—$3,542 to $2,972, but Negro deaf males (few with any college) earned an average of only $2,600 compared with $3,529, and Negro deaf females presented an even sorrier picture—$990 compared to $2,060. Some 3.9 percent of white male deaf and 3.7 percent of white female deaf were unemployed, but 15.5 percent of the Negro male deaf and 21.4 percent of the Negro female deaf were unemployed. The high rates of unemployment for Negro deaf may reflect a virtual absence of vocational training in the schools they attended.

Of the 1,132 deaf persons in the survey, 548 were male, 584 were female; 945 were white and 187 were nonwhite. The proportion white in the deaf population (83 percent) was larger than in the total population of the SMSA in 1960 (74 percent), perhaps reflecting selective inmigration. Some 291 had never married, 744 were living with a spouse, and 97 were separated, widowed, or divorced. (Only 11 percent of those ever married had ever been divorced.) Among 668 deaf persons with children present in the home, it was reported that out of 1,218 children present, 1,104, or 90.6 percent, had no hearing impairment and 114, or 9.4 percent, had a hearing impairment. Only 72 deaf persons had at least one hearing-impaired child present and more than half (45) had only one such child. In the Washington, D.C., Metropolitan Area, there was a marked tendency for deaf persons with any hearing-impaired children to have fewer children on the average than deaf persons who had only hearing children.

Deaf persons tend to mingle in the same social circles (churches, clubs, etc.) because they have many interests in common and find it easier to communicate with one another in the language of signs (few are skilled lip-readers despite extensive efforts at training during school years). Hence, it is not surprising that of 360 deaf men with wife present, 267 had a deaf wife and only 93 a hearing wife; of 380 deaf women with husband present, 267 had a deaf husband and 113 a hearing husband.

Table 2.5 presents data on children ever born to deaf women. For white women, the rates of children ever born are below those needed for replacement of the deaf population through births, but for non-white women the rates are generally well above replacement needs. For the white and nonwhite groups alike, the low rates for women aged 45-64 provide indirect evidence that deaf people were seriously affected by the economic depression of the 1930's. Judging from data for women of younger age, the nonwhite women appear to have participated in the post-World War II surge in fertility of the general population, whereas there has been little rise in the fertility of the white group.

Summary

The national maternal mortality rate per 100,000 live births has been drastically reduced from 728 in 1915-19 to 36 in 1963. That it can be reduced still further seems evident from the low rates of 6 and 10, respectively, in the District of Columbia and Rhode Island. There were only 1,466 deaths in 1963 reported to be from maternal causes, of which 797 were for white women and 619 for nonwhite women. The reduction has come about through more extensive hospitalization for maternity cases, through better prenatal and postnatal care, and through many advances in medicine. Many of the deaths could be prevented with proper care, but not all women receive such care before entering and after leaving a hospital. Only 280 of the deaths in 1963 were reported as resulting from abortion (spontaneous and induced), although estimates of the annual number of abortions run into the high hundreds of thousands. Maternal mortality is lowest at age 20-24 and increases with age. The rates decrease with order of birth up to the third child and then progressively increase. Women with high family incomes more often than those with low incomes consult specialists in obstetrics and otherwise receive more care, and there-fore are thought to have lower maternal mortality rates than women who are poor.

The belief that women who bear many children are less likely to live to advanced ages than women who bear few children, once they have completed childbearing, seems to be unfounded. Census data lend more support to the findings of Dorn and McDowell than to those of Freeman. According to the censuses of 1940, 1950, and

Table 2.5   Children ever born to deaf women, 1962, and to total women, 1960, by color, age, and marital status: Washington, D.C., Metropolitan Area

Color and age of woman	Total women	Single women		Women ever married	Children ever born	
		Number	Percent		Per woman	Per woman ever married
DEAF WOMEN, 1962						
White						
18-24	72	43	60	29	0.4	1.0
25-34	120	22	18	98	1.5	1.8
35-44	95	5	5	90	2.0	2.1
45-64	194	27	14	167	1.7	1.9
Nonwhite						
18-24	18	10	56	8	0.9	2.0
25-34	25	10	40	15	2.2	3.6
35-44	21	2	10	19	3.0	3.3
45-64	31	3	10	28	1.7	1.9
TOTAL WOMEN, 1960						
White						
18-24	69,994	30,859	44	39,135	0.6	1.0
25-34	104,566	11,663	11	92,903	1.8	2.1
35-44	124,108	11,018	9	113,090	2.0	2.2
45-64	156,181	19,062	12	137,119	1.6	1.8
Nonwhite						
18-24	25,730	11,651	45	14,079	0.9	1.7
25-34	40,218	5,950	15	34,268	2.1	2.5
35-44	38,870	3,682	10	35,188	2.1	2.4
45-64	44,330	3,626	8	40,704	1.9	2.1

Source: Data from Deaf Community Study provided by Dr. Jerome D. Schein, Gallaudet College, Washington, D.C., and from U.S. Bureau of the Census, 1960 Census of Population, Vol. I, Characteristics of the Population, Part 10, District of Columbia, Table 113.

1960, the data show a relation between nonwhite women surviving to advanced ages and high fertility. Native white women with five or more children appear to survive in larger proportion than those with fewer than five children. Possibly some of the difference reflects the effect of healthier living conditions in rural areas (where fertility is high) than in urban areas.

The level of fetal mortality in the United States is not known accurately. There are two basic difficulties in the measurement of fetal death rates: First, the failure to recognize many fetal deaths during the first ten weeks of gestation, and second, the failure to register recognized fetal deaths.

In spite of the fact that registration of fetal deaths has improved in the United States, the ratio of fetal deaths to live births has declined greatly since the 1920's. This means that the actual reduction in fetal mortality has been even greater than is indicated by data from the registration system.

Fetal death rates vary considerably according to characteristics of the mother and of the pregnancy. Fetal mortality is higher for nonwhite than for white women, for older than for younger women, and for higher-order than for lower-order pregnancies. It is higher for plural than for single deliveries, for unmarried than for married women, and it is slightly higher for male than for female fetuses.

A large majority of births in the United States (nearly 98 percent) are delivered by physicians in hospitals. This represents an important change from earlier years. In 1940 only 56 percent of births were delivered in hospitals. By 1951 the proportion had reached 90 percent, and by 1956 it had reached 95 percent. In spite of this general progress, there are some important exceptions. For example, among nonwhite births in Mississippi in 1964, only 55 percent were delivered by physicians in hospitals.

Only 0.5 percent of white women 35-44 years old and 0.9 percent of nonwhite women of like age are inmates of institutions. A much higher proportion of these women are single than in the general population. But even if comparisons are limited to women ever married, female inmates have borne fewer children than women in the general population. The majority of the inmates are in mental hospitals and places for the mentally handicapped.

The fertility of female inmates of tuberculosis sanatoriums tends to be higher than that of females of corresponding age in the general population, probably reflecting the lower socioeconomic status of tuberculosis patients. The fertility of women in correctional institutions is below that of general population, even though most prisoners have been in custody for only a short while.

About 1.1 percent of persons 18-79 years old in the United States need some amplification to understand speech or do not understand speech even with amplification. The proportion is only 0.3 percent among those 18-44 years old; it is much higher at older ages. The influence of heredity is thought to be far more common in the small minority of persons with early total deafness than in persons becoming deaf at more advanced ages. And even in this small minority, a New York State study revealed, 84 percent of fertile deaf matings produced only hearing children while 8 percent produced only deaf children.

An intensive study of the deaf noninstitutional population, 18-64 years old, of the Washington, D.C., Metropolitan Area showed that 90.6 percent of children present in the home of deaf parents have no hearing impairment. Deaf parents with any hearing-impaired children tend to have fewer children than deaf parents with only hearing children. The average number of children ever born to deaf women in the Washington, D.C., Metropolitan Area is below that needed to replace the deaf white women in the next generation, but above replacement needs for the deaf nonwhite women.

3 / The Control of Fertility

The major aim of this book is to describe the diverse relations between social structure and fertility. In the process of pursuing this goal, we often differentiate only two classes of variables: the social structure variables (such as color, educational attainment, income, occupation, etc.) and the fertility variables (such as age-specific birth rates, children ever born, intervals between births, etc.). It is obvious, however, that the relations between these two sets of variables do not arise spontaneously. On the contrary, they result from the decisions and behavior of millions of couples with respect to a third set of variables, which we shall refer to as the family planning variables. These include such characteristics as fecundity (the ability to have children), the number of children wanted, the use of contraception, and the ability to limit fertility.

We may think of this third set of variables as intermediate between the other two: social structure affects fertility through the family planning variables. In other chapters this formulation is largely implicit. In this chapter it is explicit.

The systematic study of the family planning variables began with the Indianapolis Fertility Survey, conducted in 1941. The timing of this study was especially fortunate because it provided us with a valuable record of the family planning practices of a representative segment of the white urban population during the period of relatively depressed fertility of the 1930's.

The unexpected rise in fertility during the 1940's and 1950's stimulated more research in family planning. The first large-scale postwar survey was the Growth of American Families Study of 1955. This provided us with the first information on family planning variables for a nationwide sample of couples. A second, similar study followed five years later. This chapter is intended primarily to summarize the results of these two surveys.

Another major postwar survey, the Princeton Study, conducted in 1957 and 1960, was designed to test certain hypotheses concerning social and psychological factors affecting fertility. Its aims, then, were different from those of the Growth of American Families Studies, which were intended to provide estimates of family planning variables for the entire United States.

The most recent survey of family planning variables is the National Fertility Study of 1965. Like the Growth of American Families Studies, the 1965 survey was designed to measure the family planning variables for a nationwide sample of the population of reproductive age. Some preliminary results of this survey will be presented later in this chapter.

Variations in the Ability To Have Children

The physiological ability to have children (fecundity) varies widely among couples. Some are unable to have any children, while a few can have over 20. It would be very useful to be able to rank couples with respect to some standard measure of fecundity—for example, the probability of conception during a given time period when contraception is not used. However, it is not yet possible to measure fecundity accurately.

Two nationwide surveys of married women 18-39 years old in the United States indicate that approximately one-third of married couples are below normal in the ability to reproduce. This finding is based on interviews with two independently selected samples of women, conducted in 1955 and 1960. The 1955 sample consisted of white women, 18-39 years old, married, and living with husband (or with husband temporarily absent in the Armed Forces). The 1960 sample also included nonwhite wives, who were found to differ little from similar white wives with respect to fecundity.[1]

Among white couples in the 1960 study, 11 percent could not have any more children (most of them had had at least one) and another 20 percent were below normal in their ability to have children. Together, these Subfecund[2] couples make up 31 percent of the white childbearing population. Definitions are given in the footnote to Table 3.1.

The prevalence of fecundity impairments is low among young couples (it is 13 percent for white couples with wife aged 18-24), but much higher among older couples (47 percent for wives aged 35-39; see Table 3.2).

Sterlizing Operations. In one-third of the Subfecund white couples in the 1960 study (or 10 percent of *all* white couples with the wife 18-39 years old), the wife or husband had had an operation that makes it impossible to conceive. Over half of these operations (57 percent) were performed in order to prevent further childbearing; these are called "contraceptive operations" because they were contraceptive in intent. The remaining operations were performed to correct pathological conditions and are called "remedial operations."

The dominant reason given for having a contraceptive operation is to protect the wife's health, often with a doctor's recommendation. This is the reason given for 63 percent of such operations. In other cases, the operation was performed because the couple did not want any more children for a variety of reasons—because they couldn't afford more, because they had not been able to use contraception effectively enough to prevent unwanted pregnancies, and so forth. In cases where the motive is to protect the wife's health, the operation is usually performed on the wife. Where there are other reasons for wanting to avoid conception, the husband is more likely to have the operation.

Table 3.1 Percent distribution by fecundity for white and nonwhite couples with wife aged 18–39: Growth of American Families Study, 1960

Fecundity[a]	Total	White	Nonwhite
Total	100	100	100
Subfecund	31	31	33
Definitely sterile	10	11	6
Contraceptive operation	5	6	3
Remedial operation	4	4	4
Other	1	1	–
Probably sterile	4	4	7
Possibly sterile	9	8	13
Possibly fecund	8	8	6
Fecund	69	69	67

[a]Definitely sterile: Couples who definitely cannot have children in the future; some of them have had children. Contraceptive operations were performed for the purpose of preventing pregnancy; remedial operations were performed to correct a pathological condition.

    Probably sterile: Couples who probably cannot have children in the future.

    Possibly sterile: Couples who may not be able to have children in the future, but for whom there is less evidence than for the Probably Sterile that future children are unlikely.

    Possibly fecund: Couples who probably can have children in the future, but for whom there is some reason to believe that fecundity is below normal.

    These definitions are described in detail in Pascal K. Whelpton, Arthur A. Campbell, and John E. Patterson, Fertility and Family Planning in the United States (Princeton: Princeton University Press, 1966), pp. 128–134.

The prevalence of contraceptive operations was much higher among Protestants (8 percent) than among Catholics (2 percent) in 1960 (see Table 3.3 and Fig. 3.1). This is consistent with the explicit prohibition by the Catholic Church of operations intended solely to prevent pregnancy.

Contraceptive operations are more commonly found among the less educated than among the better educated. Of the wives whose education proceeded no further than grade school or who didn't finish high school, 8 percent reported contraceptive operations; in contrast, only 3 percent of the wives who had been to college did so (see Table 3.4 and Fig. 3.2).

Table 3.2   Percent distribution by fecundity, for white couples with wife aged 18-39, by wife's age: Growth of American Families Study, 1960

Fecundity	Total	18–24	25–29	30–34	35–39
Total	100	100	100	100	100
Subfecund	31	13	21	36	47
Definitely sterile	11	3	6	13	19
Contraceptive operation	6	2	4	7	9
Remedial operation	4	1	1	4	9
Other	1	–	1	1	1
Probably sterile	4	1	2	3	7
Possibly sterile	8	4	5	9	13
Possibly fecund	8	5	8	11	8
Fecund	69	87	79	64	53

One can only speculate about the reasons for this relation, but it seems reasonable to suspect that doctors are more likely to recommend contraceptive operations to couples with less education than to other couples. In a case where pregnancy could endanger the wife's health, a doctor would probably trust a well-educated couple to use contraception effectively, but might not be as confident of a less-educated couple's ability to do so.

Four percent of the white wives reported *remedial* operations that made further childbearing impossible. These wives had borne relatively few children; their average number of births was only 2.1, compared with 3.6 for couples with contraceptive operations. About one-quarter of the wives with remedial operations had not had any children.

Table 3.3   Percent distribution by fecundity, for white couples with wife aged 18–39, by wife's religion: Growth of American Families Study, 1960

Fecundity	Total	Protestant	Catholic	Other
Total	100	100	100	100
Subfecund	31	31	30	25
Definitely sterile	11	13	5	7
Contraceptive operation	6	8	2	3
Remedial operation	4	5	3	4
Other	1	1	1	–
Probably sterile	4	3	4	4
Possibly sterile	8	7	12	9
Possibly fecund	8	8	9	5
Fecund	69	69	70	75

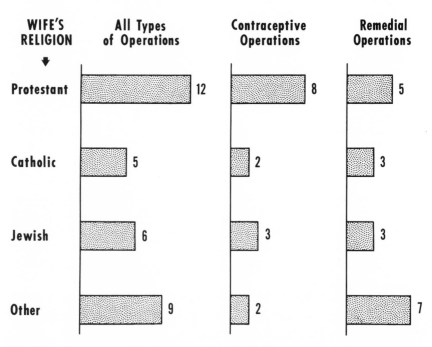

Fig. 3.1. Percentage of white couples who had contraceptive and remedial operations, by wife's religion, 1960.

Table 3.4. Percent distribution by fecundity, for white couples with wife aged 18-39, by wife's education: Growth of American Families Study, 1960

Fecundity	Total	College	High school 4	High school 1-3	Grade school
Total	100	100	100	100	100
Subfecund	31	22	28	38	40
Definitely sterile	11	5	10	14	15
Contraceptive operation	6	3	5	8	8
Remedial operation	4	2	4	5	7
Other	1	1	1	-	-
Probably sterile	4	2	3	4	7
Possibly sterile	8	8	8	8	11
Possibly fecund	8	6	7	12	7
Fecund	69	78	72	62	60

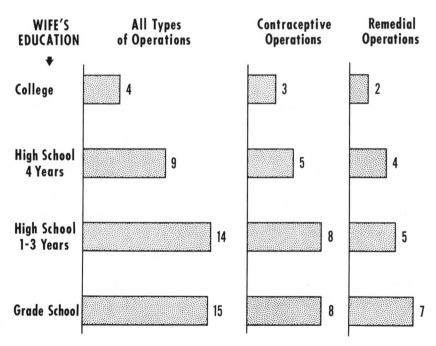

Fig. 3.2. Percentage of white couples who had contraceptive and remedial operations, by wife's education, 1960.

Other Reproductive Impairments. Two-thirds of the Subfecund (or 21 percent of white couples with wives 18-39 years old) did not have operations that prevent conception, according to the 1960 study. Within this group, the ability to have children varies greatly. At one end of the scale, 4 percent of all white couples are classified as Probably Sterile; many of these couples have been told by doctors that there is little chance that they will be able to have children in the future (although they may already have had some). Others have not conceived for ten years or more even though they have not used contraception. At the other end of the scale, 8 percent of all white couples are classified as Possibly Fecund. There is some reason for believing that these couples are below normal in their ability to reproduce (the wife's report of the doctor's opinion or her report of a moderately long period of time during which conception did not occur even though contraception was not used), but it does not seem likely that they are sterile. Between the Probably Sterile and the Possibly Fecund, there is an intermediate group called the Possibly Sterile, who comprise about 8 percent of all white couples (see definition in Table 3.1).

It is important to note that fecundity is hard to measure, and that the proportion of couples classified as Subfecund depends in part on the definition of subfecundity used. One important factor that makes it difficult to measure fecundity with accuracy is the presence of "hidden" subfecundity—that is, a subnormal ability to have children that the couple is unaware of because they have been using contraception and have not tried to have children for a long time. For example, most couples have their last wanted child before the wife is 30 years old. Then they will use contraception to try to prevent additional births. Therefore, a 35-year-old wife who has been using contraception regularly for seven years will not know whether she or her husband is now sterile unless either has some obvious impairment. There is no way of discovering such hidden subfecundity in an interview survey. This suggests that the estimate of 31 percent Subfecund, found in the 1960 study, understates the true prevalence of impairments to the reproductive system.

Even though the prevalence of subfecundity is high, there are very few couples who are prevented from having any children. If the wife is 30-34 years old, for example, only 5 percent are classified as childless *and* Subfecund (Table 3.5). There may be some couples with hidden subfecundity among another 3 percent who are childless and

Table 3.5   Percentage of couples who are childless and in specified
fecundity category, for white couples with wife aged 18-39,
by wife's age: Growth of American Families Study, 1960

Fecundity	Total	18-24	25-29	30-34	35-39
Total	12	24	10	8	10
Subfecund	6	4	4	5	8
Definitely sterile	2	1	1	2	3
Probably sterile	2	–	1	1	3
Possibly sterile	2	2	2	2	2
Possibly fecund	–	1	–	–	–
Fecund	7	20	6	3	1

Fecund, but in no case could the proportion of couples who are Subfecund and childless be above 8 percent.

The most important effect of subfecundity is to keep couples from
having as many children as they want. About half (49 percent) of the
wives in the Subfecund group said that they expected to have fewer
than the minimum number of children they wanted. The comparable
proportion for Fecund couples is 20 percent.

When the wife is close to the end of the childbearing period (aged
35-39), 26 percent of all wives are classified as Subfecund *and* report
that they want more children than they have or expect (Table 3.6).

Table 3.6   Percentage of wives who expect fewer children than wanted
and are in specified fecundity category, for white couples
with wife aged 18-39, by wife's age: Growth of American
Families Study, 1960

Fecundity	Total	18-24	25-29	30-34	35-39
Total	29	22	22	29	40
Sufecund	15	6	9	16	26
Definitely sterile	5	1	2	6	10
Probably sterile	3	1	2	2	5
Possibly sterile	4	3	3	4	7
Possibly fecund	3	2	3	3	3
Fecund	14	16	13	12	14

On the basis of the 1960 study, it was estimated that if Subfecund couples were as capable of childbearing as Fecund couples, they would have 40 percent more children altogether (usually this would mean one more child per couple), and that the number of children ever born to all couples as a group would be 17 percent higher.

Fecundity Impairments among Nonwhite Couples. There is reason to believe that in the recent past, impairments of the reproductive system were more common among nonwhite than white couples. One item of evidence is the high proportion of older nonwhite women who are childless. The 1960 census shows that among ever-married women 50-54 years old, for example, the proportion who never had any children was 28 percent for the nonwhite and 20 percent for the white.[3]

The 1960 census also shows that the percentage of ever-married women who are childless has declined to 14 percent for nonwhite women 25-29 years old—nearly as low as the 12 percent for white women in this age group. In other words, using the prevalence of childlessness as a rough indicator of the presence of fecundity impairments, it appears that young nonwhite wives are more fecund than nonwhite wives a generation earlier, and are now about as fecund as young white wives. Data from the 1960 Growth of American Families Study show no substantial white-nonwhite differences in the prevalence of fecundity impairments. The proportions Subfecund are 33 percent for nonwhite women and 31 percent for white women (Table 3.1).

Although the overall proportions with impaired fecundity are about the same for white and nonwhite couples, there appear to be some minor differences in the kinds of impairments. A higher proportion of white wives (6 percent) than of nonwhite wives (3 percent) reported that they or their husbands had undergone an operation for the purpose of preventing conception. However, the nonwhite do not seem to differ from the white in the proportion of wives reporting operations that prevent pregnancy but that were performed to correct a pathological condition. The proportion reporting such operations was the same for both groups: 4 percent.

The Use of Contraception
A large majority of married couples have or expect to have some form of limitation on their fertility. The 1960 Growth of American Families Study showed that among white couples,

81 percent had used some form of contraception (including rhythm);

7 percent expected to use contraception;

87 percent (rounded) had used or expected to use contraception;

10 percent had not used contraception and did not expect to do so, but were below normal in their physiological capacity to have children (Subfecund);

1 percent were not Subfecund and intended never to use contraception, but the wife reported that she regularly douched within one-half hour after intercourse, a practice that reduces the probability of conception;

98 percent had some form of limitation on their fertility, whether intentional or unintentional, or expected to use contraception at some time in the future;

2 percent had no limitation on their fertility and intended never to use contraception.

In other words, some form of fertility limitation is nearly universal in the United States. Values are consistent with practice in this area of married life, for the 1960 study also showed overwhelming approval of the idea that couples should exercise some control over the number of children they have.

Table 3.7 shows the distribution of couples in each age group by past and intended use of contraception. These figures indicate that

Table 3.7   Percent distribution of couples by past and expected use of contraception, for white couples with wife aged 18-39, by wife's age: Growth of American Families Study, 1960

Use of contraception	Total	18-24	25-29	30-34	35-39
Total	100	100	100	100	100
Have used or expect to use	87	92	91	88	80
Have used	81	78	84	83	77
Expect to use	7	14	7	4	2
Do not expect to use	13	8	9	12	20
Subfecund	10	4	5	10	18
Fecund					
ODFC[a]	1	1	1	-	1
Non-ODFC[a]	2	4	2	2	1

[a]The abbreviation ODFC refers to women who regularly douche within one-half hour after intercourse for reasons other than the desire to prevent conception.

the proportion of couples who do not expect to use contraception rises with age. Most of the older couples who do not expect to use contraception are Subfecund, however, and no longer have much need for contraception.

The proportion of couples who have used or intend to use contraception is a clear majority of every socioeconomic group, but the size of this majority varies. For example, it is 90 percent for Protestants and 80 percent for Catholics (Table 3.8). It is 93 percent among wives

Table 3.8   Percent distribution of couples by past and expected use of contraception, for white couples with wife aged 18-39, by wife's religion: Growth of American Families Study, 1960

Use of contraception	Total	Protestant	Catholic	Jewish	Other
Total	100	100	100	100	100
Have used or expect to use	87	90	80	95	84
Have used	81	84	70	95	77
Expect to use	7	5	10	-	7
Do not expect to use	13	10	20	5	16
Subfecund	10	8	14	5	11
Fecund					
ODFC[a]	1	1	1	-	2
Non-ODFC[a]	2	1	5	-	2

[a]The abbreviation ODFC refers to women who regularly douche within one-half hour after intercourse for reasons other than the desire to prevent conception.

with a college education and 72 percent for wives who never went beyond grade school (Table 3.9 and Fig. 3.3). What causes these variations? The main factor responsible is the fact that socioeconomic groups differ widely in *when* they begin using contraception. In certain groups it is customary for couples to delay using contraception until relatively late in the process of family growth. The longer couples put off using contraception, the more likely they are to become Subfecund before it is necessary to begin using contraception.

Delay in using contraception is most common among the less educated. For example, among grade-school educated wives who have been pregnant three times, only 18 percent began using contraception before the first pregnancy. The comparable proportion for college

Table 3.9 Percent distribution of couples by past and expected use
of contraception, for white couples with wife aged 18–39, by
wife's education: Growth of American Families Study, 1960

Use of contraception	Total	College	High school 4	High school 1-3	Grade school
Total	100	100	100	100	100
Have used or expect to use	87	93	90	85	72
Have used	81	88	83	78	66
Expect to use	7	5	7	7	6
Do not expect to use	13	7	10	15	28
Subfecund	10	4	8	12	21
Fecund ODFC[a]	1	–	–	2	2
Non–ODFC[a]	2	2	2	2	5

[a]The abbreviation ODFC refers to women who regularly douche
within one-half hour after intercourse for reasons other than the desire
to prevent conception.

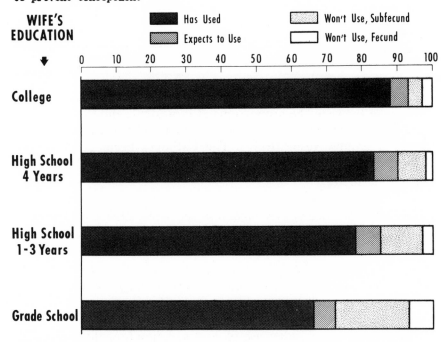

Fig. 3.3. Percent distribution of white couples by use of contraception, inten-
tion to use, and fecundity of those who will not use, by wife's education, 1960.

wives is 55 percent. By the time they had had three pregnancies, 76 percent of the grade-school wives had begun to use contraception (or their husbands had), and most of the remaining 24 percent were Subfecund and would probably never have to use contraception. By the time the college wives had three pregnancies, however, 92 percent had begun using contraception (see Table 3.10).

Table 3.10   Cumulative percentage of couples who used contraception before specified pregnancy, for white couples with wife aged 18-39 who have had three pregnancies, by wife's education: Growth of American Families Study, 1960

When contraception was used	Total	College	High school 4	High school 1-3	Grade school
Total	100	100	100	100	100
Have used	87	92	92	79	76
Before first pregnancy	38	55	42	23	18
Before second pregnancy	63	80	64	54	45
Before third pregnancy	74	88	75	66	61
After third pregnancy	87	92	92	79	76
Have not used	13	8	8	21	24
Subfecund	9	5	8	13	18
Fecund	3	3	1	8	6

A similar explanation accounts for most, though not all, of the difference between the proportions of Protestants and Catholics who have used or will use contraception (90 and 80 percent for the two religious groups, respectively). The Catholics begin contraception later, and more of them discover fecundity impairments before they have to begin use.

Trends in the Use of Contraception. Between 1955 and 1960 there was a trend toward earlier use of contraception. The proportion of white couples using contraception before the first pregnancy increased from 34 percent in 1955 to 38 percent in 1960. Also, the proportion of couples who already had used contraception by the time the wife was 18-24 years old increased from 68 to 78 percent in this five-year period (Table 3.11).

The trend toward earlier use of contraception brought about a rise in the proportion of users in the 18-39 age group as a whole. In 1955,

70 percent of white couples with wives 18-39 years old had already used contraception. By 1960 the comparable proportion was 81 percent (Table 3.11).

Table 3.11   Percentage of couples who have used or expect to use contraception, for white couples with wife aged 18-39, by wife's age: Growth of American Families Studies, 1955 and 1960

Wife's age	Have used			Have used or expect to use		
	1955	1960	Increase	1955	1960	Increase
Total	70	81	11	79	87	9
18-24	68	78	10	84	92	8
25-29	73	84	11	83	91	8
30-34	73	83	10	79	88	9
35-39	65	77	12	69	80	11

Use of Contraception among Nonwhite Couples. The use of contraception is less common among nonwhite than among white married couples. By 1960, 59 percent of the nonwhite couples had used contraception, as compared with 81 percent of the white couples. The percentages who had used or expected to use contraception were somewhat closer: 76 percent for the nonwhite group and 87 percent for the white group. The differences are statistically significant.

The distribution of nonwhite couples in each age group by past and intended use of contraception is shown in Table 3.12. These

Table 3.12   Percent distribution of couples by past and expected use of contraception, for nonwhite couples with wife aged 18-39, by wife's age: Growth of American Families Study, 1960

Use of contraception	Total	18-24	25-29	30-34	35-39
Total	100	100	100	100	100
Have used or expect to use	76	83	85	77	58
Have used	59	52	65	66	53
Expect to use	16	31	20	11	5
Do not expect to use	24	17	15	23	42
Subfecund	15	3	9	16	30
Fecund	9	13	6	6	12

figures indicate that the younger wives (those under 30 years of age) are more likely than older wives to report that they have used contraception or expect to do so.

The use of contraception among nonwhite couples is closely related to Southern farm residence. Only 36 percent of the nonwhite wives living on Southern farms reported that they or their husbands had tried to limit family size (Table 3.13). This is the lowest proportion of users found for any socioeconomic group in this study. Another 16 percent of the Southern farm residents expected to use contraception, so that slightly over half of them (52 percent, after rounding) had used contraception or expected to do so. Of the 48 percent who expected never to use contraception, 27 percent were Subfecund. Most of them would not have to use contraception to prevent additional pregnancies. The remaining 21 percent were Fecund and said they thought they would never use contraception.

Table 3.13   Percent distribution of couples by past and expected use of contraception, for nonwhite couples with wife aged 18-39, by Southern farm residence: Growth of American Families Study, 1960

Use of contraception	Total	No Southern farm residence	Some Southern farm residence, not on farm now [a]	On Southern farm now
Total	100	100	100	100
Have used or expect to use	76	78	80	52
Have used	59	65	60	36
Expect to use	17	13	20	16
Do not expect to use	24	22	20	48
Subfecund	15	17	10	27
Fecund	9	5	10	21

[a] Husband, wife, or both have lived on a farm in the South.

Nonwhite couples who have lived on a Southern farm but no longer do so are much more likely to use contraception; 60 percent of the nonwhite couples with *previous* Southern farm background have used contraception. The proportion who have used or expected to use contraception is 80 percent, which is not very far from the 87 percent for white couples (Table 3.13).

Nonwhite couples without previous Southern farm residence differ little from those who have left their Southern rural backgrounds. Slightly more of them have used contraception (65 percent instead of 60 percent), but slightly fewer have used or expect to use (78 percent instead of 80 percent). Neither of these differences is statistically significant.

Nonwhite wives with a college education report a high prevalence of use. Altogether, 95 percent of them have used or expect to use contraception, as compared with 93 percent for college-educated white wives (Table 3.14).

Table 3.14   Percent distribution of couples by past and expected use of contraception, for nonwhite couples with wife aged 18-39, by wife's education: Growth of American Families Study, 1960

Use of contraception	Total	College	High school 4	High school 1-3	Grade school
Total	100	100	100	100	100
Have used or expect to use	76	95	81	79	57
Have used	59	86	67	56	42
Expect to use	17	9	14	23	15
Do not expect to use	24	5	19	21	43
Subfecund	15	5	15	14	22
Fecund	9	-	4	7	22

It appears that better-educated nonwhite couples readily adopt the goal of moderate family size and methods of attaining it. This suggests that continued improvements in the education of nonwhite persons will bring an increase in the proportion using contraception.

How Families are Planned

As noted previously, a large majority of white couples try to exercise some control over their fertility by using contraception. However, they vary greatly in when they begin use and in how successful their efforts are. This section describes in broad outline how couples use contraception to plan their families.

First of all, nearly two out of three newlyweds do not start using contraception before the first conception, according to the 1960

Growth of American Families Study. In most cases, this is because they want to have a baby as soon as they can. Most of those who do begin contraception before the first pregnancy stop using it and conceive only 8 or 9 months later than other couples. The first child usually arrives less than 2 years after marriage.

After their first birth the typical couple wants to have another child fairly soon. Although most begin to use contraception before the second child comes along, they still feel no strong pressure to avoid conception. They may omit contraception occasionally or fail to use it properly.

This casual approach to family planning is fairly prevalent until the couple has had all the children they want. It helps to account for the fact that over half the white couples in the 1960 sample had pregnancies that were not intended to occur when they did. After they have had the two, three, or four children they want, however, most couples become more careful. Usually this means that they use contraception more regularly.[4]

By the time the wife is between 25 and 30 years old, the majority of couples consider their families complete, but they still have an average of about 13 to 16 years of potential childbearing ahead of them. Even though they now try to use contraception regularly, some couples have unwanted conceptions. But most manage to avoid having more children then they want.

How successful are couples in controlling their fertility? Success can be measured in a number of ways. It could be pointed out that 18 percent of the couples in the 1960 study had had accidental conceptions (i.e., they occurred while contraception was being used always) or that 54 percent had had conceptions that were not intended to occur when they did. But a more important measure of success is whether or not the couple avoided unwanted pregnancies—that is, pregnancies that were not wanted either when they occurred or later. To get at this, each wife with two or more births was asked whether she or her husband had wanted another child at any time shortly before their last conception occurred. If one or both partners did not want any more children, and if the conception was not deliberately planned by stopping contraception to conceive, the couple was classified as having excess fertility.

Seventeen percent of the white couples in the 1960 study are classified as having excess fertility (Table 3.15). The comparable proportion for nonwhite couples is 31 percent. Among the white couples, those with excess fertility have 3.7 births, on the average, and expect 4.1 altogether. Not all of the couples with excess fertility have or expect unusually large numbers of births: 18 percent have only two births, and 33 percent have three. In terms of expectations, 14 percent expect two births and 31 percent expect three. Thus, nearly half of the excess fertility couples expect no more births than the average white couple. Only a minority of 26 percent expect five or more births.

Table 3.15   Percentage of couples with excess fertility,[a] for white couples with wife aged 18–39, by wife's age, religion, and education, and by husband's income: Growth of American Families Study, 1960

Characteristic	Percent with excess fertility[a]	Characteristic	Percent with excess fertility[a]
Total	17	Wife's education:	
		College	11
Wife's age:		High school 4	14
18–24	8	High school 1–3	21
25–29	16	Grade school	32
30–34	23		
35–39	20	Husband's income:	
		$10,000+	15
Wife's religion:		$7,000 – $9,999	16
Protestant	19	$6,000 – $6,999	22
Catholic	15	$5,000 – $5,999	15
Jewish	10	$4,000 – $4,999	16
Other	14	$3,000 – $3,999	16
		Under $3,000	21

[a] Husband, wife, or both did not want another child at the time of the last conception, the last conception was not planned by omitting contraception in order to conceive, and the wife has had at least two pregnancies.

Excess fertility is most prevalent among couples in the lower socioeconomic categories. The greatest contrast is found when couples are classified by the wife's educational attainment: 11 percent of the white college group have excess fertility, compared with 32 percent of the white grade-school group (Table 3.15 and Fig. 3.4).

Not only do the lower-status groups include relatively more couples with excess fertility, but the degree of excess fertility is most severe among them. For example, the percentage by which the number of births expected exceeds the number of children wanted is 70 percent if the husband's income is under $3,000, but only 27 percent if his income is $10,000 or more. This means that most of the excess fertility couples in the low-income group have two or more unwanted children. The excess in the high-income group is more likely to be only one child.

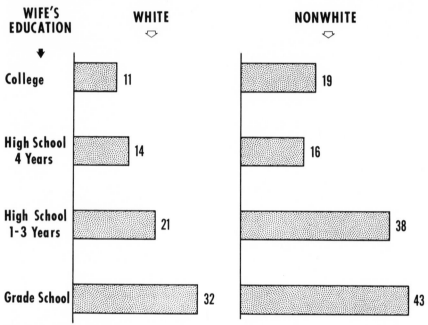

Fig. 3.4. Percentage of white and nonwhite couples with excess fertility, by wife's education, 1960.

Why do couples with lower socioeconomic status have so many unwanted pregnancies? Part of the reason is the fact that some of them do not even begin to use contraception before they have more children than they want. In the grade-school group 15 percent of the couples had unwanted pregnancies before trying to prevent conception (Table 3.16). This accounts for nearly half of the excess fertility couples in this group. There were hardly any comparable couples in the college group (only 0.2 percent).

Another reason for the high prevalence of unwanted pregnancies among less-educated couples is that after they begin to use contraception they often fail to use it regularly.

Nonwhite couples have been much less successful than white couples in planning fertility. The proportion with excess fertility is 31

Table 3.16   Percentage of couples whose last conception was unwanted[a]
and of specified contraceptive status, for white couples
with wives aged 18-39, by wife's education: Growth of
American Families Study, 1960

Wife's education	Total unwanted[a]	Before use of contraception began	Accidental[b]	Other unplanned[c]
Total	17	4	6	7
College	11	–	7	5
High school: 4	14	2	6	6
High school: 1-3	21	5	7	9
Grade school	32	15	8	10

[a]Husband, wife, or both did not want another child at the time of the last conception, the last conception was not planned by omitting contraception in order to conceive, and the wife has had at least two pregnancies.

[b]The last conception occurred while the couple was using contraception regularly.

[c]The last conception occurred when contraception was omitted for reasons other than the desire to conceive.

percent for the nonwhite group (Table 3.17), compared with 17 percent for the white group.

The white-nonwhite differences in planning family size are greatest among couples on farms in the South. Among the nonwhite couples living on Southern farms, nearly half (48 percent) have had more pregnancies than the husband or wife wanted (Table 3.17). This is the highest prevalence of excess fertility found for any socioeconomic group in this study. It compares with 20 percent for white couples on Southern farms. The only white group with a level of excess fertility anywhere near this consists of those with a poor education (the wife did not go beyond grade school) and a low income (the husband made less than $4,000 a year); such couples had 39 percent with excess fertility.

Among nonwhite couples, former residents of the rural South are more successful family planners than those who remain, but they are still not so successful as white couples. The prevalence of excess fertility is lower among nonwhite persons no longer living on Southern farms (29 percent instead of 48 percent), but this is still well above the 18 percent for the white group.

Obviously, the move from the Southern farm to other areas has brought with it a substantial improvement in the success with which nonwhite couples plan their families. But they have still not achieved the levels observed for the white population.

The extent to which nonwhite couples differ from white in their family planning practices can also be seen by comparing the different education groups. In every educational category, including the college group, nonwhite couples have shown less success in family planning than white couples (Fig. 3.4).

Table 3.17　Percentage of couples with excess fertility,[a] for nonwhite couples with wife aged 18–39, by wife's age and education and couple's Southern farm residence: Growth of American Families Study, 1960

Characteristic	Percent with excess fertility[a]	Characteristic	Percent with excess fertility[a]
Total	31		
Wife's age:		Couple's Southern farm residence:	
18–24	22		
25–29	37	No Southern farm	
30–34	30	residence	28
35–39	35	Some Southern	
		farm residence,	
Wife's education:		not on farm now[b]	29
College	19	On Southern farm	
High school: 4	16	now	48
High school: 1–3	38		
Grade school	43		

[a]Husband, wife, or both did not want another child at the time of the last conception, the last conception was not planned by omitting contraception in order to conceive, and the wife has had at least two pregnancies.

[b]Husband, wife, or both have lived on a farm in the South.

Methods of Contraception

According to the 1955 and 1960 studies, the two most effective methods of contraception then available (condom and diaphragm) were those most commonly used by white couples. In 1960, 50 percent of the white couples using any method had used condom and 38 percent had used diaphragm. Rhythm was the third most popular method (35 percent), douche was fourth (24 percent), and withdrawal was fifth (17 percent). Only relatively small proportions had used spermicidal jelly alone (without diaphragm), vaginal suppositories, abstinence, or other methods (Table 3.18).

The Catholic prohibition of certain methods of contraception has had a substantial influence on the methods selected by Catholic couples. Among Catholic wives reporting any use of contraception, 67 percent said that they had used rhythm. This was by far the most popular method among Catholics. The second choice (condom) was reported by only 28 percent of the Catholic wives in 1960 (Table 3.18).

Table 3.18   Percentage of users who have used specified method of contraception, for white couples with wife aged 18-39, by wife's religion: Growth of American Families Study, 1960

Method	Total	Protestant	Catholic	Jewish
Total[a]	186	201	157	156
Condom	50	56	28	74
Diaphragm	38	46	12	51
Rhythm	35	27	67	9
Douche	24	28	17	8
Withdrawal	17	18	17	4
Jelly alone	11	14	4	8
Suppositories	6	8	3	–
Abstinence	4	3	9	2
Other	1	1	–	–

[a]The total exceeds 100 because many couples used two or more methods.

Although rhythm is the most popular method among Catholic couples, a substantial proportion of them have used methods not approved by their Church. Among couples using any method, Catholic wives in 1960 reported that 55 percent had used methods other than rhythm or abstinence. Since 70 percent of all Catholic wives reported using any method, this means that 38 percent of them admitted that they and their husbands had failed to conform to Catholic teachings on contraception some time during their married lives. This was a significantly higher proportion than the 30 percent observed in the 1955 study.

Nonwhite couples tend to use less effective methods than white couples. One of the most important differences is the greater reliance of nonwhite couples on douche, a method that is relatively low in effectiveness. Half of the nonwhite users of contraception have used this method, as compared with only about a quarter of white users. Among nonwhite couples, it is the second most common method, while among white couples, it ranks fourth (compare Tables 3.18 and 3.19).

Table 3.19   Percentage of users who have used specified method of contraception, for nonwhite couples with wife aged 18–39: Growth of American Families Study, 1960

Method	Percent who have used
Total[a]	215
Condom	58
Diaphragm	30
Rhythm	18
Douche	50
Withdrawal	21
Jelly alone	19
Suppositories	16
Abstinence	2
Other	1

[a]The total exceeds 100 because many couples used two or more methods.

Condom is the most popular method among nonwhite users, as it is among the white. In fact, the proportion using this highly effective method may be somewhat greater for the nonwhite than for the white group, but it is not possible to be sure because the white-nonwhite differences are not quite large enough to be significant.

The proportions of couples using diaphragm and rhythm are both lower for the nonwhite than for the white group.

It is important to note that nonwhite couples show higher proportions trying to control fertility with the most readily available "female" methods: douche, jelly, and vaginal suppositories. Unlike diaphragm, these three methods may be obtained without a doctor's prescription, and like diaphragm, they are applied by the wife. In other words, it appears that in many nonwhite families, the wife feels that she must take the chief responsibility for contraception; and she tries to do this without medical advice, which is generally less available to nonwhite than to white wives.

New Methods of Contraception

Since the 1960 Growth of American Families Study, two highly effective methods of contraception have become available: the contraceptive pill and the intrauterine device. By 1966 the pill was being used by a large number of women in the United States. The intrauterine device had not yet attained the wide acceptance of the pill.

The number of women using the contraceptive pill was not known accurately before 1965. The following estimates are based on pharmaceutical company records:[5]

1961	500,000
1962	1,370,000
1963	2,280,000

Informed guesses for later years varied between 3 and 4 million.[6]

By 1966, however, preliminary results of the 1965 National Fertility Study had become available. They showed that among 24.6 million married women under age 45 in the United States, 6.4 million (or 26 percent) had ever used the contraceptive pill; of these, 3.8 million (or 15 percent of the total) were still using the pill at the time of the survey. These estimates are provisional and subject to revision.[7]

There has been some speculation that the decline in annual measures of fertility which occurred during the period when the use of the pill was rapidly increasing was due to the greater effectiveness of this method of contraception. The decline in fertility was considerable. By 1963 the decline of the fertility rate (births per 1,000 women 15-44 years of age) from its 1957 peak was 11 percent; by 1964 it was 14 percent; by 1965, it was 20 percent. To what extent might the pill have been responsible for these declines?

It is impossible to tell with any degree of assurance what effect the pill has had, but there are certain considerations that must be taken into account in arriving at an informed opinion about its impact on fertility. In the first place, the pill was not permitted to be used as a contraceptive until June 1960 and probably did not come into wide use until a year or more later. This means that if it did have any major influence on fertility, it would not be felt until 1962, at the earliest, when children conceived in 1961 were born. The decline in fertility, however, started in 1958, so it was not possible for the pill to have initiated the downward trend or to have contributed to its early progress.

Another important consideration is that the use of the pill is still confined to a minority of the childbearing population. The preliminary estimates cited above indicate that 26 percent of the married women of reproductive age had used the pill, and that 15 percent were using it at the time of the 1965 National Fertility Survey. Even if it is assumed that the pill has helped these women reduce their fertility by a substantial amount (say, 20 or 30 percent), this would result in a relatively small change in the number of births for the entire childbearing population.

Another consideration is the fact that fertility is still high relative to levels prevailing in the period 1933-39. With the methods of control then in use, couples were able to maintain the total fertility rate within the narrow range between 2,100 and 2,200.[8] The comparable rate for 1965 is 2,922. In other words, couples could have achieved levels of fertility observed recently without using methods of control that were any more effective than those available 30 years ago. Therefore, it would be difficult, and perhaps impossible, to prove that the increased use of the pill has caused any reduction in fertility that would not otherwise have taken place.

However, there is a plausible reason for believing that the pill has had some effect. The incidence of unintended pregnancies may be regarded as a function of three variables: the strength of couples' desire to prevent pregnancy, the effectiveness of the methods they use, and the convenience (or acceptability) of the methods. The pill is more effective than any other method in common use, and is generally regarded as more convenient. Therefore, the substitution of the pill for other methods of family limitation would reduce the incidence of unintended conceptions without any necessary increase in the strength of couples' motivation to prevent pregnancy.

Inasmuch as many unintended conceptions are simply conceptions that occur somewhat sooner than they are wanted, it is also possible to speculate that one of the pill's major effects may be to help couples delay births for longer periods of time. If so, some of the recent shift toward later childbearing may be aided by widespread use of the pill.

In addition, the pill is undoubtedly helping some couples avoid unwanted conceptions—that is, conceptions that occur when the couple does not want to have any more children. Whether or not this will have very much effect on the total fertility rate is impossible to foresee at the present time.

In summary, we can be certain that the recent decline in fertility was not initiated by the introduction of the contraceptive pill. To a considerable extent the decline is the expected result of certain shifts in the ages at which women bear children. The recent tendency for couples to have their children somewhat later in life and, possibly, to have fewer children altogether may have been aided by the use of the pill.

Summary
A large majority of wives and husbands in the United States agree that the control of fertility is desirable, and most couples who are able to have children either make some attempt to prevent pregnancy or intend to do so. Couples who have never used contraception and do not expect to begin usually have impairments of the reproductive system.

Most couples want two, three, or four children, and they want them within the first 10 years of marriage. A majority do not use contraception before the first conception. After beginning use, but before having all the children they want, some couples do not use contraception very effectively. Most of those who have had all the children they want, however, are able to prevent unwanted conceptions.

An important minority of couples (17 percent), however, have had more children than the husband, wife, or both partners wanted. Although excess fertility is experienced in all socioeconomic groups, it is most common among couples with low educational attainment and low income. The 1960 Growth of American Families Study shows that the most important reasons for excess fertility in the lower socioeconomic groups are the failure of some couples to use contraception after they have all the children they want, and the tendency of other couples to use contraception irregularly.

Preliminary results of the 1965 National Fertility Survey indicate that about one-quarter of the married women under age 45 have used the contraceptive pill. However, it has not yet been possible to estimate the independent effect of the increasing use of the pill on trends in fertility.

Approximately 20 million people, or about 11 percent of the total population in the conterminous United States, were classified as nonwhite in the 1960 census. The great majority of these, about 94 percent, were Negroes. These are, for the most part, descendants of slaves. The next largest number, the American Indians, are descendants of the aborigines from whom the white settlers wrested land. Most of the remaining nonwhite persons are of Asiatic origin—Japanese, Chinese, Filipinos, Koreans, and Asian Indians. They descended from people who migrated to this country before, or who managed to come here after, the establishment of an Asiatic Barred Zone in our immigration laws.

The circumstances surrounding the origins of the nonwhite people in this country, and the record of their early experiences here, are not a part of our national history of which conscientious whites can be proud. However, a full century after the emancipation of their ancestors, the Negroes are gaining at least some improvement in educational and employment opportunities and in their citizenship status. Gains have also been realized by the other nonwhite groups.

Because of the burgeoning increase of the nonwhite population in the United States, and its rapid urbanization, it is manifestly important to learn more about the levels and trends of nonwhite fertility. The first and largest part of this chapter deals with white-nonwhite comparisons. The second part is concerned with the fertility of specific ethnic groups: Negroes, Puerto Ricans, and other Spanish-speaking people in the Southwest; and with specific nationality groups of our "foreign white stock."

The White-Nonwhite Dichotomy

The nonwhite group, which, as has been mentioned, is composed largely of Negroes, has long been more fertile than the white group in this country. One reason for this is that the characteristics generally associated with high fertility tend to characterize the nonwhite population to a greater extent than the white population. Until fairly recently nonwhite persons were concentrated largely in the rural South. They were sharecroppers, tenant farmers, owners of small farms, and unskilled laborers of low economic and educational status. Legally, the Civil War broke the chains of slavery, but the ex-slaves continued to be bound by the persistence of repressive attitudes on the part of Southern white people, and hence by poverty, illiteracy, and lack of occupational skills and opportunities.

The above is not to say that no Negroes resided outside the South during the Reconstruction Period. Some, in fact, had lived in large Northern cities either as slaves or as free men prior to the Civil War, and others drifted northward later in small but growing numbers.

It was not until the close of World War I, however, that a virtual flood of Negro migration from the rural South to the urban areas of the North began. Data of that period suggest that Negroes migrating to large cities either were a highly selective group with respect to low fertility or that they experienced sharp reductions in fertility. At all events, during the 1930's and early 1940's the average fertility of Negro marriages in large cities was low and the proportions childless were exceedingly high. A frequent and a plausible explanation was the high rate of venereal infection among Negroes in large cities. But, whereas the interwar levels of fertility of urban Negroes were *conspicuously low* in an era of low fertility, the fertility of Negroes is now *conspicuously high* in an era of high fertility. An important fact regarding nonwhite families since World War II has been the sharper rise in their fertility than in that of white families. Moreover, since that time, the nonwhite group have exceeded the white group in the proportions of its people living in cities. The greater increase in the fertility of nonwhite than of white families is possibly due in part to the reduction in cases of sterility following the suppression of venereal infections after World War II.[1]

The crude birth rates by color point up the increases in fertility (Table 4.1). From 1915 to 1947 the birth rates per 1,000 white and nonwhite population were remarkably parallel; the rates for the non-white group were about 8 points above those for the white group during most of this period. Both groups experienced sharp increases in 1946 and 1947 following demobilization of servicemen at the end of World War II. However, whereas the white crude birth rate reached a peak in 1947 and remained virtually stationary at about 24 during the years 1951-57, the nonwhite rate continued to increase almost without exception each year until it reached about 35 in 1956. Since 1957 the crude birth rates for the white and nonwhite groups have declined, being respectively about 18 and 28 in 1965.

The general fertility rates,[2] shown in Table 4.1 for the period 1925-65 point up still more sharply the greater increase in the annual fer-

Table 4.1   Crude birth and death rates and general fertility rates, by color: United States, 1925-64

Year	Birth rate		Death rate		Fertility rate	
	White	Nonwhite	White	Nonwhite	White	Nonwhite
1965	18.3	27.6	9.4	9.6	91.4	133.9
1964	20.0	29.1	9.4	9.7	99.9	141.7
1963	20.7	29.7	9.5	10.1	103.7	144.8
1962	21.4	30.5	9.4	9.8	107.5	148.7
1961	22.2	31.6	9.3	9.6	112.2	153.5
1960	22.7	32.1	9.5	10.1	113.2	153.6
1959	23.1	34.2	9.3	9.9	114.6	162.2
1958	23.3	34.3	9.4	10.3	114.9	160.5
1957	24.0	35.3	9.5	10.5	117.7	163.0
1956	24.0	35.4	9.3	10.1	116.0	160.9
1955	23.8	34.7	9.2	10.0	113.8	155.3
1954	24.2	34.9	9.1	10.1	113.6	153.2
1953	24.0	34.1	9.4	10.8	111.0	147.3
1952	24.1	33.6	9.4	11.0	110.1	143.3
1951	23.9	33.8	9.5	11.1	107.7	142.1
1950	23.0	33.3	9.5	11.2	102.3	137.3
1949	23.6	33.0	9.5	11.2	103.6	135.1
1948	24.0	32.4	9.7	11.4	104.3	131.6
1947	26.1	31.2	9.9	11.4	111.8	125.9
1946	23.6	28.4	9.8	11.1	100.4	113.9
1945	19.7	26.5	10.4	11.9	83.4	106.0
1944	20.5	27.4	10.4	12.4	86.3	108.5
1943	22.1	28.3	10.7	12.8	92.3	111.0
1942	21.5	27.7	10.1	12.7	89.5	107.6
1941	19.5	27.3	10.2	13.5	80.7	105.4
1940	18.6	26.7	10.4	13.8	77.1	102.4
1939	18.0	26.1	10.3	13.5	74.8	100.1
1938	18.4	26.3	10.3	14.0	76.5	100.5
1937	17.9	26.0	10.8	14.9	74.4	99.4
1936	17.6	25.1	11.1	15.4	73.3	95.9
1935	17.9	25.8	10.6	14.3	74.5	98.4
1934	18.1	26.3	10.6	14.8	75.8	100.4
1933	17.6	25.5	10.3	14.1	73.7	97.3
1932	18.7	26.9	10.5	14.5	79.0	103.0
1931	19.5	26.6	10.6	15.5	82.4	102.1
1930	20.6	27.5	10.8	16.3	87.1	105.9
1929	20.5	27.3	11.3	16.9	87.3	106.1
1928	21.5	28.5	11.4	17.1	91.7	111.0
1927	22.7	31.1	10.8	16.4	97.1	121.7
1926	23.1	33.4	11.6	17.8	99.2	130.3
1925	24.1	34.2	11.1	17.4	103.3	134.0

Source: National Center for Health Statistics, Vital Statistics of the United States, 1965, Vol I, Natality, Table 1-2; Vol. II, Mortality, Part A, Table 1-1; and Monthly Vital Statistics Report, Vol. 15, No. 11, p. 4; Vol. 16, No. 1, p. 2. (See text for definitions of rates.)

tility of nonwhite than of white women during the years 1950-57. Thus, in 1950, the number of births per 1,000 women 15-44 years old was 102 for white women and 137 for nonwhite women. In 1957 the two figures were respectively 118 and 163. In 1965 they were 91 and 134.

The gross and net reproduction rates exhibit approximately the same contrasts. In 1947 the net reproduction rate of white females was about 50 percent above replacement requirement and that for nonwhite females about 60 percent above this requirement. In 1957 the white net reproduction rate was about 70 percent above replacement requirement, and nonwhite women were reproducing at a rate more than sufficient to double their numbers in one generation.[3] In 1965 the net reproduction rate for white women was below its 1947 level (31 percent above replacement requirements), and that for nonwhite women was 80 percent above this requirement (Table 4.2).

The trends in intrinsic birth and death rates by color are analogous to those of general fertility and gross reproduction rates (Table 4.2). The intrinsic birth and death rates express the numbers of births and deaths per year per 1,000 population that eventually would be yielded in a closed population with continuation of given schedules of age-specific fertility and mortality rates. During the period 1946-57 the increases in intrinsic birth rates were more persistent and more marked for nonwhite than for white persons. In 1946 the intrinsic birth rates were 20.6 and 25.6 for white and nonwhite respectively. In 1957 they were 27.0 (white) and 38.2 (nonwhite). Since 1957 there have been continuous declines in the intrinsic birth rates for both groups; in 1965 the rates were 20.3 for white persons and 31.5 for nonwhite persons.

In contrast to the widening of the difference by color in the intrinsic birth rate during 1946-57, there has been a marked similarity by color in levels and trends of the intrinsic death rate. The slightly lower intrinsic death rate for nonwhite than for white persons in 1962-65 reflects the younger age structures of the nonwhite group in the stable population.

The trends described above reflect a widening of the difference by color in the intrinsic rate of natural increase (intrinsic birth rate minus the intrinsic death rate). In 1946 the intrinsic rate of natural increase was 10.5 for white persons and 14.0 for nonwhite persons. In 1957 the respective rates were 20.4 and 31.3. And in 1965 they were 10.4 and 23.1.

The data presented thus far have been based upon the annual registration of births and deaths. The crude birth and death rates relate to total populations, and the general fertility and reproduction rates relate to women of childbearing age regardless of marital status. The trends in all these rates are affected by trends in marriage as well as fertility.

We may turn now to data on children ever born from the censuses of 1960 and earlier years for further indication of trends in fertility by color and for suggestions regarding the relevance of differences

Table 4.2   Gross and net reproduction rates and intrinsic rates of birth and death, by color: United States, 1940–65

| Year | Reproduction rate | | | | Intrinsic rate | | | |
| | Gross | | Net | | Birth | | Death | |
	White	Nonwhite	White	Nonwhite	White	Nonwhite	White	Nonwhite
1965	1,357	1,919	1,314	1,802	20.3	31.5	9.9	8.4
1964	1,495	2,051	1,447	1,923	22.8	33.7	8.8	8.0
1963	1,556	2,102	1,506	1,973	23.2	33.8	7.7	7.1
1962	1,630	2,170	1,577	2,033	24.6	34.8	7.1	6.9
1961	1,704	2,240	1,648	2,100	25.8	35.9	6.7	6.7
1960	1,720	2.241	1,662	2,093	26.2	36.1	6.7	6.9
1959	1,737	2,360	1,679	2,200	26.4	37.8	6.6	6.6
1958	1,735	2,339	1,675	2,178	26.4	37.7	6.7	6.9
1957	1,764	2,371	1,701	2,206	27.0	38.2	6.6	6.9
1956	1,724	2,339	1,665	2,184	26.3	37.7	6.8	6.8
1955	1,675	2,255	1,617	2,101	25.4	36.4	7.1	7.0
1954	1,660	2,216	1,601	2,062	25.1	35.8	7.2	7.2
1953	1,607	2,118	1,546	1,959	24.2	34.4	7.7	7.8
1952	1,579	2,062	1,516	1,897	23.7	33.7	8.0	8.2
1951	1,534	2,027	1,472	1,865	23.0	33.2	8.3	8.4
1950	1,446	1,940	1,387	1,780	21.3	31.8	9.0	8.9
1949	1,462	1,906	1,397	1,743	21.7	31.3	9.1	9.2
1948	1,469	1,845	1,400	1,679	21.9	30.3	9.2	9.6
1947	1,568	1,766	1,492	1,594	23.6	28.8	8.6	10.3
1946	1,406	1,600	1,331	1,435	20.6	25.6	10.1	11.6
1945	1,175	1,493	1,106	1,323	----	----	----	----
1944	1,214	1,520	1,139	1,334	----	----	----	----
1943	1,294	1,543	1,211	1,348	----	----	----	----
1942	1,250	1,487	1,171	1,293	----	----	----	----
1941	1,131	1,458	1,052	1,242	----	----	----	----
1940	1,082	1,422	1,002	1,209	----	----	----	----

Source: National Center for Health Statistics, Vital Statistics of the United Statistics of the United States, 1965, Vol. I, Natality, Tables 1-4, 1-5. (See text for definitions of rates.)

by color in proportions married to the fertility rates. Table 4.3 presents the average number of children ever born per 1,000 ever-married women for 1950 and 1960. The data are shown by age, type of residence, and color. As expected, the rates were rather considerably higher for the nonwhite than for the white group for both census years. For both dates and for both color groups, the rates were lowest in urban areas and highest in rural-farm areas.

Table 4.3 Children ever born per 1,000 ever-married women 15-49 years old, by color and age of woman: United States, urban and rural, 1960 and 1950

Residence and age	White			Nonwhite			Percent excess nonwhite over white	
	1960	1950	Percent change 1950-60	1960	1950	Percent change 1950-60	1960	1950
UNITED STATES								
15-19	729	548	33.0	1,234	917	34.6	69.3	67.3
20-24	1,370	1,028	33.3	1,992	1,473	35.2	45.4	43.3
25-29	2,171	1,620	34.0	2,766	1,932	43.2	27.4	19.3
30-34	2,559	2,034	25.8	3,138	2,272	38.1	22.6	11.7
35-39	2,629	2,218	18.5	3,147	2,476	27.1	19.7	11.6
40-44	2,516	2,329	8.0	2,977	2,660	11.9	18.3	14.2
45-49	2,354	2,456	- 4.2	2,824	2,803	0.7	20.0	14.1
URBAN								
15-19	709	502	41.2	1,219	901	35.3	71.9	79.5
20-24	1,292	910	42.0	1,899	1,320	43.9	47.0	45.1
25-29	2,067	1,454	42.2	2,585	1,632	58.4	25.1	12.2
30-34	2,444	1,821	34.2	2,860	1,806	58.4	17.0	- 0.8
35-39	2,481	1,943	27.7	2,761	1,879	46.9	11.3	- 3.3
40-44	2,330	2,022	15.2	2,504	2,057	21.7	7.5	1.7
45-49	2,133	2,141	- 0.4	2,323	2,263	2.7	8.9	5.7
RURAL NONFARM								
15-19	768	612	25.5	1,272	946	34.5	65.6	54.6
20-24	1,550	1,218	27.3	2,289	1,687	35.7	47.7	38.5
25-29	2,381	1,857	28.2	3,370	2,469	36.5	41.5	33.0
30-34	2,781	2,325	19.6	4,072	2,930	39.0	46.4	26.0
35-39	2,924	2,543	15.0	4,351	3,255	33.7	48.8	28.0
40-44	2,877	2,661	8.1	4,306	3,328	29.4	49.7	25.1
45-49	2,787	2,776	0.4	4,072	3,166	28.6	46.1	14.0
RURAL FARM								
15-19	773	589	31.2	1,270	927	37.0	64.3	57.4
20-24	1,609	1,304	23.4	2,442	1,902	28.4	51.8	45.9
25-29	2,587	2,167	19.4	3,843	2,947	30.4	48.6	36.0
30-34	3,083	2,732	12.8	4,914	3,963	24.0	59.4	45.1
35-39	3,265	3,137	4.1	5,462	4,508	21.2	67.3	43.7
40-44	3,260	3,403	- 4.2	5,584	4,719	18.3	71.3	38.7
45-49	3,161	3,582	-11.8	5,307	4,869	9.0	67.9	35.9

Source: U. S. Bureau of the Census, 1960 Census of Population, Vol. I, Characteristics of the Population, Part 1, U. S. Summary, Table 190; 1950 Census of Population, Fertility, P-E, No. 5C, Table 1.

In urban areas and in the United States as a whole the fertility differential by color in 1960 tended to be inversely related to age: it was most pronounced at the youngest ages and least pronounced at ages 40-44.

Table 4.3 points up the fact that the 1950-60 percent increases in fertility were larger for nonwhite than for white women within each type of residence and at each age of ever-married women considered, but especially at ages 25 and over. Hence the differentials by color were wider in 1960 than in 1950, especially at ages 25 and over. Also, the differentials by type of residence were larger among the nonwhite than among the white group. After age 25 the differentials by color were lowest in urban areas and largest in the rural-farm areas (Fig. 4.1).

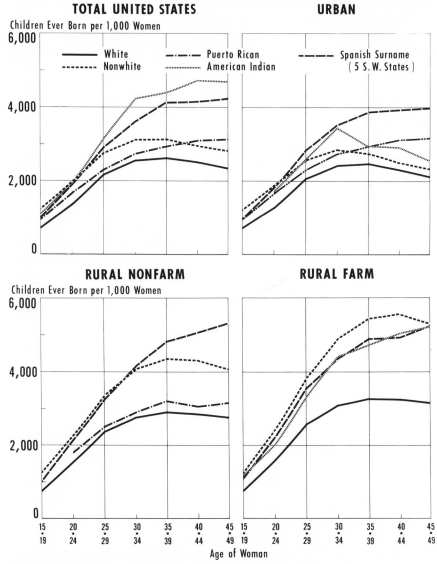

Fig. 4.1. Number of children ever born per 1,000 ever-married women 15-49 years old, by age, color, ethnic group, and type of residence of the woman: United States, 1960.

However, relatively few of either the white or nonwhite people are now classified as "rural-farm."

The disparity of fertility rates by color was greater in the South than in other regions. Also, it may be noted that regional differences in fertility were greater among the nonwhite than among the white group. Both of these situations may be due to the relatively high fertility of rural Negroes in the South and to the higher proportion of nonwhite residents in rural areas in the South than in other regions. In other regions virtually all of the nonwhite population was concentrated in urban areas, where fertility rates were relatively low. In the Northeast and North Central regions the fertility rates were lower for nonwhite than for white ever-married women 35-49 years of age.[4]

It may also be noted that the differentials in fertility rates by size of urbanized area were greater for nonwhite than for white women. This held true for the total urbanized areas and for the central cities and the urban fringe considered separately. For both white and nonwhite women the fertility rates tended to be higher in the urban fringes than in central cities of urbanized areas of each size. However, the fertility rates for nonwhite women in central cities tended to be higher than those for white women in the urban fringes of urbanized areas.[5]

The fertility rates for the years 1940-60 permit one to follow certain cohorts through two decades, that is, three census reports. They indicate that the greater excess of nonwhite over white fertility at younger rather than older ages held true for cohorts as well as for cross-cohort comparisons. Thus for the cohort of women born in 1920-24, the excess of nonwhite over white fertility was 32 percent at ages 15-19 in 1940, 19 percent at ages 25-29 in 1950, and 20 percent at ages 35-39 in 1960. For the 1915-19 cohort, the excess was 31 percent, 11 percent, and 18 percent at ages 20-24, 30-34, and 40-44, respectively. For the 1910-14 cohort the percentage excesses for the nonwhite group were 27 percent, 12 percent, and 20 percent at ages 25-29, 35-39, and 45-49, respectively.[6]

There are differences by color in proportions married at young ages and also in stability of marriage; Chapter 7 presents much of the analysis of marital characteristics in relation to fertility by color.

For both white and nonwhite women under 25 years old and described as "married and husband present," the fertility rates were generally about the same as (sometimes even lower than) those for the "other ever-married" women. However, at older ages of the childbearing period the fertility rates for the women classified as "married and husband present" were higher than those for the "other ever-married" women. Since broken marriages are more frequent among nonwhite couples than among white couples, the excesses in fertility of the nonwhite over white tended to be enhanced at the older ages when the analysis is restricted to the "married and husband present" group.

Distributions of White and Nonwhite Women by Number of Children Ever Born

The preceding discussion has concerned the *average* number of children ever born, by age and color of the women. Table 4.4 presents the *distributions* of ever-married women in the United States in 1960, by number of children ever born, color, age, and type of residence. The data for urban women point up the higher proportions childless among white than among nonwhite women under 25 years old but lower proportions at later ages. The conspicuously high proportions childless among nonwhite women 40-49 years old reflect the conditions of low fertility and high proportions childless among urban Negro couples a quarter of a century ago. At all ages the proportion of women reporting five or more children ever born was higher for the nonwhite than for the white women.

The 1950-60 increase in the fertility of white women was achieved not by major increases in proportions of wives with five or more children but by decreases in proportions with fewer than two children and increases in proportions with two, three, and four children. Thus, among white ever-married women 25-29 years old, the proportions reporting two to four live births were about 46 percent in 1950 and 62 percent in 1960. Among nonwhite women, however, there were appreciable increases in proportions reporting five or more children as well as increases in proportions reporting two to four children. The decline in proportions reporting under two children was also more pronounced among the nonwhite than among the white women.

For both white and nonwhite women, the proportion childless was higher in 1940 than in 1910 for each age and type of residence. Since 1940, there have been marked declines in proportions childless for both white and nonwhite women. The declines have been especially marked for urban nonwhite women under 25 years old. Thus, in 1940, the proportion childless among urban ever-married women 20-24 years old was 47 percent for white women and 46 percent for non-

Table 4.4 Percent distribution of ever-married women 15-49 years old, by number of children ever born, by age and color: United States and urban areas, 1960

Residence, color, and age	Total women	Children ever born						
		None	1	2	3	4	5 and 6	7 or more
UNITED STATES								
White								
15-19	100.0	46.0	39.7	11.4	2.2	0.4	0.2	0.1
20-24	100.0	25.0	33.7	26.4	10.5	3.2	1.0	0.1
25-29	100.0	12.3	19.6	31.3	21.1	9.8	5.1	0.7
30-34	100.0	9.7	14.5	28.9	23.4	12.8	8.5	2.2
35-39	100.0	10.2	14.9	28.0	21.7	12.5	9.2	3.4
40-44	100.0	13.0	17.2	27.5	19.0	10.8	8.4	4.0
45-49	100.0	17.1	19.5	25.9	16.4	9.1	7.6	4.4
Nonwhite								
15-19	100.0	26.7	40.3	22.4	7.4	2.0	0.9	0.4
20-24	100.0	17.7	25.5	24.1	16.5	9.3	6.0	0.9
25-29	100.0	14.4	17.5	19.2	16.2	12.5	14.6	5.6
30-34	100.0	15.6	15.7	16.7	14.2	11.2	15.1	11.5
35-39	100.0	18.9	16.8	15.6	12.5	9.6	12.9	13.8
40-44	100.0	23.6	18.2	14.8	10.7	8.1	10.8	13.8
45-49	100.0	26.7	19.1	14.1	9.9	7.3	9.6	13.3
URBAN								
White								
15-19	100.0	47.2	39.1	11.0	2.1	0.4	0.2	0.1
20-24	100.0	27.5	34.1	25.2	9.5	2.7	0.8	0.1
25-29	100.0	13.7	20.8	31.6	20.2	8.9	4.2	0.6
30-34	100.0	10.6	15.4	29.9	23.2	11.9	7.3	1.7
35-39	100.0	11.0	15.9	29.4	21.7	11.7	7.9	2.4
40-44	100.0	14.0	18.3	29.1	18.9	9.9	7.0	2.8
45-49	100.0	18.3	20.9	27.5	16.2	8.2	6.1	2.8
Nonwhite								
15-19	100.0	26.9	40.6	22.0	7.2	2.0	0.8	0.4
20-24	100.0	19.0	26.5	24.3	15.8	8.5	5.2	0.8
25-29	100.0	15.6	18.9	20.1	16.3	11.8	12.8	4.5
30-34	100.0	16.9	16.9	17.9	14.7	11.2	13.6	8.7
35-39	100.0	20.8	18.2	16.9	13.1	9.5	11.8	9.7
40-44	100.0	26.2	19.9	16.0	11.1	7.9	9.7	9.2
45-49	100.0	29.7	20.9	15.1	10.3	7.0	8.4	8.6

Source: Derived from U. S. Bureau of the Census, 1960 Census of Population, Vol. I, Characteristics of the Population, Part 1, U. S. Summary, Table 190.

white women. In 1950 the respective proportions were 38 and 32 percent. In 1960 they were 27.5 and 19 percent, respectively. As noted
in Table 4.5, the 1950-60 declines in proportion childless were larger
for nonwhite than for white women for each age group under 40.

Table 4.5   Percent childless among ever-married urban women, by color
and age: United States, 1960 and 1950

Age	Percent childless				Percent change, 1950 to 1960	
	White		Nonwhite		White	Nonwhite
	1960	1950	1960	1950		
15-19	47.2	58.0	26.9	38.4	-18.6	-30.0
20-24	27.5	38.3	19.0	32.1	-28.2	-40.8
25-29	13.7	22.5	15.6	33.9	-39.1	-54.0
30-34	10.6	17.7	16.9	34.8	-40.1	-51.4
35-39	11.0	19.5	20.8	37.2	-43.6	-44.1
40-44	14.0	20.7	26.2	33.7	-32.4	-22.3
45-49	18.3	21.3	29.7	31.7	-14.1	- 6.3

Source: Derived from U. S. Bureau of the Census, 1960 Census of
Population, Vol. I, Characteristics of the Population, Part 1, U. S. Sum-
mary, Table 190; and 1950 Census of Population, Fertility, P-E, No. 5C,
Table 2.

When white and nonwhite cohorts of ever-married women are followed through time, however, the attenuation of childlessness with
age is more marked for the white than for the nonwhite. This could
be due partly to a higher proportion of involuntary childlessness
among the nonwhite women and partly to a higher proportion of
broken marriages. Examples for the total United States follow.

Percent childless among:

	White	Nonwhite
1920-24 cohorts		
At ages 15-19 in 1940	56.2	47.0
At ages 25-29 in 1950	20.1	29.6
At ages 35-39 in 1960	10.2	18.9
1915-19 cohorts		
At ages 20-24 in 1940	40.1	38.3
At ages 30-34 in 1950	15.8	30.2
At ages 40-44 in 1960	13.0	23.6
1910-14 cohorts		
At ages 25-29 in 1940	29.5	34.1
At ages 35-39 in 1950	17.5	31.9
At ages 45-49 in 1960	17.1	26.7

Fertility of Specific Nonwhite Groups

Since Negroes numerically dominate the nonwhite group, the levels and trends of fertility for the total nonwhite group are substantially those for Negroes. As indicated in Table 4.6 and Fig. 4.1, American Indians have the highest age-specific fertility rates except at ages under 25, in which case the rates are highest for Negroes. The Japanese exhibit the lowest rates and the Chinese the next lowest.

Table 4.6 Children ever born per 1,000 ever-married women 15-49 years old, by nativity of white women and by ethnic group of nonwhite women, by residence and age of woman: United States, 1960

Residence and age of woman	White		Nonwhite				Other races
	Native	Foreign-born	Negro	American Indian	Japanese	Chinese	
UNITED STATES							
15-19	724	815	1,258	1,092	a	a	992
20-24	1,376	1,177	2,030	1,952	940	1,151	1,756
25-29	2,189	1,706	2,835	3,170	1,469	1,688	2,526
30-34	2,584	2,149	3,190	4,238	1,968	2,578	3,206
35-39	2,643	2,298	3,139	4,402	2,379	2,547	3,652
40-44	2,525	2,285	2,949	4,733	2,625	2,836	3,974
45-49	2,365	2,191	2,761	4,709	3,013	2,875	3,884
URBANIZED AREAS							
15-19	706	813	1,252	a	a	a	1,107
20-24	1,269	1,077	1,890	1,743	860	1,133	1,609
25-29	2,047	1,614	2,601	2,602	1,381	1,657	2,283
30-34	2,434	2,046	2,797	3,473	1,865	2,547	2,852
35-39	2,445	2,196	2,650	2,982	2,314	2,540	3,278
40-44	2,277	2,149	2,339	2,936	2,469	2,816	3,297
45-49	2,065	2,072	2,157	2,570	2,834	2,852	2,939
OTHER THAN URBANIZED							
15-19	739	820	1,267	1,192	a	a	895
20-24	1,486	1,447	2,299	2,017	1,126	a	1,909
25-29	2,346	1,980	3,340	3,335	1,643	a	2,895
30-34	2,757	2,460	4,042	4,443	2,157	a	3,729
35-39	2,876	2,641	4,177	4,755	2,523	a	4,168
40-44	2,818	2,790	4,133	5,052	2,973	a	4,794
45-49	2,705	2,686	3,769	5,237	3,349	a	5,189

Source: U. S. Bureau of the Census, 1960 Census of Population, Women by Number of Children Ever Born, PC(2)-3A, Table 8. (The rates for "other than urbanized" areas were derived.)

a Rate not shown where base is less than 1,000.

The relatively high rate for the American Indians in the United States as a whole is due in part to their concentration in rural areas. Similarly, the concentration of the Chinese and Japanese in urban areas is doubtless a factor in their relatively low fertility. In urbanized areas the fertility rates for American Indian wives 35 years of age and over are not conspicuously higher than those for the other nonwhite groups. Other factors, however, are the low economic status of the American Indians and the relatively high economic and educational status of the younger Japanese and Chinese in this country. Reflecting the conditions of a generation ago, the fertility rates of the Japanese and Chinese women 40-49 years old surpassed those of Negro women of those ages in urbanized areas.

Puerto Rican Fertility

Fertility rates are available from the 1960 census data for ever-married women in the United States of Puerto Rican birth or parentage. The data in Table 4.7 are shown by type of residence and for the Chicago and New York SMSA's separately.

Table 4.7   Children ever born per 1,000 Puerto Rican women 15–49 years old ever married, by age and nativity of woman: United States, urban and rural nonfarm, and Chicago and New York Standard Metropolitan Statistical Areas, 1960

Area and nativity of woman	15–19	20–24	25–29	30–34	35–39	40–44	45–49
UNITED STATES							
Puerto Rican, total	960	1,692	2,311	2,754	2,974	3,115	3,160
Born in Puerto Rico	977	1,722	2,351	2,784	2,985	3,132	3,155
Puerto Rican parentage	808	1,422	1,992	2,457	2,814	2,748	3,252
URBAN							
Puerto Rican, total	957	1,688	2,306	2,748	2,966	3,117	3,156
Born in Puerto Rico	976	1,718	2,348	2,781	2,981	3,132	3,161
Puerto Rican parentage	785	1,411	1,961	2,423	2,741	2,741	3,034
RURAL NONFARM							
Puerto Rican, total	a	1,825	2,516	2,933	3,201	3,061	3,164
Born in Puerto Rico	a	1,880	2,457	2,880	3,104	3,136	2,772
Puerto Rican parentage	a	a	a	a	a	a	a
CHICAGO SMSA							
Puerto Rican, total	975	1,866	2,661	3,241	3,443	4,136	4,251
Born in Puerto Rico	992	1,859	2,703	3,280	3,409	4,206	4,285
Puerto Rican parentage	a	a	a	a	a	a	a
NEW YORK SMSA							
Puerto Rican, total	951	1,649	2,221	2,667	2,910	3,058	3,102
Born in Puerto Rico	966	1,678	2,265	2,701	2,937	3,069	3,112
Puerto Rican parentage	816	1,368	1,851	2,234	2,291	2,483	a

Source: U. S. Bureau of the Census, 1960 Census of Population, Women by Number of Children Ever Born, PC(2)-3A, Table 10.

[a]Rate not shown where base is less than 200.

The age-specific fertility rates of women of Puerto Rican birth or parentage were consistently higher than those for native white or foreign-born white women in the United States. However, the fertility rates of the Puerto Ricans fell below those of nonwhite women except at ages 40 and over. In urban areas the fertility of Puerto

Rican women was below that of nonwhite women at ages under 35 and above that of nonwhite women at ages 35 and over (Fig. 4.1). Among urban ever-married women of completed fertility (ages 45-49), the average number of children ever born per woman was 2.1 for the white, 2.3 for the nonwhite, and 3.2 for the Puerto Rican group.

Among the Puerto Ricans in this country, the fertility rates tended to be higher for the relatively few living in rural-nonfarm areas than for those in urban areas. Those living in the New York SMSA exhibited fertility rates a little lower than those of the total urban women.

The fertility rates of Puerto Ricans in the New York SMSA were conspicuously lower than those of Puerto Ricans in the Chicago SMSA. This was due partly to the higher proportion in Chicago than in New York of those born in Puerto Rico. In all areas and types of residence in the United States the fertility rates were higher for women of Puerto Rican birth than for those of Puerto Rican parentage. However, the marked contrast between Chicago and New York persists with respect to the fertility of the women born in Puerto Rico. It is likely that since those living in Chicago are more recent migrants from Puerto Rico they are of lower socioeconomic status.

Persons of Spanish Surname

The 1960 census identified white persons of Spanish surname in five Southwestern States. These are largely the Spanish and Mexican Americans in Arizona, California, Colorado, New Mexico, and Texas. It is possible to present fertility rates for these and also for persons of non-Spanish surname in the same five Southwestern states. The age-specific fertility rates for the women of non-Spanish surname in the five Southwestern states were of about the same magnitudes as those for all white women in the United States (compare Tables 4.3 and 4.8). In both cases the data reflect the postwar increases, insofar as women aged 30-39 have higher fertility than those aged 40-49.

The rates of fertility for women of Spanish surname were much higher than those for women of non-Spanish surname (Fig. 4.1). Thus, among ever-married women 30-34 years of age, the fertility rates were approximately 2.4 children ever born per woman of non-Spanish surname and about 3.6 for those of Spanish surname. Among the latter there was a marked differential according to rural-urban residence. The lowest rate was consistently found in urban areas and the highest tended to be found in rural farm areas. That most of the ever-married women of Spanish surname and of childbearing age in the

five Southwestern states are now classified as urban is attested to by
the similarity of the rate for the urban areas and that for the total
Spanish-surname group.

Table 4.8   Spanish surname in relation to children ever born per
1,000 ever-married white women 15-49 years old in five
Southwestern states,[a] by age and residence of woman: 1960

Age of woman	Total white, five states[a]	Spanish surname				Other surname
		Total	Urban	Rural nonfarm	Rural farm	
15-19	750	997	983	1,028	1,127	706
20-24	1,446	1,907	1,852	2,141	2,241	1,375
25-29	2,245	2,937	2,852	3,267	3,554	2,137
30-34	2,584	3,643	3,526	4,170	4,387	2,428
35-39	2,605	4,029	3,856	4,843	4,905	2,435
40-44	2,426	4,140	3,936	5,085	4,943	2,257
45-49	2,243	4,246	3,994	5,336	5,245	2,053

Source: U. S. Bureau of the Census, 1960 Census of Population,
Women by Number of Children Ever Born, PC(2)-3A, Table 11.

[a]The five states are Arizona, California, Colorado, New Mexico,
and Texas

Fertility of Foreign Stock by Country of Origin

The foreign stock by census definition consists of the foreign born
and the natives of foreign of mixed parentage. Because of the nature
of our immigration history the persons of foreign stock in this country are mainly white and are concentrated in the older age groups.
The natives of foreign or mixed parentage are younger on the average
than the foreign-born.

Among ever-married women of foreign stock of given age and country of origin, the average number of children ever born was conspicuously high for those of Mexican origin (Table 4.9). For women under
45 years of age, those of Canadian origin stood in second place. This
probably reflects the influence of the French Catholics among the
migrants from Canada to the United States.

Among ever-married women of foreign white stock under 45 years
of age, those of foreign birth with few exceptions exhibited lower
average number of children ever born than did the natives of foreign
or mixed parentage of similar age and country of origin.[7] In fact, at
young ages the foreign-born in this country are now notable for their

Table 4.9   Country or origin of the foreign stock in relation to children ever born per 1,000 ever-married women 25-54 years of age, by age and nativity of the woman: United States and urbanized areas, 1960

Country of origin and nativity of woman	United States			Urbanized areas		
	25-34	35-44	45-54	25-34	35-44	45-54
Total Foreign Stock	2,208	2,392	2,163	2,106	2,272	2,022
Foreign-born	1,949	2,296	2,226	1,864	2,180	2,103
Foreign or mixed parentage	2,280	2,412	2,143	2,175	2,292	1,992
United Kingdom	2,215	2,402	1,976	2,131	2,307	1,882
Foreign-born	2,023	2,249	1,850	1,902	2,170	1,805
Foreign or mixed parentage	2,304	2,467	2,023	2,235	2,369	1,916
Ireland	2,347	2,725	2,294	2,318	2,715	2,280
Foreign-born	1,997	2,539	2,539	2,014	2,513	2,549
Foreign or mixed parentage	2,410	2,749	2,223	2,377	2,743	2,190
Norway	2,398	2,587	2,275	2,104	2,285	1,916
Foreign-born	1,589	2,167	1,774	1,427	2,018	1,507
Foreign or mixed parentage	2,489	2,627	2,330	2,216	2,323	1,985
Sweden	2,277	2,426	1,921	2,118	2,283	1,703
Foreign-born	1,509	2,094	1,718	1,313	1,947	1,555
Foreign or mixed parentage	2,328	2,447	1,942	2,187	2,309	1,723
Germany	2,006	2,320	2,012	1,870	2,120	1,750
Foreign-born	1,613	1,815	1,565	1,543	1,744	1,461
Foreign or mixed parentage	2,299	2,490	2,121	2,135	2,282	1,844
Poland	2,105	2,247	2,081	2,058	2,191	2,007
Foreign-born	1,946	2,015	1,972	1,893	1,999	1,934
Foreign or mixed parentage	2,123	2,269	2,107	2,078	2,212	2,027
Czechoslovakia	2,136	2,297	2,175	2,052	2,165	1,986
Foreign-born	1,890	1,953	2,073	1,824	1,972	1,955
Foreign or mixed parentage	2,173	2,341	2,194	2,093	2,195	1,993
Austria	2,023	2,133	1,930	1,914	2,021	1,788
Foreign-born	1,623	1,746	1,781	1,501	1,712	1,671
Foreign or mixed parentage	2,077	2,166	1,959	1,969	2,050	1,813
U.S.S.R.	2,059	2,151	1,878	1,970	2,052	1,735
Foreign-born	2,144	2,011	1,850	2,116	1,945	1,768
Foreign or mixed parentage	2,055	2,163	1,886	1,962	2,062	1,725
Italy	2,022	2,233	2,233	1,991	2,218	2,215
Foreign-born	1,893	2,317	2,554	1,863	2,316	2,529
Foreign or mixed parentage	2,036	2,225	2,145	2,006	2,208	2,125
Canada	2,385	2,554	2,215	2,272	2,424	2,059
Foreign-born	2,159	2,415	2,127	2,038	2,275	1,987
Foreign or mixed parentage	2,477	2,640	2,271	2,381	2,533	2,112
Mexico	3,276	4,148	4,580	3,101	3,758	4,127
Foreign-born	3,150	3,982	4,631	2,935	3,516	4,153
Foreign or mixed parentage	3,311	4,221	4,508	3,148	3,866	4,088
Other countries	2,059	2,322	2,123	1,965	2,195	1,979
Foreign-born	1,763	2,157	2,121	1,729	2,093	2,031
Foreign or mixed parentage	2,199	2,368	2,124	2,088	2,228	1,953

Source: U. S. Bureau of the Census, 1960 Census of Population, Women by Number of Children Ever Born, PC(2)-3A, Table 9.

relatively low fertility. The situation is in marked contrast to that existing 50 years ago and reflects in part a change of national origins but mainly a marked decline in fertility levels abroad and among immigrants to this country.[8]

Conspicuously low fertility rates were observed for the foreign-born women reporting Norway, Sweden, Germany, and Austria as countries of birth. The rates were low compared with those for foreign-born women from other countries and those for natives of foreign or mixed parentage representing these four countries. Those born in Austria and Germany probably are in large part refugees of Jewish ancestry and of middle- and upper-educational status. Those from the Scandinavian countries may include an appreciable proportion who came to this country to work as maids, a group that has tended to marry relatively late and to have relatively few children.

Summary
In summary, fertility rates for nonwhite women tend to surpass those for white women in this country. Among the nonwhite ever-married women, the American Indians exhibit highest fertility rates at ages 25 and over and the Negroes at ages under 25. The Japanese and Chinese tend to have the lowest fertility rates among nonwhite women under 40 years of age.

The numerically predominant nonwhite group, the Negroes, tend to surpass the white group with respect to fertility at all ages and in each type of residence. The increase in the fertility of young Negro marriages has tended to surpass that of white marriages since World War II, especially since 1950. As a consequence, the differential in fertility by color has widened. The greater increase in the fertility of nonwhite than of white women and the resulting increase in the excess of the fertility of nonwhite over that of white women, in 1960 as compared with 1950, occurred despite the handicap of larger proportions of broken marriages among the nonwhite couples (described in Chapter 7). In fact, the fertility differential apparently widened despite a widening differential by color in marriage instability during the 1950-60 decade.[9] Several factors may be responsible for these seemingly incompatible trends. As indicated in Chapters 7 and 8, illegitimate births and premarital conceptions among young nonwhite women probably increased substantially during the decade. Also, despite improvements in educational attainment and occupational opportunity, nonwhite women are still more concentrated in the lower socioeconomic groups than are white women. As shown in Chapter 3, family planning had made less impact on nonwhite than on white couples of low economic status by 1960. As indicated in Chapters 9 to 11, the relatively few nonwhite ever-married women 25 years of age and over who attended college and the relatively few of these ages who married men of professional status tended to be characterized by lower fertility than white women of similar age and socioeconomic status. The sharpest increases in fertility of nonwhite women were those for the groups of low educational, occupational, and income status. An important element in the increase in fertility of nonwhite women has been the sharp reduction in childlessness among urban Negro marriages, which may have been due in part to the suppression of venereal infection during and after World War II.

The Puerto Ricans in this country and the women of Spanish surname in five Southwestern states were also characterized by relatively high fertility. As for women of foreign white stock, the average number of children ever born per ever-married woman of specific age within the childbearing period tended to be a little lower for women born abroad than for women born in this country of foreign or mixed parentage. The fertility rates were conspicuously low for women born in Scandinavian countries, Austria, and Germany. The relatively low fertility of the foreign-born stands in marked contrast to the situation 50 years ago.

5 / Residence

Regions[1]

Significant changes have been occurring in the characteristics of the United States population by regions that may, in the long run, bring about considerable differences in traditional fertility patterns. For many years the South has been the region with the highest average number of children ever born to women, reflecting in part the larger proportion of its population residing in rural areas and its considerable nonwhite population. The Northeast has been the region with the lowest fertility, reflecting in part its high proportion of urban population. However, something more than white-nonwhite and urban-rural differences are coming to the fore, as will be evident from data presented below.

As of 1960, regional rates of children ever born per 1,000 women of childbearing age (all races, all marital classes combined) were generally closer to the national averages than they were in 1950 and in 1940, indicating a trend towards a narrowing of fertility differences (Table 5.1). In particular, the North Central region and the West have been gradually overtaking the South with respect to highest fertility. This has happened even though the South still has the lowest proportion of urban population of any region and also contains a relatively larger nonwhite population of high fertility. Probably the rates shown in Table 5.1 for women 30-34 years old in 1960 are better indicators of evolving patterns than those for women of older age. The women 30-34 years old have had full experience from age 15 onwards with high birth rates prevailing in the post-World War II period, whereas some of the older women began childbearing during or before World War II, when birth rates at young ages were lower.

Were it not for the many fertile nonwhite people in the South, the North Central and West regions would already have surpassed the South by 1960 in respect to average number of children ever born to women in some age groups (Tables 5.2 and 5.3). In the 1960 census, for the first time since frontier days, the white population of middle childbearing ages (25-29 and 30-34) in the North Central and West regions was more fertile than that of the South, and this pattern is expected to extend to older ages in the future as the cohorts presently of middle ages advance to those older ages. As recently as the 1950 census, the reverse situation of highest fertility in the South was very much in evidence at all ages.

Nonwhite women in the South have had large increases in fertility since 1950, or since 1940, depending on which age groups of women are compared. But through outmigration of nonwhite persons to other regions, the proportion nonwhite in the total population of the South declined from 24.0 percent in 1940 to 20.9 in 1960, whereas in other regions the proportion increased from 3.8 percent to 7.2.

Table 5.1 Regional variations in children ever born per 1,000 women of childbearing age: 1940-60

Year and age	Rate per 1,000					Regional rate as percent of corresponding U.S. rate			
	United States	North-east	North Central	South	West	North-east	North Central	South	West
1960									
15-19	127	83	112	164	144	65.4	88.2	129.1	113.4
20-24	1,030	799	1,045	1,137	1,127	77.6	101.5	110.4	109.4
25-29	2,007	1,711	2,091	2,114	2,103	85.3	104.2	105.3	104.8
30-34	2,452	2,157	2,560	2,584	2,493	88.0	104.4	105.4	101.7
35-39	2,518	2,234	2,589	2,694	2,531	88.7	102.8	107.0	100.5
40-44	2,407	2,119	2,452	2,648	2,373	88.0	101.9	110.0	98.6
1950									
15-19	105	49	83	154	122	46.7	79.0	146.7	116.2
20-24	738	497	711	912	834	67.3	96.3	123.6	113.0
25-29	1,436	1,152	1,433	1,652	1,509	80.2	99.8	115.0	105.1
30-34	1,871	1,605	1,882	2,101	1,867	85.8	100.6	112.3	99.8
35-39	2,061	1,787	2,026	2,378	1,956	86.7	98.3	115.4	94.9
40-44	2,170	1,885	2,127	2,540	2,015	86.9	98.0	117.1	92.9
1940									
15-19	61	28	49	97	65	45.9	80.3	159.0	106.6
20-24	505	318	461	691	554	63.0	91.3	136.8	109.7
25-29	1,129	858	1,077	1,413	1,125	76.0	95.4	125.2	99.6
30-34	1,678	1,401	1,614	2,025	1,595	83.5	96.2	120.7	95.1
35-39	2,156	1,832	2,041	2,644	1,954	85.0	94.7	122.6	90.6
40-44	2,501	2,201	2,405	3,055	2,201	88.0	96.2	122.2	88.0
Increase 1950-60									
15-19	22	34	29	10	22	...	...	...	...
20-24	292	302	334	225	293	...	...	...	...
25-29	571	559	658	462	594	...	...	...	...
30-34	581	552	678	483	626	...	...	...	...
35-39	457	447	563	316	575	...	...	...	...
40-44	237	234	325	108	358	...	...	...	...
Increase 1940-50									
15-19	44	21	34	57	57	...	...	...	...
20-24	233	179	250	221	280	...	...	...	...
25-29	307	294	356	239	384	...	...	...	...
30-34	193	204	268	76	272	...	...	...	...
35-39	- 95	- 45	- 15	-266	2	...	...	...	...
40-44	-331	-316	-278	-515	-186	...	...	...	...

Source: U. S. Bureau of the Census, 1960 Census of Population, Women by Number of Children Ever Born, PC(2)-3A, Table 1; 1950 Census of Population, Fertility P-E, No. 5C, Tables 1 and 32; and 1940 Census of Population, Differential Fertility, 1940 and 1910—Fertility for States and Large Cities, Tables 3 and 17.

There are some elements of noncomparability in the data shown in Tables 5.2 and 5.3. The 1960 census data include the new states of Alaska and Hawaii, whereas they are not included in 1950 and 1940. Also, the definition of urban and rural residence has been modified since 1940, and the definition of a farm has been changed since 1950. Inclusion of data for Alaska and Hawaii has little effect on the fertility of the white population but reduces slightly that of the nonwhite population in the West. Tabulations of fertility data in the 1950 census by both the old and new definition of urban and rural indicated that the change in definition had little effect on fertility rates.

Table 5.2 Children ever born per 1,000 white women of childbearing age, by age of woman: Regions, urban and rural, 1940-60

Area and year	Age of woman						Age of woman					
	15-19	20-24	25-29	30-34	35-39	40-44	15-19	20-24	25-29	30-34	35-39	40-44
	Total						Urban					
United States												
1960	117	995	1,959	2,392	2,475	2,364	111	900	1,835	2,260	2,314	2,170
1950	92	701	1,409	1,847	2,030	2,132	75	582	1,234	1,625	1,752	1,825
1940	54	472	1,088	1,640	2,112	2,459	37	347	843	1,325	1,725	2,047
Northeast												
1960	74	777	1,694	2,149	2,247	2,136	67	702	1,588	2,057	2,153	2,045
1950	44	475	1,154	1,613	1,807	1,897	34	410	1,063	1,507	1,711	1,780
1940	26	310	851	1,402	1,839	2,207	20	261	754	1,281	1,709	2,069
North Central												
1960	105	1,025	2,074	2,535	2,596	2,463	104	923	1,937	2,387	2,420	2,263
1950	76	692	1,431	1,901	2,046	2,137	71	590	1,274	1,690	1,786	1,849
1940	47	452	1,074	1,617	2,055	2,414	39	364	879	1,348	1,732	2,051
South												
1960	154	1,073	1,996	2,423	2,547	2,506	153	976	1,884	2,275	2,333	2,196
1950	136	859	1,588	2,021	2,291	2,445	124	710	1,332	1,664	1,784	1,879
1940	85	647	1,358	1,969	2,590	3,008	66	449	934	1,404	1,836	2,158
West												
1960	139	1,124	2,096	2,479	2,519	2,352	134	1,046	1,988	2,373	2,394	2,214
1950	121	831	1,513	1,867	1,951	2,010	102	732	1,377	1,694	1,722	1,783
1940	64	549	1,109	1,581	1,931	2,165	47	425	887	1,276	1,592	1,811
	Rural Nonfarm						Rural Farm					
United States												
1960	148	1,280	2,246	2,670	2,815	2,762	84	1,171	2,365	2,933	3,141	3,147
1950	135	962	1,710	2,193	2,393	2,492	98	980	1,972	2,559	2,977	3,241
1940	82	668	1,396	1,962	2,413	2,742	68	705	1,672	2,484	3,159	3,498
Northeast												
1960	103	1,104	2,075	2,461	2,576	2,468	70	1,026	2,235	2,827	3,046	3,021
1950	81	745	1,475	1,965	2,120	2,257	75	784	1,826	2,443	2,683	2,943
1940	44	493	1,208	1,780	2,207	2,588	51	501	1,348	2,152	2,797	3,184
North Central												
1960	134	1,323	2,359	2,790	2,891	2,778	61	1,211	2,479	3,061	3,211	3,138
1950	105	915	1,664	2,205	2,317	2,408	61	925	1,900	2,467	2,826	3,036
1940	73	630	1,340	1,917	2,330	2,658	45	596	1,528	2,291	2,883	3,351
South												
1960	174	1,275	2,182	2,650	2,855	2,912	107	1,108	2,170	2,740	3,057	3,185
1950	170	1,055	1,834	2,302	2,628	2,726	123	1,046	2,044	2,678	3,173	3,528
1940	112	777	1,560	2,121	2,688	3,051	87	810	1,816	2,690	3,568	4,160
West												
1960	171	1,475	2,489	2,848	2,972	2,839	100	1,381	2,646	3,105	3,207	3,132
1950	181	1,108	1,846	2,238	2,384	2,505	120	1,085	2,044	2,583	2,898	2,929
1940	102	778	1,401	1,985	2,311	2,543	68	730	1,731	2,438	3,009	3,271

Source: U. S. Bureau of the Census, 1960 Census of Population, Vol. I, Characteristics of the Population, state reports, Table 113 and estimates for states with no color detail for urban-rural parts; 1950 Census of Population, Fertility, P-E, No. 5C, Table 32; and 1940 Census of Population, Differential Fertility, 1940 and 1910--Fertility for States and Large Cities, Tables 3 and 17.

Table 5.3 Children ever born per 1,000 nonwhite women of childbearing age, by age of woman: Regions, urban and rural, 1940-60

Area and year	Age of woman — Total						Age of woman — Urban					
	15-19	20-24	25-29	30-34	35-39	40-44	15-19	20-24	25-29	30-34	35-39	40-44
United States												
1960	200	1,287	2,332	2,836	2,909	2,787	212	1,244	2,186	2,587	2,548	2,340
1950	195	1,012	1,654	2,079	2,310	2,509	192	906	1,391	1,643	1,749	1,936
1940	122	769	1,463	2,011	2,509	2,915	105	574	1,060	1,475	1,826	2,225
Northeast												
1960	186	1,045	1,825	2,171	2,144	1,911	190	1,042	1,810	2,145	2,107	1,863
1950	128	782	1,114	1,499	1,489	1,677	126	774	1,097	1,451	1,437	1,627
1940	79	507	1,005	1,393	1,699	2,082	81	492	983	1,368	1,644	2,014
North Central												
1960	219	1,359	2,329	2,677	2,560	2,303	226	1,361	2,322	2,652	2,517	2,236
1950	210	997	1,463	1,575	1,728	1,970	218	984	1,418	1,456	1,631	1,862
1940	116	707	1,158	1,545	1,777	2,218	104	672	1,075	1,459	1,638	2,056
South												
1960	202	1,366	2,581	3,216	3,382	3,281	223	1,323	2,377	2,839	2,818	2,612
1950	207	1,093	1,892	2,404	2,683	2,893	207	949	1,539	1,819	1,918	2,126
1940	130	819	1,580	2,214	2,807	3,216	114	582	1,079	1,519	1,951	2,367
West												
1960	176	1,181	2,096	2,597	2,704	2,641	176	1,113	1,976	2,449	2,529	2,430
1950	136	890	1,440	1,864	2,064	2,122	147	859	1,295	1,638	1,743	1,664
1940	75	675	1,604	2,106	2,670	3,305	74	406	1,083	1,492	2,028	2,357
	Rural Nonfarm						Rural Farm					
United States												
1960	188	1,453	2,839	3,668	4,027	4,021	151	1,369	3,100	4,426	5,140	4,349
1950	233	1,196	2,133	2,696	3,008	3,110	177	1,270	2,556	3,715	4,292	4,526
1940	136	844	1,655	2,244	2,844	3,183	136	1,049	2,251	3,211	4,065	4,430
North and West												
1960	159	1,390	2,521	3,216	3,520	3,641	117	1,259	2,597	3,487	3,731	4,066
1950	146	1,048	1,893	2,871	3,211	3,088	103	918	2,306	3,972	3,640	3,814
1940	119	732	1,491	1,829	2,492	2,845	87	886	2,133	2,836	3,334	4,317
South												
1960	193	1,467	2,921	3,780	4,141	4,094	153	1,377	3,145	4,518	5,283	5,456
1950	247	1,220	2,173	2,664	2,976	3,115	181	1,292	2,570	3,699	4,322	4,561
1940	139	852	1,657	2,277	2,843	3,177	139	1,051	2,246	3,205	4,071	4,400

Source: U. S. Bureau of the Census, 1960 Census of Population, Vol. I, Characteristics of the Population, state reports, Table 113 and estimates for states with no color detail for urban-rural parts; 1950 Census of Population, Fertility, P-E, No. 5C, Table 32; and 1940 Census of Population, Differential Fertility, 1940 and 1910—Fertility for States and Large Cities, Tables 3 and 17.

Unfortunately, the change in the definition of a farm may introduce an appreciable difference in fertility data for rural nonfarm and rural farm areas for 1960 as compared with those for earlier censuses. One reason for the change was to make the definition of farm residence essentially consistent with the definition of a farm used in the 1959 census of agriculture. The net effect of the change is to exclude from the farm population persons living on places considered farms by the occupants but from which agricultural products are not sold or from which sales are below a specified minimum. (Some lived where they could grow food for their large family only.) A test conducted in the Current Population Survey of April 1960 indicated that at that time the change in the definition of the farm population resulted in a net reduction of about 21 percent in the farm population.[2] A cohort comparison of data from the 1950 and 1960 censuses can be used to obtain an idea of the combined effect on fertility rates of changes in the definition of a farm, net migration from farms between 1950 and 1960, and mortality. For example, the 1950 census found 676,500 women 40-44 years old (all races) residing in rural farm areas of the United States; these women had an average of 3,391 children ever born per 1,000 women. The 1960 census found only 397,758 women 50-54 years old in rural farm areas, who represent in a sense the rural farm women surviving from those 40-44 years old in 1950; these women in 1960 had an average of 3,160 children ever born per 1,000 women. Thus, the rural farm cohort apparently *lost* 231 children per 1,000 women between 1950 and 1960, or 7 percent of the rate of 3,391 in 1950, by the time of the 1960 census. In contrast, similar computations for the rural nonfarm women aged 40-44 in 1950 and aged 50-54 in 1960 indicated a *gain* of 203 children per 1,000 women, or 8 percent of the rate of 2,544 in 1950.

The loss to rural farm fertility from changes in definition of a farm and from net outmigration of farm population can only be measured by following a cohort of completed or virtually completed fertility from one census to the next, as was done above. It cannot be measured by comparing data for women of the *same* age group in two censuses, as such data involve different cohorts of women. The 1960 census generally shows much higher fertility among rural farm women of each 5-year age group through 35-39 than the 1950 census shows for *other* women of the *same* age. Rural farm white women in the South are an exception; they have had little apparent change. However, rural farm nonwhite women in the South have had very large increases, in terms of comparisons for identical age groups in 1950 and 1960.

It is not known whether the change in the definition of a farm was the main cause, but as of 1960 the traditional pattern of higher fertility among white women in the South than in other regions was reversed among rural farm women at ages from 20-24 through 30-34, whereas the traditional pattern was very strong in 1950. In urban areas the traditional pattern of highest fertility in the South was strong for urban white women in 1940, was weaker in 1950, and by 1960 the South had a slightly less fertile urban white population than the North Central and West regions. Possibly, the South would have fallen even further behind the other regions had movement of population from rural to urban areas of the South not bolstered the urban fertility of that region.

Although nonwhite women are generally much more fertile than white women, an exception may be noted for the Northeast region in 1960. In some age groups the nonwhite women in urban areas of the Northeast were less fertile than the white women.

Most of the above discussion of data for regions has been based on rates for women aged 25-29 and older. The South still has a pattern of early marriage that causes the fertility rates for women 15-19 years old to be higher there than in other regions, for white and nonwhite alike. By age 25-29 the basic differences emerging in lifetime fertility are more apparent.

Perhaps one of the most significant changes in the fertility of the white population has occurred in urban areas of the various regions. This was a transition from fertility inadequate for replacement of population to fertility that is more than adequate. Given a sex ratio at birth of 105.8 male babies per 100 female babies and a survival proportion for daughters from birth to age 27 (the mean age of child-bearing), according to United States life tables for 1959-61, white women need a *lifetime* average of about 2,130 children ever born per 1,000 women in order that 1,000 of these children will be daughters surviving to the mean age of childbearing in turn to replace the 1,000 women. As of 1960 the white women 30-34 years old in urban areas already had rates of 2,057 in the Northeast and 2,275 to 2,387 in the other three regions; these rates will increase considerably by the time the women complete their childbearing. (A rough idea of the possible further increase can be obtained by subtracting the rate for women 30-34 years old in 1950 from the rate for women 40-44 in 1960; this procedure yields a further increase of about 500 per 1,000 women, or ultimate rates ranging from about 2,600 to 2,900 in the urban parts of regions.)

In contrast to the more than adequate fertility in 1960 among urban white women 30-34 years old, the less fertile urban white women 40-44 years old had fertility rates that were of border-line replacement magnitude, and data from the 1950 and the 1940 censuses indicate that some older cohorts of urban white women fell far short of replacement needs. A higher replacement quota than 2,130 should be used for censuses prior to 1960, because the white women bore most of their children at a time when mortality was higher. (A corresponding quota computed from 1939 to 1941 life tables is 2,220.)

Usually, there is more variation in fertility rates between the urban and rural parts of regions than there is among regions within any one type of urban-rural residence. This means that other things being equal, there is an *underlying* tendency for urban-rural residence to be more important than region of residence in explaining levels of fertility.

Another way of examining the situation is to study the contribution of various factors to changes over time in national fertility in a manner that takes population distribution into account. For example, the following type of information is obtained by conventional standardization procedures:

Children ever born per 1,000 white women 30-34 years old

Year:	
1960	2,392
1950	1,847
Increase	545
Change due to:	
Changing distribution of population[a] by regions	+ 5
Changing distribution of population by urban-rural residence	− 40
Increase in fertility of urban population	+ 436
Increase in fertility of rural nonfarm population	+ 97[b]
Increase in fertility of rural farm population	+ 42[b]
Interaction of above factors	+ 5
Total	+ 545

[a]The term population, as used here, refers to white women aged 30-34.

[b]The figures for the rural nonfarm and rural farm population unavoidably include the effect of the change in definition of a farm. Were it possible to use a comparable definition, the rural nonfarm figure would be somewhat lower than the one shown and the rural farm figure would be somewhat higher, but rough tests indicate that the rural nonfarm figure would still exceed the rural farm figure.

The above components of change were obtained by permitting only one characteristic to vary at a time, all others being held constant.[3] The results are only illustrative, because different magnitudes would be obtained from similar computations for the other age groups, but the figures given illustrate the general principle that between 1950 and 1960 increases in urban fertility accounted for the bulk of the increase in national fertility, in substance reflecting the fact that a large proportion of the population resides in urban areas.

States

Certain states west of the Mississippi River and in the deep South have the most fertile populations, whereas states with the least fertile populations are in the Northeast. Because the ranking of the states varies with different measures of fertility and the date to which the measure relates, no one state can be characterized as having the most fertile or the least fertile population except in terms of a specific measure and date. This is illustrated by the brief table below.

Crude birth rate

Five most fertile states: 1960		Five most fertile states: 1950	
Alaska	33.4	New Mexico	34.5¹
New Mexico	32.3	Alaska	31.2
Utah	29.5	Utah	31.1
Arizona	28.2	Arizona	30.7
Louisiana	27.7	Mississippi	30.4
Five least fertile states: 1960		Five least fertile states: 1950	
West Virginia	21.2	Connecticut	20.2
Pennsylvania	21.3	New Jersey	20.3
New York	21.4	New York	20.4
Rhode Island	21.4	Rhode Island	20.5
Oregon	21.7	Massachusetts	20.6

Total fertility rate: 1960
(Sum of age-specific birth rates)

Five most fertile states		Five least fertile states	
Alaska	4,881	West Virginia	3,297
New Mexico	4,566	New York	3,298
North Dakota	4,399	Tennessee	3,336
South Dakota	4,371	Pennsylvania	3,359
Utah	4,332	North Carolina	3,396

Children ever born per 1,000
women 30-34 years old: 1960

Five most fertile states		Five least fertile states	
Utah	3,121	New York	2,049
Mississippi	3,110	New Jersey	2,094
Idaho	3,079	Rhode Island	2,160
North Dakota	3,057	Connecticut	2,174
South Dakota	2,980	Pennsylvania	2,221
		(District of Columbia	1,860)

Alaska ranks high in terms of the crude birth rate and the total fertility rate for 1960. Several other states have more children ever born per 1,000 women 30-34 years old, although Alaska is well above the national average. Alaska's Eskimos and American Indians are among the most fertile ethnic groups, but in 1960 only 23 percent of the population was nonwhite. The annual crude birth rate is high in Alaska partly because it has relatively many young white couples and relatively few older ones as compared with the situation in some other states. Some couples live temporarily in Alaska while the husband is in military service, have children there, are later rotated back home and replaced by other couples who repeat the process.

West Virginia ranks low in terms of the crude birth rate in 1960 but that state has rates of children ever born to women of various ages that are above the national average. Possibly net outmigration of young adults from West Virginia had something to do with the deviant patterns in fertility. Again, the District of Columbia's women are among the nation's least fertile in respect to children ever born, but the District usually has an annual birth rate above the national average.

In the preceding section on regions it was pointed out that women 30-34 years old, nationally, might increase their average number of children ever born by about 500 children per 1,000 women by the time they reach age 45. If 500 is added to the average number of children ever born per 1,000 women aged 30-34 in each state in 1960 and if the resulting sum is compared with corresponding total fertility rate from vital statistics for the year 1960, the latter turns out to be much higher than the former. The situation holds for the most fertile states and the least fertile states alike. It is believed, therefore, that the total fertility rates in 1960 were temporarily high, not indicative of likely magnitudes of lifetime childbearing by women.

Presented below are tallies of states and the District of Columbia by (1) the crude birth rate and (2) children ever born per 1,000 women 30-34 years old, for specified dates. The crude birth rate tallies indicate that in 1960 the states were more concentrated in the range from 21.0 to 26.9 than they were in 1950 and 1940, reflecting a trend towards homogeneity. In the section on regions it was noted that there was also a trend over time towards more homogeneity in data on children ever born; but when individual states are tallied (below) an opposite pattern emerges, with wider distribution in 1960 than in 1950. This simply means that large groups of states, such as regions, are less subject to deviation than individual states. Many of the states that in 1950 had rates of children under 2,600 per 1,000 women aged 30-34 moved up by 300 to 400 points by 1960, but a few of the less populous states had even greater increases.

It may also be of interest to note from the tallies that only 8 states in 1960 had rates of less than 2,300, whereas in 1910 there were 21 states with fertility that low, although nationally the women aged 30-34 in 1910 were more fertile than women of the same ages in 1960.

Tally of states and the District of Columbia
(New states of Alaska and Hawaii included in 1960)

Crude birth rate	1960	1950	1940	
Under 21	-	5	29	
21.0-22.9	13	4	4	
23.0-24.9	17	16	5	
25.0-26.9	14	10	7	
27+	7	14	4	
Total	51	49	49	
Children ever born per 1,000 women 30-34	1960	1950	1940	1910
Under 2,000	1	23	34	9
2,000-2,299	6	17	12	12
2,300-2,599	17	9	3	7
2,600-2,899	20	-	-	5
2,900+	7	-	-	16
Total	51	49	49	49

In 1960 New York had the lowest rate (2,049) of children ever born per 1,000 women 30-34 years old among the states. The chances were excellent that these women would augment that rate by more than 400 per 1,000 by age 45 and thus eventually exceed by a considerable margin a replacement rate of about 2,130. Hence, no state in 1960 was falling short of replacement needs in terms of data for women 30-34 years old. In contrast, 12 states in 1960 had rates of less than 2,130 per 1,000 women 45-49 years old, indirectly reflecting the effect of the economic depression of the 1930's, when annual birth rates were very low.

Some correlations. In terms of data for states and the District of Columbia, there is high correlation ($r = .90$) between the crude birth rate and the total fertility rate for the one year, 1960. These two measures involve the same births but differ in the extent to which the age-sex composition of the population is taken into account. (The crude birth rate uses the total population as a base without regard to its sex or age distribution, whereas the total fertility rate involves the sum of birth rates specific for age of women and thus holds age and sex constant.)

The correlation between the total fertility rate for 1960 and the 1960 census ratio of population under 5 years old to women 15-49 years old is only .79. The "low" correlation of .79 does not mean that the two measures of fertility are inconsistent with one another; it rather reflects the effect of the different time periods involved. There is generally good agreement, at least for white persons, between 1960 census data for states on population under 5 years old and vital statistics for the 5-year period ending on the 1960 census date; that is, the population under 5 years old as counted by the census in each state compares quite well with the number expected from data on births in the 5-year period according to vital statistics after allowance is made for mortality and migration between the time the children were born and the date of the census. Because mortality and migration are of relatively minor importance, the "low" correlation of .79 just cited is thought to reflect chiefly the difference between fertility conditions in the one year 1960 and conditions in the 5-year period ending April 1, 1960.

The correlation between the 1960 census ratio of population under 5 to women aged 15-49 and the 1960 census rate of children ever born per 1,000 women aged 30-34 is .81. Further evidence of the instability of correlations when different measures of fertility are used is given by the following data. It will be noted that the crude birth rates for any one year are less well correlated with the proportion of population that is urban than are rates of children ever born per 1,000 women aged 30-34. The fact that these correlations fall far short of unity indicates that fertility conditions vary depending on the point of view and no one type of measure will serve all viewpoints.

Crude birth rate correlated with
percent urban, for states, by color

Year	White	Nonwhite
1960	-.14	-.37
1950	-.52	-.52
1940	-.72	-.78

Children ever born per 1,000 women
aged 30-34 correlated with percent
urban, for states

Year	
1960	-.79
1950	-.86
1940	-.85

Metropolitan Areas

Except in New England, a standard metropolitan statistical area (SMSA) consists of one or more counties which are metropolitan in character and which meet certain criteria of social and economic integration, such as movement of persons to work, telephone services, marketing distributions, and so forth. In New England, where towns (townships) are administratively more important, SMSA's are delineated in terms of towns rather than counties. The largest city in an SMSA is always a central city, but any other large city in the area is not classified as a central city unless it meets special rules for classification as such. All 313 cities of 50,000 or more inhabitants according to the 1960 census are in SMSA's, but only 208 are primary or secondary central cities. A few SMSA's have twin central cities (26 such cities in all) that are individually of smaller size but in combination have at least 50,000 population.

In 1960, 212 SMSA's were delineated in the United States. They contained 63.0 percent of the nation's population. Within SMSA's, 51.4 percent of the population resided in central cities and 48.6 percent in the SMSA "rings."

Since SMSA's have predominately urban populations, they have a less fertile population than nonmetropolitan areas. This is exemplified by the data presented in Table 5.4. Whereas women ever married 35-

44 years old in SMSA's in 1960 averaged 2,433 children ever born per 1,000, those outside SMSA's averaged 3,003. Within SMSA's, nationally, the women who lived in the urban parts of rings had fertility nearly as low as that of women living in central cities, suggesting that people in the suburbs have a tendency towards large-city fertility patterns. Even the women living in the rural parts of SMSA's have somewhat lower fertility than those living in rural areas outside SMSA's who are not as close to a large city.

Table 5.4 Children ever born per 1,000 women ever married 35–44 years old, by metropolitan-nonmetropolitan residence: United States, 1960

Area	Women ever married, 35–44	Children ever born per 1,000 women
METROPOLITAN		
Total	7,635,251	2,433
Central cities	3,752,748	2,347
Other urban	3,024,790	2,429
Rural nonfarm	757,170	2,771
Rural farm	100,543	3,236
NONMETROPOLITAN		
Total	3,952,324	3,003
Urban	1,593,369	2,657
Rural nonfarm	1,655,200	3,124
Rural farm	703,755	3,499

Source: U. S. Bureau of the Census, 1960 Census of Population, Vol. I, Characteristics of the Population, Part 1, U. S. Summary, Table 101.

On a national basis, fertility varies inversely with the size of the SMSA's. That is, fertility in terms of average number of children ever born to women is lowest in SMSA's of 3 million or more, intermediate for those of 1 million to 3 million, and highest for those with less than 1 million population.

The population of SMSA's increased by 26.4 percent between 1950 and 1960, using their 1960 boundaries. Within SMSA's the population in central cities increased by 10.7 percent, of which 9.3 percent is a result of annexation of territory by central cities. Outside central cities the population of the "rings" had a net increase of 48.5 percent despite a loss of 13.1 percent through annexation of territory to central cities. Population growth between 1950 and 1960 of course reflected the balance of births, deaths, and net migration (including annexations as a form of "migration"). A considerable excess of births over deaths, and hence a considerable natural increase, usually exists even in areas where the average number of children ever born to women is low. Annual births and deaths are partly a function of the age and sex distribution of the population. Most parts of the country, urban and rural alike, have large proportions of population of childbearing age and relatively few elderly persons as compared with the distribution that would eventually exist were migration to cease and were age-specific birth rates and death rates to remain unchanged for many years.

Table 5.5 presents a brief summary of the balance of births, deaths, and net migration for the 12 largest SMSA's listed in order of size, and for their central cities. (Data on children ever born to women 35-44 years old appear in Table 5.7.) For reasons of space, Table 5.5 does not show deaths separately, but the number of deaths can be determined by subtraction of natural increase from the number of births. When that is done, the ratio of births to deaths turns out to range from 2.0 in the New York SMSA to 3.4 in the Washington SMSA. The ratio generally is a little over 2.0 in central cities and around 3.0 in most rings.

SMSA's vary considerably in the extent to which they attract inmigrants in search of economic opportunity. In fact, a few SMSA's lose population through net outmigration, but most have net inmigration. Vital statistics do not differentiate between events occurring to new residents and those occurring to residents long present in an area. Hence, some of the natural increase in an SMSA is an indirect result of migration, because these migrants are generally concentrated in the child-rearing ages when mortality is low. In many of the largest SMSA's, however, population growth over the short run, such as the period from 1950 to 1960, comes more largely from an excess of births over deaths than from net inmigration from outside the SMSA. The same may also be true of the smaller SMSA's. The discussion here is of the SMSA as an entity and not of what happens within an SMSA through movement of population from central cities to the suburbs. With relatively few exceptions, natural increase is of greater magnitude than net migration for large SMSA's as *entities,* but the reverse situation usually applies for components *within* an SMSA.

Table 5.5 Components of population change, 1950–60, for the
12 largest Metropolitan Areas and their central cities

(Numbers in thousands)

Area	Popu-lation 1960	Increase or decrease in population, 1950-60	Natural increase[a]	Births	Net migra-tion[b]
METROPOLITAN AREAS					
New York, N. Y.	10,695	1,139	1,029	2,067	109
Los Angeles-Long Beach	6,743	2,375	790	1,287	1,585
Chicago, Ill.	6,221	1,043	782	1,362	261
Philadelphia, Pa.-N. J.	4,343	672	496	914	176
Detroit, Mich.	3,762	746	649	928	97
San Francisco-Oakland	2,783	543	348	580	195
Boston, Mass.	2,589	179	c	c	c
Pittsburgh, Pa.	2,405	192	296	525	-104
St. Louis, Mo.-Ill.	2,060	341	291	485	50
Washington, D.C.-Md.-Va.	2,002	538	330	468	208
Cleveland, Ohio	1,797	331	240	399	91
Baltimore, Md.	1,727	322	233	385	89
CENTRAL CITIES					
New York, N. Y.	7,782	-110	708	1,562	-818
Los Angeles-Long Beach	2,823	602	291	555	311
Chicago, Ill.	3,550	- 71	447	864	-518
Philadelphia, Pa.	2,003	- 69	210	454	-279
Detroit, Mich.	1,670	-179	276	450	-455
San Francisco-Oakland	1,108	- 52	97	235	-149
Boston, Mass.	697	-104	c	c	c
Pittsburgh, Pa.	604	- 72	107	190	-180
St. Louis, Mo.	750	-107	106	210	-212
Washington, D. C.	764	- 38	119	205	-158
Cleveland, Ohio	876	- 39	136	237	-174
Baltimore, Md.	939	- 11	126	235	-137

Source: U.S. Bureau of the Census, 1960 Census of Population, and National Center for Health Statistics, Vital Statistics of the United States, annual reports 1950-60

[a]Excess of registered births over deaths, April 1, 1950, to March 31, 1960.

[b]Difference between increase in population, 1950 to 1960, and natural increase.

[c]Vital statistics not available separately for Boston area or city, 1958.

Among the 12 largest SMSA's, the Los Angeles-Long Beach SMSA is the only one in which net migration for the SMSA as a whole exceeded natural increase in the period from 1950 to 1960. The Los Angeles-Long Beach SMSA gained 1,585,000 from net inmigration as compared with 790,000 from natural increase. In contrast, the nation's largest SMSA, New York, gained only 109,000 from net inmigration but 1,029,000 from natural increase. The Pittsburgh SMSA had net outmigration but that was more than offset by natural increase, so some population growth occurred. Vital statistics and net migration are not available for the Boston SMSA, but that area had a rather small total population growth between 1950 and 1960 so it probably also had net outmigration of population (like the Pittsburgh SMSA) that was more than offset by natural increase.

In 11 of the 12 largest SMSA's the central cities lost population between 1950 and 1960 through more net outmigration than natural increase. By subtraction of data shown in Table 5.5 for central cities from data shown for SMSA's as entities, it can be determined that the SMSA rings generally had considerable net inmigration (mostly from central cities) and that this net inmigration was generally of greater magnitude than the natural increase of the population within the ring. The Pittsburgh SMSA was an exception; its ring gained 76,000 from net inmigration but 189,000 from natural increase.

The loss of population from central cities in 11 of the 12 largest SMSA's should not be taken as an indication that smaller SMSA's also had as extensive a pattern of losses from their central cities. As is noted later, in the section on urbanized areas, only about a third of all central cities lost population between 1950 and 1960.

Many large cities have lost white population through net outmigration to the suburbs, but in some instances this was partly offset by increase in nonwhite population through net inmigration to central cities from areas outside the SMSA. Some idea of color differences in population change in large cities may be obtained from the data presented in Table 5.6.

Table 5.7 presents rates of children ever born per 1,000 women ever married 35-44 years old in 1960, for component parts of the 12 largest SMSA's. The central cities of Boston and Pittsburgh have considerably higher rates than New York, Los Angeles-Long Beach, San Francisco-Oakland, and Washington, indicating that even large cities vary considerably in fertility. The rings also vary among one another in respect to fertility, in a manner that is not well correlated with the pattern of variation for central cities. That is, an SMSA with a relatively high or low rate for a central city does not necessarily have a relatively high or low rate for the ring. Although the rings do tend to have higher fertility than the central cities, the former appear to be somewhat more similar in respect to fertility than the central cities, but there are some exceptions. In none of the 12 largest SMSA's is the rate for the ring more than 15 percent different from that for the central city.

Table 5.6   Women 25–34 years old, by color: Selected cities, 1940, 1950, and 1960

(Numbers in thousands)

City	White			Nonwhite		
	1960	1950	1940	1960	1950	1940
Boston	37	60	64	6	4	2
Chicago	161	272	296	71	56	31
Cleveland	38	71	74	22	16	8
Los Angeles	136	154	129	37	25	10
Philadelphia	86	143	146	43	39	26
Pittsburgh	30	52	55	7	7	6
Washington	20	52	50	34	32	22

Source: U. S. Bureau of the Census, 1960, 1950, and 1940 Censuses of Population.

Urbanized Areas by Size

An urbanized area may be regarded as generally comprising a central city of 50,000 or more inhabitants plus the contiguous thickly populated territory or "urban fringe." Urbanized areas differ from SMSA's mainly in that the former are restricted to thickly settled areas whereas the SMSA's include the remainder of the counties involved. Generally, a central city of an urbanized area is also a central city of an SMSA.

Urbanized areas are determined separately in each census, with boundaries changed from one census to another as the thickly populated area expands. In 1960, 53.5 percent of the nation's population resided in 213 urbanized areas. Between 1950 and 1960 the population classified as residing in urbanized areas increased by 38.4 percent. Two-thirds of the increase occurred in the urban fringe and one-third in central cities. Despite an increase in the number of urbanized areas, from 157 in 1950 to 213 in 1960, in the aggregate they gained more population from territory that formerly was rural than they did from territory that formerly was urban outside urbanized areas. In some urbanized areas the population in central cities decreased between 1950 and 1960, while that in the fringe areas grew, reflecting net movement of population to the suburbs. That happened in 50 of the 157 urbanized areas existing in 1950. Nationally, the fertility of the population in urbanized areas varies inversely with the size of the area. This is illustrated by the data in Table 5.8.

Table 5.7 Children ever born per 1,000 women 35-44 years old, ever married, for the 12 largest Metropolitan Areas: 1960

Metropolitan Area	Total	Central cities	Ring
New York, N.Y.	2,152	2,066	2,343
Los Angeles–Long Beach, Calif.	2,226	1,829	2,503
Chicago, Ill.	2,344	2,251	2,455
Philadelphia, Pa.-N.J.	2,349	2,271	2,410
Detroit, Mich.	2,523	2,377	2,634
San Francisco–Oakland, Calif.	2,225	2,020	2,338
Boston, Mass.	2,566	2,581	2,562
Pittsburgh, Pa.	2,441	2,422	2,447
St. Louis, Mo.-Ill.	2,461	2,397	2,491
Washington, D.C.-Md.-Va.	2,270	2,069	2,366
Cleveland, Ohio	2,329	2,289	2,361
Baltimore, Md.	2,394	2,391	2,397

Source: U.S. Bureau of the Census, 1960 Census of Population, Standard Metropolitan Statistical Areas, PC(3)-1D, Table 2.

Individual urbanized areas differ from one another, with small areas sometimes having lower fertility than large areas. On a regional basis there is still a tendency for fertility to vary inversely with the size of urbanized area, but exceptions occur. In terms of the data shown in Table 5.8, in three regions the urbanized areas of 1 million to 3 million population have fertility rates that are out of line with the otherwise inverse relation of fertility with size of area. In the Northeast and the North Central regions the rates are higher for areas of 1 million to 3 million population than for urbanized areas of next larger and next smaller size, whereas in the West the reverse situation occurs.

A large part of the urban fringe consists of urban places of 2,500 to 50,000 population. In incorporated urban places of 2,500 or more in fringe areas, women ever married, 35-44, had 2,392 children ever

Table 5.8   Children ever born per 1,000 women 35-44 years old, ever married, for urbanized areas by size, central **cities, and urban fringe: United States and regions,** 1960

Region and size of urbanized area	Total urbanized area	Central cities	Urban fringe	
			Incorporated places of 2,500 or more	Other urban
UNITED STATES				
All urbanized areas	2,375	2,346	2,392	2,441
3,000,000 or more	2,256	2,167	2,332	2,408
1,000,000 to 3,000,000	2,391	2,345	2,438	2,409
250,000 to 1,000,000	2,430	2,418	2,443	2,445
Less than 250,000	2,515	2,520	2,472	2,519
NORTHEAST				
3,000,000 or more	2,194	2,119	2,251	2,339
1,000,000 to 3,000,000	2,478	2,479	2,468	2,488
250,000 to 1,000,000	2,368	2,353	2,424	2,364
Less than 250,000	2,393	2,446	2,296	2,312
NORTH CENTRAL				
3,000,000 or more	2,398	2,312	2,476	2,662
1,000,000 to 3,000,000	2,474	2,451	2,494	2,505
250,000 to 1,000,000	2,455	2,442	2,469	2,482
Less than 250,000	2,588	2,583	2,559	2,637
SOUTH				
1,000,000 to 3,000,000	2,307	2,284	2,390	2,322
250,000 to 1,000,000	2,403	2,416	2,366	2,385
Less than 250,000	2,503	2,500	2,472	2,537
WEST				
3,000,000 or more	2,217	2,068	2,274	2,469
1,000,000 to 3,000,000	2,180	2,020	2,272	2,377
250,000 to 1,000,000	2,493	2,429	2,535	2,611
Less than 250,000	2,607	2,556	2,784	2,717

Source: U.S. Bureau of the Census, 1960 Census of Population, Size of Place, PC(3)-1B, Tables 1 to 5, and Vol. I, Characteristics of the Population, Part 1, U. S. Summary, Table 100.

born per 1,000 women. A comparable fertility rate computed from data for women in all urban places of 2,500 to 50,000, including those outside urbanized areas, is 2,546. Apparently, fertility tends to be lower for the urban places of 2,500 to 50,000 when they are close to large cities than when they are not. It is definitely known from other data that the fertility of the rural population is lower when the rural population is close to a large city than when it is not.[4] In the case of urban fringes, however, some of the residents migrated from the large cities, and therefore already had some experience with large-city ways of life.

Urban Places

The count of urban places in 1960 includes all incorporated and unincorporated places of 2,500 or more inhabitants. There were 5,445 such places in 1960, which contained 91.6 percent of the nation's urban population. Not included are places of less than 2,500 that are urban because they are located in the urban fringe part of urbanized areas.

A previous section gave data on fertility by size of urbanized areas (fringes included) but not by color. Table 5.9 presents data by color for urban places by size (fringes excluded). In terms of children ever born per 1,000 women 35-44 years old (including single women as well as ever-married women), the inverse relation of fertility with size of place is stronger for nonwhite than for white women. On a national basis white women are more homogeneous than nonwhite women with respect to fertility by size of place. In urban places of 1 million or more population, nonwhite women are only slightly more fertile than white women but the differences by color increase as size of place decreases. The near-equality of fertility for nonwhite and white women in urban places of 1 million or more inhabitants provides some basis for speculating that in time the nonwhite women in smaller urban places may also tend to approach the lower fertility of the white population, with a consequent narrowing of the nation's overall differences in fertility by color.

Among women 35-44 years old in 1960, fertility was close to replacement needs for the white and nonwhite in urban places of 1 million or more population. The women 35-44 years old had completed roughly 95 percent of their eventual lifetime fertility, and in the cited urban places appeared unlikely to exceed an ultimate rate of about 2,130 children per 1,000 women required for replacement of their generation. It should be kept in mind, however, that the women 35-44 years old in 1960 are being followed through the childbearing ages by some younger cohorts whose ultimate fertility in all probability will considerably exceed that of the women currently 35-44 years old. Large cities may be regarded as a barometer in a fashion, as they should be the first to have fertility below replacement needs if the nation's overall fertility heads in that direction.

Table 5.9 Children ever born per 1,000 women 35-44 years old, in urban places of 2,500 or more, by size of place, color, and marital status of woman: United States, 1960

Color and size of place	Women (thousands)		Children per 1,000 women	
	Total	Ever married	Total	Ever married
WHITE				
Total	7,171	6,656	2,230	2,403
1,000,000 or more	1,021	907	1,904	2,143
250,000 to 1,000,000	1,211	1,103	2,131	2,340
50,000 to 250,000	1,632	1,515	2,223	2,394
2,500 to 50,000	3,307	3,131	2.371	2,504
NONWHITE				
Total	1,011	938	2,436	2,626
1,000,000 or more	274	251	2,022	2,214
250,000 to 1,000,000	318	297	2,354	2,520
50,000 to 250,000	194	181	2,558	2,738
2,500 to 50,000	224	209	2,955	3,175

Source: U.S. Bureau of the Census, 1960 Census of Population; unpublished data from 25-percent sample.

Individual urban places vary considerably in the characteristics of their population, and of course in fertility, in a manner that is often unrelated to their size. There are some small urban places, such as Williamsburg, Virginia, where fertility is lower than in the nation's largest cities, and there are some large cities, notably Salt Lake City, Utah, where fertility is quite high. The following is a tally of the distribution of urban places of 10,000 or more by number of children ever born per 1,000 women ever married 35-44 years old in 1960, for the United States and for several selected states:

Children ever born per 1,000 women ever married 35-44 years old, 1960	United States	Utah	California	New Jersey	Indiana	Louisiana
Total	1,899	9	196	128	46	29
Under 2,000	47	-	17	11	-	-
2,000-2,299	371	-	50	76	1	-
2,300-2,599	880	-	84	39	32	4
2,600-2,899	428	-	35	2	13	12
2,900+	173	9	10	-	-	13

Fertility is not necessarily low in communities in which the average educational attainment is high. This is illustrated in Table 5.10, which presents data on some characteristics of the population and on fertility for individual urban places of 10,000 or more selected on the basis of a median of at least 16 years of school completed by males 25 years old and over. Many "blue chip" areas with high income averages, high educational attainment, and so forth, have fertility that is well above replacement needs, notwithstanding a national tendency for fertility to vary inversely with socioeconomic status. The places listed in Table 5.10 with "manufacturing" as the principal industry of employed are generally wealthy residential suburbs of large industrial areas, and those with "education" as the principal industry are seats of large universities. Bethesda, Maryland, is a suburb of the nation's capital. Perhaps the main value of these selected places is to serve as a caution against a facile assumption that fertility will always decline nationally as the average socioeconomic status increases. More likely, fertility will only decline to a point and then level off, or even increase, thereafter.

Counties

In the 1960 census, for the first time in any decennial census, data on children ever born were tabulated on a county basis. Several measures of period fertility, such as annual births by counties from past and present vital statistics reports and ratios of young children to women from decennial census reports on population by age and sex, are also available. There is a need for both data on short-run or period fertility and data on children ever born, because data of one type are not necessarily indicative of the other. Such factors as variations in the timing of births and in the composition of the population by age and sex produce a relatively low correlation between the two types of data.

Table 5.10 Specified social and economic characteristics for urban places of 10,000 or more, with males 25 years old and over having a median of 16 or more years of school completed: United States, 1960

Place	Median family income	Principal industry of employed	Males in labor force: percent under 35 years old	Married women, husband present: percent of women in labor force	Total population: percent moved into house after 1958
Scarsdale, N. Y.	$22,177	Manufacturing	17.4	16.3	14.0
Winnetka, Ill.	20,166	Manufacturing	18.2	16.2	15.8
Glencoe, Ill.	20,136	Manufacturing	18.0	17.2	15.3
San Marino, Calif.	16,728	Manufacturing	16.4	13.3	14.7
Mountain Brook, Ala.	14,689	Manufacturing	21.0	20.9	20.6
Bethesda, Md.	12,357	U. S. Gov't.	28.9	27.1	27.4
Princeton, N. J.	8,833	Education	49.8	40.1	40.2
West Lafayette, Ind.	8,068	Education	55.6	28.5	37.8
East Lansing, Mich.	7,152	Education	64.3	39.5	50.7
State College, Pa.	6,689	Education	64.9	32.9	55.7
Chapel Hill, N. C.	6,173	Education	62.4	44.3	46.8
Pullman, Wash.	5,981	Education	68.6	47.8	46.5
College Station, Texas	4,733	Education	66.4	44.8	51.1

	Women ever married					
	15-24 years old		25-34 years old		35-44 years old	
	Number	Children ever born per 1,000 women	Number	Children ever born per 1,000 women	Number	Children ever born per 1,000 women
Scarsdale, N. Y.	83	a	736	2,319	1,454	2,573
Winnetka, Ill.	84	a	437	2,261	1,003	2,641
Glencoe, Ill.	73	a	520	2,496	948	2,526
San Marino, Calif.	16	a	415	2,330	986	2,563
Mountain Brook, Ala.	173	a	763	1,995	1,104	2,349
Bethesda, Md.	519	892	3,261	2,011	5,042	2,308
Princeton, N. J.	140	a	461	1,738	526	2,342
West Lafayette, Ind.	320	728	559	1,911	595	2,422
East Lansing, Mich.	1,525	661	1,539	1,834	1,108	2,432
State College, Pa.	687	639	870	1,805	675	2,391
Chapel Hill, N. C.	428	533	536	1,757	478	1,954
Pullman, Wash.	651	803	550	1,825	475	2,421
College Station, Texas	721	723	634	2,181	337	2,525

Source: U. S. Bureau of the Census, 1960 Census of Population, Vol. I, Characteristics of the Population, selected state reports, Tables 32, 33, 72, 73 and 75.

aRate not shown where base is less than 200.

For reasons of space, only brief summary-type data on fertility will be presented here for counties. Readers who want a scholarly analysis in depth may wish to read the forthcoming Beegle-Hathaway-Bryant census monograph tentatively titled *The People of Rural America, 1960.*[5] The authors have used 1960 census data on children ever born to women for urban and rural parts of counties as units of measurement. These fertility data have been related to other characteristics of the population by regression techniques and other procedures, with findings summarized for geographic division and regions.

Over the years there have been numerous reports, monographs, and articles involving data on short-run fertility for various geographic areas in relation to social and economic characteristics of the population. An Irishman, Michael Sadler,[6] is credited with having been the first writer to make extensive use of ratios of young children to women from United States census data to prove that newly settled areas had more rapid increase from fertility than long-settled areas, but the memoirs of President John Quincy Adams indicate that the usefulness of such ratios was known in 1822, if not earlier.[7] Perhaps the best known reports making extensive use of ratios of young children to women are the 1920 census monograph *Ratio of Children to Women* by Warren S. Thompson[8] and the report on population problems issued in the 1930's by the National Resources Committee.[9] Donald J. Bogue of the University of Chicago is currently directing a monograph that will make extensive use of data from the 1960 census on women by own children under 5 and 5-9 years old.

Figure 5.1 presents a map with counties shaded according to the number of children ever born per 1,000 women ever married 35-44 years old in the 1960 census. Counties with relatively low fertility (light shadings) are chiefly in a band extending westward from the Middle Atlantic States to Kansas, down to Texas. Another band with relatively low fertility is along the Pacific coast. Counties with relatively high fertility (dark shadings) are chiefly in the deep South, in some western states, and in the far North. Only vestiges remain of a more or less traditional tendency for high-fertility counties to be in the far North, deep South, connecting in the West to form a horseshoe-shaped pattern. The traditional pattern appeared in data on ratios of young children to women in several past censuses.

The map has shadings that bear a strong resemblance to another map (not shown) for counties classified by proportion of families with incomes under $3,000 in 1959. The strong resemblance suggests there is still some relation between poverty and high fertility. Were the fertility map to be compared with one on relative increase or decrease in population between 1950 and 1960, it would be noted that counties of relatively high fertility in the far North and the deep South were often ones that decreased in population, suggesting there is considerable net outmigration from areas where economic opportunities are relatively limited, more than offsetting high fertility.

Table 5.11 presents data for counties (or county equivalents), with counties grouped according to magnitudes of rates of children ever born. The groupings were designed to provide approximately equal

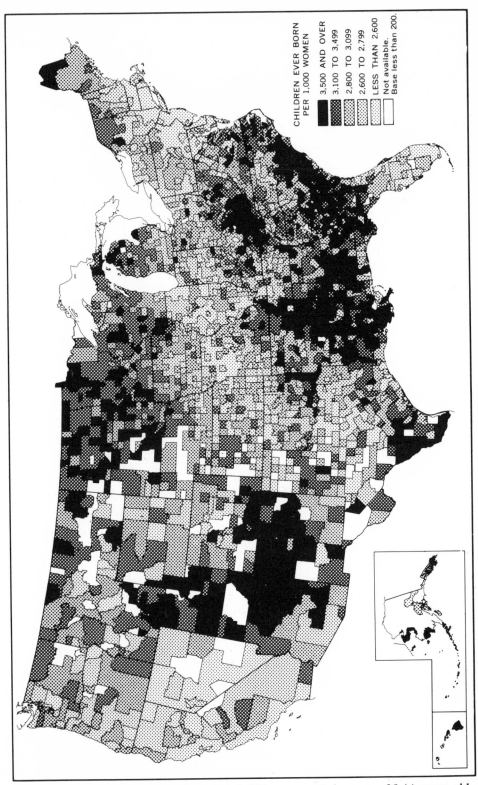

CHILDREN EVER BORN
PER 1,000 WOMEN

3,500 AND OVER
3,100 TO 3,499
2,800 TO 3,099
2,600 TO 2,799
LESS THAN 2,600
Not available.
Base less than 200.

Fig. 5.1. Children ever born per 1,000 ever-married women 35-44 years old, by counties: 1960.

numbers of counties in each group. For each group, averages are shown for selected socioeconomic characteristics. The averages are simply the sum of the individual county values for a given characteristic, divided by the number of counties in the group. That is, each county has equal weight regardless of whether it has many or few inhabitants.

It will be evident from even a casual inspection of Table 5.11 that many socioeconomic characteristics appear to be highly correlated with the level of fertility. But since the data for each group are averages of county data, a very high correlation between fertility and a given socioeconomic characteristic does not mean that a similarly high correlation would also be found from data for individual counties. Rather, the data should be viewed as merely indicating general tendencies that come to light when grouped data are used. As an example of how grouped data mask certain tendencies, it may be of interest to note that almost half of the 3,134 counties in the United States lost population between 1950 and 1960, whereas no such tendency for extensive losses appears in the item on percent change in population, 1950 to 1960, for groups of counties. Yet Table 5.11 does bring out the important point that the percent change in population between 1950 and 1960 tends to be inversely related to rates of children ever born. That is, counties with high fertility often had actual population decreases (from outmigration) and counties with successively lower fertility rates tended to have successively larger percent increases in population (reflecting inmigration). Those with high fertility tended to have the youngest median age of population (reflecting more children present) and those with low fertility tended to have the highest median age of population (reflecting fewer children but many adults of middle age). The ratio of population under 5 to women 15-49 is more strongly correlated (in terms of grouped data) with rates of children ever born than are the crude birth rates for the year 1960. Average family income and median years of school completed varies inversely with fertility, as expected.

It may be noted from Table 5.11 that a range of 1,723 to 2,653 for the rate of children ever born is used for the one-fifth of counties with lowest rates. The upper limit of 2,653 is much above the rate needed for replacement of women through births, so most counties in the United States have more than adequate fertility. Among the least fertile 593 counties, only 13 had ratios below 2,100, 50 had ratios of 2,100 to 2,299, and 530 had ratios of 2,300 to 2,653.

Table 5.11   Characteristics of the population of counties grouped by
number of children ever born per 1,000 women ever married
35-44 years old: United States, 1960

(Data exclude 173 counties with fewer than 200 women ever married
35-44 years old)

Subject	Counties with specified rate of children ever born				
	3,487 to 5,784	3,121 to 3,486	2,874 to 3,120	2,654 to 2,873	1,723 to 2,653
Number of counties	592	592	592	592	593
Children ever born (average)	3,920	3,281	2,974	2,762	2,484
Crude birth rate, 1960	25.4	22.9	22.3	21.7	21.9
Fertility[a]	590	532	507	485	463
Infant mortality rate[b]	35.0	28.7	25.4	24.6	24.5
POPULATION					
Average per county	18,866	21,233	30,843	46,952	183,840
Per square mile	29.8	33.1	51.3	88.2	931.9
Percent change, 1950-1960	-4.2	-2.0	6.4	12.2	22.4
Percent urban	18.4	-23.4	31.1	40.0	57.1
Percent nonwhite	25.4	10.3	7.9	5.7	7.5
Per household	3.82	3.47	3.35	3.24	3.18
Median age (years)	24.7	28.7	29.9	31.0	31.4
Percent migrant[c]	13.4	16.0	18.2	19.5	20.8
Median family income	$3,013	$3,817	$4,247	$4,636	$5,460
LABOR FORCE					
Nonworker/worker ratio[d]	2.24	1.88	1.76	1.68	1.57
Percent in white collar occ.	25.9	28.7	30.8	33.6	38.5
Percent in manufacturing	15.8	17.5	20.0	21.0	23.6
Wives in labor force, percent	26.1	27.2	28.3	29.2	31.3
Percent unemployed	6.2	5.5	5.0	5.0	4.8
HOUSING					
Dwelling unit sound, w/plumbing facilities, percent	40.6	52.1	58.5	63.6	70.8
1.01 or more persons per room, percent	23.5	15.4	13.2	11.1	10.1
Amenities index[e]	65.0	75.1	78.0	80.6	80.5

Source: U.S. Bureau of the Census, County and City Data Book,
1962, and 1960 Census of Population; National Center for Health
Statistics, Vital Statistics of the United States, 1960.

[a] Ratio of population under 5 to women 15-49, 1960.

[b] Deaths in first year of life per 1,000 live births, 1960.

[c] Persons 5 years old and over who did not live in this county
in April 1955.

[d] Ratio of persons of all ages not in labor force to persons
14 and over in labor force.

[e] Index is one-fourth the sum of the percentages of housing units
that have (1) clothes-washing machine, (2) television set, (3) telephone,
and (4) one or more automobiles. An index value of 100.0 would mean
that all housing units in the counties have all amenities.

Ecological Correlation

To some extent, the fertility of the population is affected by the environment in which people live or in which they grew up. Evidence on this point is of a varied nature.

The lesser fertility of the urban than of the rural population is one example of the effect of environment. So also is the tendency for the fertility of the population to vary inversely with size of place, and for the rural people in the vicinity of large cities to be less fertile than those further removed. Beegle, Hathaway, and Bryant in their 1960 census monograph on *The People of Rural America*[10] found not only a negative relation between the fertility of the rural farm population and proximity to a large SMSA but also that in some geographic divisions only the level of education outranked the proximity variable in terms of its contribution to explaining the observed variance in rural farm white birth rates.

Goldberg studied a sample of couples in the Detroit Metropolitan Area, with wife at least 40 years old and the couple classified into "two-generation urbanites" and "farm migrants" on the basis of whether the husband's father had a nonfarm occupation or a farm occupation while the husband was growing up.[11] The data were collected between 1952 and 1958 and comprised 1,072 cases of two-generation urbanites and 442 farm migrants. Goldberg found far weaker differentials in the average number of children ever born to the two-generation urbanites by socioeconomic characteristics than for the farm migrants. In this sample, the couples with some farm background were more concentrated in the lower socioeconomic classes than the two-generation urbanites but the farm migrants were more fertile than the two-generation urbanites at comparable socioeconomic levels, especially when the level of education or income was low. Goldberg suggested that in the coming years, as the nation becomes increasingly composed of two-generation urbanites, differential fertility by socioeconomic characteristics will diminish in importance.

Duncan reexamined data from the Indianapolis Study of 1941 for a special study of ecological correlation.[12] He cross-classified data for each couple by rent paid for their own dwelling unit with the median rent for all dwelling units in the census tract in which the couple lived. He found a high degree of correlation between fertility variations in terms of areal data on tract median rent and in terms of data on rent paid by the couples themselves and concluded: "This exploration, therefore, serves to bolster our confidence in the general validity of studies in differential fertility where areal variation was the sole source of information on socioeconomic differentials. At this time, analyses in which areal classification of socioeconomic characteristics suggest that areal differences in fertility may not be completely reducible to the areally clustered effects of some conventional individual variables."

In one of his tables, Duncan presented cross-classified data on median rent and couples' own rent. As he stated, allowance must be made for the small frequencies in some cells, but where the frequencies are substantial, one generally finds a pattern of decreasing fertility as rent of either type (tract average or rent for own dwelling unit) increases. Implied, but not specifically stated, by Duncan is a tendency for poor people who live in poor areas to have higher fertility than equally poor people who live in wealthy areas, and for wealthy people who live in poor areas to have higher fertility than wealthy people who live in wealthy areas. Few wealthy people live in poor areas, however, and conversely. The figures in Duncan's table do suggest that environment or the place where people live has some effect over and above that of the person's own characteristics.

Summary

In 1960, as in prior censuses, the Northeast was the region with the least fertile population. In 1950 and 1940 rates of children ever born per 1,000 women in that region were well below those needed for replacement of the women in the next generation, whereas they were already above replacement levels in 1960 for women aged 30-34 and 35-39, who still had some years of childbearing left. The North Central and West had overtaken the South by 1960 in respect to the fertility of the *white* population at ages under 40; only the presence of many nonwhite persons in the South enabled that region to maintain a slight lead in terms of data for all races. Except in the Northeast, the nonwhite population is considerably more fertile than the white population.

A large proportion (63 percent) of the nation's population resides in metropolitan areas. Between 1950 and 1960 the excess of births over deaths was a greater factor than net inmigration in population increase for most large metropolitan areas. *Within* metropolitan areas, however, many central cities lost more population through net outmigration to the suburbs than they had natural increase and some suburbs gained more through net inmigration from central cities than they gained from natural increase.

Nationally, there is a tendency for the fertility of the population to vary inversely with the size of the community and for the rural population to be less fertile when located near a large city than when not located near a large city. There are wide variations in fertility for individual places of any given size. Within a city, fertility varies from neighborhood to neighborhood, with perhaps some tendency for poor people in wealthy areas to have fewer children than poor people in poor areas, and for wealthy people in poor areas to have more children than wealthy people in wealthy areas. The data on ecological correlations are for only one city, circa 1940, and thus are only suggestive, not conclusive, evidence.

It was also pointed out that certain communities with a well-educated population of high income had rates of children ever born that were above replacement needs. Fertility is not always low when the socioeconomic status is high.

Migration is a prominent fact of life in the modern United States. Nearly one-fifth (17.5 percent) of persons 5 years of age and over in the 1960 census were living in a different county 5 years previously. The proportion having migrated varied by age; it was highest (35 percent) for persons 20-24 years old, and it was under 10 percent for persons 55 or more years of age.[1]

Unlike the other two components of population change, births and deaths, the migration of an individual can occur a large number of times during his lifetime. One can be born and die but once, but one can—and frequently does—move over and over again.

Fertility, mortality, and migration are generally regarded as the components of population change. Migration is frequently an important factor in the rapid growth of certain areas as compared with population loss in other areas. The present concern, however, is with the interrelation of two of the components of population change, migration and fertility.

There is no doubt about the existence of a reciprocal relation between these variables. This interrelation operates at different levels, and through selective as well as determinative channels. The selective factors, in particular, may sometimes yield a direct and sometimes an inverse relation of fertility to migration.

To illustrate the intricacies of the interrelation one may note first of all that rapid population growth resulting from high fertility rates in rural areas, and particularly in poor rural areas, is generally regarded as a stimulus to migration *out of* the area. In complementary fashion, the low fertility rates of urban areas, particularly of the economically healthy areas, are commonly regarded as stimuli to migration *into* the cities.

At another level, it may be noted that persons involved in the rural-urban migration tend to be young unmarried adults, childless couples, and small families. Unencumbered by large families, they are relatively free to move. This is a selective factor conducive to an inverse relation of fertility to migration.[2]

An example of a selective factor operating in the other direction is the stimulus that the arrival or impending arrival of a baby gives a young couple to move out of their parents' home into a home of their own, to move out of an apartment into a house, to move from the central city to the suburbs, or simply to find a larger house. Factors of this type doubtless were responsible, in part at least, for the finding in the second phase of the Princeton Fertility Study (1960) that the onset of a pregnancy within 3 years after the birth of the second child was more frequent among couples living in a different house than among couples still living in the same house at the end of a 3-year period.[3]

Data from the first phase of the Princeton Fertility Study (1957) relating to couples' experience prior to the birth of the second child also illustrate the manner in which study design, and the nature of classifications and definitions, may affect the findings on the relation of migration to fertility behavior. It will be recalled that the couples originally selected for the Princeton Fertility Study were those that had had their second birth in September 1956. Among data collected in the first interviews 6 months later were those concerning number of moves since marriage and interval between marriage and the second births. Among Protestant couples, the interval from marriage to second birth was relatively long for couples reporting a large number of migrations since marriage and relatively short for those reporting a large number of *migrations per year.* In explanation, the author stated:

> Selective factors enter into the cross-classification of the present data by migration and duration of marriage. Thus, the longer a couple has been married the longer the opportunity they have had to move several times . . .
>
> However, [the classification by average number of moves per year] was accompanied by an opposite type of bias with respect to duration of marriage. Whereas couples reporting *a large number of moves since marriage* tended to be unduly weighted with long duration of marriage, those with a high frequency of *moves per year* tended to be those with short durations of marriage.[4]

Census Data on Migration Status and Fertility

Although mobility is a basic characteristic of man, arbitrary definitions must be set up to measure migration. Thus, in census usage, migration is first of all a change of *residence.* Persons who commute to work 50 miles by train, crossing a dozen county lines and a state line or even an international boundary, are not necessarily migrants in the census meaning. A person might tour Europe during the summer, go on an extended business trip to South America, take a trip around the world, or even orbit the globe a thousand times and still not be classified as a migrant. But if he reported in the 1960 census that 5 years previously, on April 1, 1955, he lived in a county different from the one in which he was currently being enumerated, he would be regarded as a migrant.[5] If he lived in a different house but in the same county, that fact too would be recorded and tabulated, but in that case he would be considered a "mover," not as a bona fide migrant.

Specifically, the 1960 census contained the question, "Did he live in this house on April 1, 1955?" The enumerator was asked to check one of the three possible replies:

1. Born April 1955 or later.
2. Yes, this house
3. No, different house.

For persons living in a different house, the additional question was asked, "Where did he live on April 1, 1955?" The replies permitted classification of persons 5 years of age and over into the following categories:

Same house.
Different house—same county.
Different county—same state.
Different state.
Abroad.
Moved—residence in 1955 not reported.

Fertility and Migration
Except for the low fertility of women who moved to this country from abroad during the 5 years preceding 1960, there was not a marked variation in fertility by migration status as described above. However, among the native white ever-married women, the differential that did exist was an inverse relation of fertility to degree of migration during the preceding 5 years. Within the narrow limits of the variation, the inverse relation was rather complete for ever-married women under 35 years of age. The highest average fertility tended to be that for women reporting that they had lived in the same house in 1955 as in 1960. In descending order were the rates for those reporting previous residence in a different house but in the same county, in a different county but in the same state, and lowest rates for those

reporting residence in a different state 5 years earlier (Table 6.1).

Among white women, the excess fertility of the nonmovers over that of movers tended to be more pronounced at ages 25-29 than at other ages. Perhaps the selective factor implicit in a woman changing houses at the time of her marriage was more relevant at these ages than in any other age group. The relatively low fertility of the interstate migrants tended to be more pronounced at the older ages. Among the white women, the interstate migrants may be more heavily weighted by wives of white-collar workers than the intrastate migrants.

Table 6.1 Residence in 1955 in comparison with 1960 in relation to number of children ever born per 1,000 ever-married women 15-49 years of age, by color, age of woman, and type of residence: United States

Residence in 1960 and age of woman	White					Nonwhite				
	Same house in 1955	Same county	Different county, same state	Different state	Abroad	Same house in 1955	Same county	Different county, same state	Different state	Abroad
UNITED STATES										
15-19	850	732	674	667	703	1,285	1,274	1,039	1,168	[a]
20-24	1,530	1,411	1,302	1,288	1,180	2,131	2,101	1,859	1,687	1,069
25-29	2,405	2,169	2,136	2,038	1,618	3,029	2,843	2,637	2,333	1,414
30-34	2,651	2,548	2,567	2,455	1,972	3,325	3,188	3,147	2,633	1,786
35-39	2,661	2,607	2,665	2,554	2,279	3,245	3,128	3,384	2,667	1,998
40-44	2,545	2,492	2,569	2,397	2,249	3,050	2,971	3,223	2,573	2,128
45-49	2,362	2,380	2,411	2,195	2,233	2,842	2,810	3,193	2,636	2,188
URBANIZED AREAS										
15-19	825	726	648	634	677	1,234	1,281	980	1,193	[a]
20-24	1,371	1,317	1,170	1,176	1,090	1,896	1,970	1,683	1,641	982
25-29	2,249	2,040	1,990	1,900	1,507	2,710	2,609	2,292	2,246	1,408
30-34	2,505	2,394	2,383	2,348	1,851	2,833	2,811	2,681	2,531	1,776
35-39	2,473	2,393	2,425	2,407	2,194	2,700	2,648	2,733	2,514	2,012
40-44	2,301	2,229	2,262	2,258	2,242	2,353	2,379	2,559	2,433	2,295
45-49	2,077	2,047	2,111	2,029	2,269	2,131	2,209	2,584	2,748	2,159
OTHER URBAN										
15-19	818	711	613	645	786	1,401	1,186	1,008	1,110	[a]
20-24	1,516	1,445	1,260	1,308	1,306	2,211	2,219	1,808	1,833	[a]
25-29	2,384	2,245	2,106	2,102	1,773	3,015	3,137	2,713	2,497	1,519
30-34	2,624	2,610	2,551	2,507	2,077	3,517	3,557	2,958	2,865	1,630
35-39	2,602	2,696	2,658	2,627	2,481	3,366	3,413	3,441	2,812	[a]
40-44	2,491	2,600	2,591	2,437	2,387	3,189	3,344	3,587	2,582	[a]
45-49	2,306	2,534	2,385	2,268	2,492	2,780	3,228	2,872	2,039	[a]
RURAL NONFARM										
15-19	877	758	741	746	758	1,261	1,281	1,142	1,099	[a]
20-24	1,715	1,550	1,500	1,512	1,468	2,439	2,379	2,082	1,780	1,241
25-29	2,564	2,366	2,341	2,286	1,950	3,683	3,513	2,985	2,643	1,336
30-34	2,812	2,799	2,803	2,640	2,387	4,260	4,349	3,751	2,828	1,936
35-39	2,917	2,986	2,954	2,805	2,479	4,336	4,717	3,699	2,997	2,097
40-44	2,882	2,976	2,872	2,645	2,158	4,342	4,676	3,612	3,062	[a]
45-49	2,754	3,001	2,688	2,487	1,745	4,111	4,312	3,312	2,578	[a]
RURAL FARM										
15-19	934	725	754	759	[a]	1,433	1,362	1,039	[a]	[a]
20-24	1,759	1,591	1,537	1,641	[a]	2,818	2,554	2,350	2,216	[a]
25-29	2,684	2,532	2,455	2,381	1,744	3,804	3,935	3,556	[a]	[a]
30-34	3,083	3,146	3,104	2,960	[a]	4,949	5,394	4,560	[a]	[a]
35-39	3,220	3,375	3,371	3,274	[a]	5,267	5,959	5,749	[a]	[a]
40-44	3,220	3,449	3,534	3,212	[a]	5,517	6,029	4,622	[a]	[a]
45-49	3,114	3,467	3,340	3,057	[a]	5,269	5,527	5,447	[a]	[a]

Source: U.S. Bureau of the Census, 1960 Census of Population, Women by Number of Children Ever Born, PC(2)-3A, Table 13.

[a] Rate not shown where base is less than 1,000.

The inverse relation of fertility to degree of migration during the years 1955-60 also holds for nonwhite couples. Among the nonwhite group, however, the relatively high rates obtained almost equally for those reporting 1955 residence as "same house" and for those reporting "different house—same county," and also for "different county—same state." The differentials in fertility by migration status were especially marked for the nonwhite women in rural nonfarm areas.

Region of Residence in Relation to Region of Birth

In addition to the data on fertility according to migration status as described above, the 1960 census provided data on fertility according to geographic region of residence in relation to region of birth. In recording the data, the enumerators indicated "country of birth" for the foreign-born and "state of birth" for those born in the United States.[6] For the fertility tabulations the Census Bureau used the four broad geographic regions rather than specific states in the cross-classification by region of residence and region of birth of women born in the United States.

It should be emphasized that when broad regions are taken as the points of reference, those residing in the region of their birth may have been involved in much *intraregional* migration, including intercounty and even interstate migration. Some may have had periods of residence in other regions and then returned to their native region. The time of such migration is indeterminate; the move occurred some time during the life of the individual. Nevertheless, the data yield comparisons of fertility of those involved in various streams of interregional or generally long distance change of residence and those not so involved.

Despite their manifest limitations, the data reveal several points of interest. They point up the fact that the relative position of the fertility rates for those living in the region of their birth (underlined in Table 6.2) as compared with those of inmigrants or outmigrants varies by specific region of residence considered, as well as by color and age.

Little variation in fertility by region of birth was found for the native white ever-married women residing in the Northeast in 1960 (horizontal comparisons in Table 6.2). Among those residing in the North Central region, those born in the Northeast were characterized by relatively low fertility at all ages and those born in the South were characterized by relatively high fertility, especially at ages 40-49. Probably the South-born residents of the North Central states were weighted by the rural-born persons of low economic status.

The differentials in fertility by region of birth are somewhat more pronounced for native white residents of the South and the West than for those of the two northern regions. In each of these two instances the migrants from the Northeast tended to exhibit lowest fertility and those from the North Central region the next lowest. In the South the native white ever-married women born in the South ranked with those born in the West with respect to fertility at ages under 40 and exhibited highest rates at later ages. Probably the South-born residents of the South were more highly weighted by rural dwellers than were the migrants, especially the migrants from the North.

Table 6.2 Region of residence by region of birth in relation to children ever born per 1,000 ever-married native women, 15-49 years of age, by color and age of woman: 1960

Age of woman and region of residence in 1960	Color of woman and region of birth							
	White				Nonwhite			
	Northeast	North Central	South	West	Northeast	North Central	South	West
15-19								
Northeast	**736**	697	754	a	**1,144**	a	1,353	a
North Central	674	**708**	760	696	a	**1,230**	1,369	a
South	625	611	**717**	717	a	a	**1,267**	a
West	625	703	798	**754**	a	a	1,140	**1,141**
20-24								
Northeast	**1,227**	1,177	1,250	1,282	**1,662**	a	1,794	a
North Central	1,212	**1,404**	1,516	1,432	1,860	**1,928**	2,054	a
South	1,134	1,298	**1,403**	1,299	1,617	1,759	**2,192**	a
West	1,196	1,406	1,588	**1,490**	a	1,763	1,881	**1,732**
25-29								
Northeast	**2,006**	1,912	2,070	2,012	**2,268**	1,848	2,474	a
North Central	2,070	**2,305**	2,285	2,190	2,237	**2,672**	2,839	1,789
South	1,940	2,069	**2,195**	2,194	2,071	2,419	**3,116**	a
West	1,897	2,209	2,356	**2,408**	a	2,345	2,642	**2,514**
30-34								
Northeast	**2,412**	2,460	2,507	2,530	**2,558**	2,093	2,529	a
North Central	2,565	**2,740**	2,681	2,764	2,567	**2,862**	3,105	2,598
South	2,383	2,481	**2,576**	2,677	2,631	3,183	**3,648**	a
West	2,334	2,544	2,603	**2,778**	a	2,529	2,794	**3,040**
35-39								
Northeast	**2,477**	2,593	2,417	2,576	**2,499**	2,102	2,474	a
North Central	2,614	**2,776**	2,729	2,814	2,178	**2,731**	2,793	2,227
South	2,479	2,554	**2,702**	2,628	2,856	3,089	**3,691**	a
West	2,301	2,501	2,612	**2,824**	a	2,113	2,741	**3,157**
40-44								
Northeast	**2,359**	2,358	2,298	2,353	**2,198**	1,928	2,086	a
North Central	2,374	**2,629**	2,760	2,561	1,869	**2,500**	2,467	2,594
South	2,215	2,300	**2,695**	2,404	2,272	a	**3,540**	a
West	2,167	2,290	2,461	**2,619**	a	2,255	2,294	**3,504**
45-49								
Northeast	**2,181**	2,081	2,148	2,161	**2,195**	a	2,029	a
North Central	2,141	**2,437**	2,577	2,346	a	**2,478**	2,165	s
South	1,857	2,056	**2,646**	2,204	1,667	a	**3,296**	a
West	1,838	2,073	2,323	**2,374**	a	1,765	1,978	**3,821**

Source: U.S. Bureau of the Census, 1960 Census of Population, Women by Number of Children Ever Born, PC(2)-3A, Table 12.

a Rate not shown where base is less than 1,000.

Among the native white ever-married women residing in the West in 1960, the fertility of those born in the West was exceeded by those born in the South at ages under 25; at later ages the fertility of the indigenous white women was higher than that of white women born in other regions of the United States.

As for nonwhite women, the variations in fertility by region of birth tended to be more erratic than those for the white. Among the nonwhite in the Northeast, those born in the South exhibited higher fertility than those born in the Northeast at the youngest ages but the reverse was true at ages 30-49. The lowest rates found for nonwhite women in the Northeast were uniformly those for women born in the North Central region.

The fertility rates of the nonwhite women residing in the North Central states were somewhat analogous to those just described for the Northeast. At ages under 40 the fertility of migrants from the South exceeded that of women born in the North Central states. At ages 40-49 the fertility of the indigenous group stood highest. The rates were relatively low for women born in the Northeast and West.

As for nonwhite residents of the South, the fertility rates were uniformly highest for those born in that area and lowest for those born in the Northeast. The fertility rates for women born in the North Central states were in intermediate position. Nonwhite natives of the West are not shown because of inadequate numbers. It is likely that the conspicuously high fertility rate for the nonwhite women born and living in the South is associated in part with higher proportions in rural areas.

Among nonwhite women residing in the West in 1960, the fertility of those born in the South stood highest at ages under 30 but the fertility of those born in the West stood much the highest at later ages. The Western nonwhite women who were born in the West and were 30 years of age and over in 1960 are largely non-Negro. Among the nonwhite residents of the West, the lowest fertility rates shown in Table 6.2 are those for natives of the North Central region. Possibly this position would have been occupied by natives of the Northeast had they been represented.

Origin and Destination

A question is sometimes raised regarding the relative influence of places of origin and destination on the fertility of migrants. The present data by region of birth and residence can hardly be expected to yield definitive answers to this question. Regions are too large to be used as units for this type of analysis. One would need comparability with respect to type of residence. One would also need more control over time and age at migration and type of residence and duration of residence in the places of origin and residence.

The present data do suggest, however, that the relative influence of origin and destination may vary according to circumstances. Thus the data in Table 6.2 indicate that the average number of children of white or nonwhite ever-married women migrating from the South to the Northeast (born in the South—residing in the Northeast) tended to be more similar to the rates for those born and residing in the Northeast than to those born and residing in the South. This may seem to suggest a stronger influence of the region of destination than the region of origin. However, there is a maxim that "it is a poor rule that doesn't work both ways." Thus, Table 6.2 also shows that the white and nonwhite women migrating from the Northeast to the South tended to have families more nearly the size of those in the region of origin (born and living in the Northeast) than of those in the region of destination (born and living in the South).

A similar situation was found for white and nonwhite women in the migration from the North Central to the Northeast region. However, the fertility of migrants from the West to the Northeast as well as that of migrants from the Northeast to the West tended to be nearer those of the region of destination than of the region of origin.

For a total of 83 possible comparisons of the age-specific fertility rates of white migrants in specific types of migration routes with those of the region of origin and region of destination as illustrated above, the fertility rates of the migrants were nearer those of the region of origin in 36 cases, nearer those of the region of destination in 46 cases, and equidistant in one case. Among 50 possible comparisons for nonwhite women, 22 favored the area of origin and 28 the area of destination.

Although comparisons of the type considered above yield only negative results on the question of relative influence of region of origin and region of destination, they do serve to point up the relatively low fertility of the migrants. Thus, in the 83 comparisons for white women, in only six cases were the rates for the migrants higher than those for both the region of origin and region of destination. In 26 cases the rates for migrants were in intermediate position, and in 51 cases they were lower than those for both region of origin and region of destination. Among the 50 possible comparisons for nonwhite women, the rates for the migrants were higher than those for both the region of origin and region of destination in two cases, in intermediate position in 16 cases, and lower than those for both region of origin and region of destination in 32 cases.

Thus, instead of a rule that areas of destination exert more or less influence than areas of origin on the fertility of migrants, we may have the twofold situation that (1) because of selective or determinative influences, or both, interregional migrants tend to be people of relatively low fertility, and (2) whether the fertility level of the migrants is more similar to that of the area of origin or destination tends to depend on which of these is lower, or on the specific stream of migration considered.

Summary

In summary, it is rather clear that the relation of migration to fertility is not a simple one. Change in county or state of residence during the preceding 5 years appears to be associated with lower fertility than residence in the same house or in the same county.

The limitations of data on fertility by region of residence in relation to region of birth were emphasized. The results were found to vary by age, color, and specific region considered. For both white and nonwhite women, the fertility rates of inter-regional migrants tend to be relatively low. The data provide no evidence as to whether region of origin or region of destination has more influence on the fertility of migrants. They suggest that this may depend in part on route and direction of migration considered.

7 / Marital Characteristics

This chapter concerns mainly the marital characteristics of women of childbearing age. The fertility of women is affected by the proportion of women who ever marry, their age at marriage, and the stability of marriages. For the most part, cross-sectional data for women enumerated in a given census or survey are studied here; longitudinal data for marriage cohorts are discussed in Chapter 13.

Trends in Proportion of Women Ever Married

A considerable part of the baby boom that began after World War II resulted from an increase of unprecedented magnitude in the proportion of women of childbearing age who had ever married. As may be seen from the data presented in Table 7.1, the decennial censuses of 1950 and 1960 found much larger age-specific proportions of women

Table 7.1 Percent ever married among women 14-44 years old, by age: Conterminous United States, 1920-60

Age at census	1960	1950	1940	1930	1920	Increase, 1940 to 1960
14	1.1	0.7	0.3	0.4	0.6	0.8
15	2.3	2.1	1.2	1.3	1.4	1.1
16	5.8	6.2	3.9	4.5	4.3	1.9
17	12.2	13.2	9.0	10.3	10.1	3.2
18	24.4	24.6	17.7	20.0	20.0	6.7
19	40.3	37.6	27.0	29.8	29.7	13.3
20	54.0	50.2	37.2	39.5	40.0	16.8
21	65.4	61.1	45.6	47.1	47.5	19.8
22	74.4	69.6	53.8	55.0	55.1	20.6
23	80.6	76.0	61.3	61.9	61.7	19.3
24	84.3	80.4	67.1	67.6	67.0	17.2
25	86.9	83.4	71.4	71.7	71.0	15.5
26	88.6	85.2	74.9	75.8	74.7	13.7
27	89.8	87.2	78.0	79.2	78.0	11.8
28	90.7	88.4	79.9	81.2	79.8	10.8
29	91.3	89.6	82.3	84.4	82.5	9.0
30-34	93.1	90.7	85.3	86.8	85.1	7.8
35-39	93.9	91.6	88.8	89.6	88.6	5.1
40-44	93.9	91.7	90.5	90.5		3.4

Source: U.S. Bureau of the Census, 1960 Census of Population, Vol. I, Characteristics of the Population, Part 1, U.S. Summary, Tables 177 and 179.

ever married than those of 1920 to 1940, especially at ages from 19 to 29 years. Censuses back to 1890, the first census in which data on marital status were tabulated, exhibited slightly lower proportions ever married than those shown for 1920 to 1940. Thus, the percentages shown for 1950 and 1960 are the highest on record for the 70-year period for which data on marital status are available.

It may be of some interest to note from Table 7.1 that over 50 percent of the women 20 years old in 1960 had ever been married, whereas in the censuses of 1920 to 1940 such a high percentage was exceeded only by women 22 years old and above. Furthermore, over 74 percent of the women 22 years old in 1960 had ever been married, whereas in the censuses of 1920 to 1940 such a high percentage was exceeded only by women 26 years old and above. Taken together, these patterns suggest that the rise in proportions ever married by age drew heavily from women who under former conditions would have married after age 22, if at all.

Data from the Current Population Survey indicate that the rise in the proportion ever married for women under age 25 reached a peak around 1956, and that declines have since occurred in this age group. Pertinent figures are presented in Table 7.2.

Table 7.2   Percent ever married, by age, for women 14-44 years old: United States, 1954-65

Age at survey date	1965	1964	1960	1957	1956	1954
14-17	3.5	3.0	4.6	5.1	6.2	5.0
18-19	26.6	27.9	29.1	30.3	34.0	29.8
20-24	67.5	68.9	71.1	71.0	71.4	69.3
25-29	91.6	90.6	90.5	88.8	89.1	89.0
30-34	94.7	95.4	93.1	92.7	93.2	91.3
35-44	95.2	95.5	94.1	93.6	92.8	93.1

Source: U. S. Bureau of the Census, Current Population Reports, Series P-20, Nos. 144, 135, 105, 81, 72, and 56.

At this point, it seems advisable to present some illustrative data for selected birth cohorts of women, although data for cohorts properly belong in Chapter 13. Changes in proportions ever married as women pass through life are more precisely measured from longitudinal data than from data for a cross-section of women enumerated at a given date. In the August 1959 Current Population Survey women were asked their date of birth, and those who had ever been married were asked their date of first marriage. The information obtained permitted tabulations of the proportions of women who had married by successive ages as a birth cohort of women passed through life, up to the age attained by August 1959. The tabulations were made up to the midpoint of each year of age, to match as nearly as possible the kind of age detail normally available from a census or survey. In a census or survey, women normally are classified by age at last birthday, and those 21 years old, for example, would be anywhere between exact age 21.0 and exact age 21.9, but of midpoint age 21.5.

Table 7.3 presents pertinent data for white women born in 1935-39

Table 7.3   Percent married by successive ages, for white women born in 1935-39 and in 1920-24: United States, August 1959

Retro-spective age (x)	Percent ever married		Percent married between age $x - 1$ and age x[a]	
	1935-39	1920-24	1935-39	1920-24
15	3.3	1.5	3.3	1.5
16	8.4	5.0	5.1	3.5
17	16.5	10.6	8.1	5.6
18	30.2	19.1	13.7	8.5
19	44.0	29.9	13.8	10.8
20	56.9[b]	41.1	12.9	11.2
21	70.3[b]	52.1	13.4	11.0
22	78.9[b]	61.5	8.6	9.4
23	83.6[b]	69.2	4.7	7.7
24	86.4[b]	75.2	2.8	6.0
25	...	80.3	...	5.1
26	...	84.2	...	3.9
27	...	86.7	...	2.5
28	...	89.3	...	2.6
29	...	90.8	...	1.5
30	...	91.7	...	0.9
31 & over	...	94.6	...	2.9

Source: U.S. Bureau of the Census, Current Population Reports, Series P-20, No. 108, Table 5.

[a]Figures obtained by differencing percent ever married. The results show the percent who married between the midpoint of age x - 1 and the midpoint of age x, e.g., between exact age 21.5 and exact age 22.5.

[b]Percent adjusted for the part of the cohort that has not attained the stated age.

and for those born in 1920-24. These typify some of the changes in proportions ever married by age that have occurred over time on a cohort basis. The women born in 1935-39 were 20-24 years old in 1959 and those born in 1920-24 were 35-39 years old. Women born around 1935, in particular, appear to have a history of earlier marriages than earlier and later cohorts. It seems also that the percent of women in this cohort that will eventually marry is higher than that of earlier and later cohorts. The birth cohort of 1920-24 had slightly earlier marriages than most earlier cohorts but it is nonetheless generally representative of marriage patterns prevailing prior to the end of World War II. These statements are based on an examination of data (not shown) for birth cohorts dating back to 1880.[1]

It is evident from the table that the cohort of 1935-39 had larger proportions ever married by each age from 15 to 29 than the cohort of 1920-24. For example, 70 percent of the 1935-39 cohort had ever been married by the midpoint of age 21 as compared with 52 percent of the 1920-24 cohort. The younger cohort had higher marriage rates than the latter at each age, up to the midpoint of age 21, but lower marriage rates thereafter, up to the midpoint of age 24, which is as far as age comparisons can be made.

Table 7.4 Percent distribution by age at first marriage, for selected marriage cohorts and for white women 35-44 years old in 1960: United States

Age at first marriage	Year of first marriage			White women 35-44, years old, ever married, 1960
	White women		Nonwhite women	
	1955-59	1935-39	1950-59	
Total	100.0	100.0	100.0	100.0
14-17	20.7	15.3	25.5	14.9
18-19	27.0	20.5	21.7	20.0
20-21	23.6	19.2	16.7	21.0
22-24	14.2	21.0	16.1	23.4
25-29	8.5	16.4	11.1	14.8
30 and over	5.9	7.5	8.9	6.0
Median age at marriage	20.2	21.4	20.3	21.4

Source: U. S. Bureau of the Census, Current Population Reports, Series P-20, No. 108, Tables 14 and 15, and 1960 Census of Population, Women by Number of Children Ever Born, PC(2)-3A, Table 18.

Age at First Marriage

Table 7.4 presents selected data on the distribution of women by age at first marriage. The first three columns are based on the August 1959 Current Population Survey and relate to women surviving in August 1959 who first married in specified prior years. The data in those columns correspond in principle to a distribution of brides by age at marriage such as could be shown by marriage registration data.

The data for white women married in 1955-59 reflect the marriage age patterns prevailing at a time when marriage rates for young ages were the highest on record. Those for white women married in 1935-39 reflect the relatively fewer marriages at young ages in the economic depression of the 1930's. It may be noted that the 1955-59 white marriage cohort had a higher proportion married at ages 14-17, 18-19, and 20-21 than the cohort of 1935-39, and a lower proportion married at ages over 21. The median age of white brides was 20.2 years in the 1955-59 cohort and 21.4 years in the 1935-39 cohort, reflecting a drop of 1.2 years in the median age at marriage. Three-fourths of the white brides in 1955-59 were under age 22.8 as compared with a third quartile age of 24.7 in 1935-39—a decline of 1.9 years.

Fertility by Age at First Marriage

Some demographers believe that in these days of widespread birth-control practices, changes in the average age at marriage mainly result in women having their children earlier or later than they otherwise would have had them, with little effect on the eventual size of completed families. The underlying theory is that most couples want a certain number of children, and that changes in marriage age patterns do not have much effect on the ultimate number because nearly all women marry at ages that are sufficiently young to permit them to have as many children as they want. As is noted in Chapter 13, the white marriage cohort of 1935-39 completed its childbearing with more children on the average than the cohort of 1930-34 despite an older average marriage age for the cohort of 1935-39. Small families may result from being at the height of childbearing ages at depression time rather than just getting married and then having children later when economic conditions improve. Hence, there is some evidence that postponement of marriage does not always reduce the ultimate average number of children. But tabulations of fertility by specific ages at first marriage invariably show that fertility varies inversely with the age at marriage. That suggests that either the age at marriage has some effect on the number of children women want, or the women who have a desired number of children earlier are more likely to have unplanned pregnancies thereafter because of the longer period of risk that remains. Probably both elements are involved.

The general inverse relation between age at first marriage and the number of children ever born is typified by the following data from Tables 18 and 19 of the 1960 census report on *Women by Number of Children Ever Born.*

Age at first marriage	Children ever born per 1,000 women 35-44 years old, married once and husband present: United States, 1960	
	White	Nonwhite
All ages	2,634	3,364
14-17	3,485	5,005
18-19	2,989	4,175
20-21	2,741	3,590
22-24	2,530	2,905
25-26	2,281	2,476
27-29	2,008	2,147
30-44	1,292	1,514

It may be noted from these data that the rates for all marriage ages combined are intermediate between the rates for marriage ages 20-21 and marriage ages 22-24, among white and nonwhite women alike. Perhaps the rates of 2,741 and 2,530 for white women at marriage ages 20-21 and 22-24 may be used as a very rough guide to the maximum range in which shifts in marriage age may affect the ultimate fertility of white women in general, other things being equal. The former rate is only 8 percent higher than the latter. Among nonwhite women, the rate of 3,590 for marriage ages 20-21 is 24 percent higher than the rate for marriage ages 22-24.

Age of Husband by Age of Wife

It is known from various studies that on the average, husbands tend to be about 3 years older than their wives. About 90 percent of women who marry for the first time have a husband who had no previous marriage. Data for married couples living together in 1960, with husband 35-54 years old, will be cited here for illustrative purposes only, but they are thought to represent the general patterns prevailing in the population. As may be seen from the data in Table 7.5, the median age difference was 2.8 years for all couples with husband 35-54 years old. Among couples where *both* the husband and wife had been married only once, the difference was 2.7 years, and among those where *both* had been married more than once, it was 3.0 years.

Table 7.5 Difference between ages of husband and wife, for couples with husband 35-54 years old: United States, 1960

Times married for husband and wife	Couples (thousands)	Percent distribution						Median age difference (years)
			Husband older			Same or husband 1 year younger	Husband 2 or more years younger	
		Total	10+ years	5-9 years	1-4 years			
Total	18,507	73.8	8.8	24.2	40.8	15.2	11.0	2.8
Both married once	14,714	75.4	6.5	24.2	44.7	15.9	8.7	2.7
Husband once, wife more than once	1,243	52.9	7.0	17.2	28.7	16.5	30.6	0.9
Husband more than once, wife once	1,227	84.5	29.8	32.0	22.7	8.0	7.5	6.3
Both married more than once	1,323	66.2	17.0	23.5	25.7	12.7	21.1	3.0

Source: U. S. Bureau of the Census, 1960 Census of Population, Marital Status, PC(2)-4E, Table 9.

In contrast to the nearly equal age difference of 2.7 and 3.0 years just cited for both married once and both married more than once, fairly large variations occurred when *one* spouse or the other, but not both, was in a remarriage. Among couples with husband married more than once, wife only once, the median age difference was 6.3 years. Among those with husband married once, but wife more than once, the median difference was 0.9 years. There appears to be a tendency for a remarried person of either sex to seek out a partner who is relatively young. Less than 9 percent of couples where the wife had been married only once involved husbands 2 or more years younger than the wife, but 31 percent of couples with wife married more than once and husband married once involved husbands 2 or more years younger than the wife. A substantial minority (21 percent) of couples with both husband and wife married more than once also involved husbands 2 or more years younger than the wife. Thus, women married more than once are far more likely than women married only once to have husbands who are 2 or more years younger than themselves. Men married more than once are also more likely to have wives considerably younger than themselves as compared with men married only once. Among couples with both husband and wife married more than once, there is wider diffusion of age differences between husband and wife than among couples with both husband and wife married only once.

It may be of some interest to note that the average differences between age of husbands and wives decline with advancing age of wife at first marriage, up to about age 24. According to a Current Population Survey made in June 1954, among couples at first marriages of both husband and wife who married between January 1947 and June 1954, the median age of husband at time of marriage for wives who were 16 years old at marriage was 20.9 years, reflecting an age difference of about 4.4 years between husband and wife if the wives 16 years old are taken as of average midpoint age 16.5. Among wives 24 years old at marriage, the median age of husband was 26.4 years, reflecting a difference of about 1.9 years between age of husband and wife. Marriage registration data for the year 1962 show smaller differences between ages of bride and groom than those found in the June 1954 survey but still a pattern of decline with advancing age at first marriage of the wives. It appears from the 1962 data, however, that the decline with advancing age of wife at first marriage terminates at about age 24; thereafter the differences either level off or slowly increase with age of bride.

Table 7.6 presents data on fertility for women 35-39 years old in 1960, with both husband and wife married only once, by age of husband. These data indicate the effect on fertility of age differences between husband and wife. The great majority of wives 35-39 years old in first marriages had husbands who were either 35-39 years old or 40-44 years old (81 percent of white wives and 73 percent of nonwhite wives). Larger proportions of nonwhite wives than of white wives 35-39 years old in intact first marriages had husbands who were either younger or much older than themselves.

The average number of children ever born per 1,000 wives 35-39 years old was lowest in the relatively few cases in which the husband was 14-29 years old; these probably consisted largely of wives 35 years old with husbands 29 years old, or about 6 years younger than themselves. Women with husbands younger than themselves were mainly women who married relatively late in life and who had a marriage duration (as of the survey date) that was well below the average for all wives 35-39 years old. Most fertile, overall, were wives with a husband 40-44 years old.

Nearly as fertile were the women with husbands 45-49 years old, and among whites only, those with husbands 35-39 years old. Even the women with husbands 50 years old and over had average numbers of children ever born that were within 10 percent of the average for all wives 35-39 years old. However, the last group had a proportion of women childless that was far above the average for all wives 35-39. In terms of data that exclude women who were childless, the women with husbands over age 50 had higher fertility than the average for women with husbands of all ages. Perhaps childless women with husbands over age 50 were somewhat selective of those marriages in which husband and wife married at a very advanced age and did not want family responsibilities; but reduced fecundity with advancing age may also have been an important factor.

Table 7.6 Fertility by age of husband, for white and nonwhite women 35-39 years old, married and husband present, both husband and wife married once: United States, 1960

Color of wife and age of husband	Percent distribution	Percent childless	Children ever born	
			Per 1,000 wives	Per 1,000 mothers
WHITE				
Total	100.0	8.2	2,721	2,964
14-29	0.5	25.6	1,775	2,385
30-34	5.9	12.7	2,383	2,729
35-39	44.1	7.3	2,718	2,932
40-44	36.4	7.3	2,788	3,006
45-49	9.9	9.8	2,775	3,077
50 and over	3.2	15.4	2,609	3,082
NONWHITE				
Total	100.0	16.1	3,498	4,167
14-29	1.4	31.4	2,207	3,216
30-34	7.6	21.2	2,858	3,627
35-39	40.3	14.7	3,407	3,995
40-44	32.8	14.2	3,780	4,406
45-49	11.7	16.9	3,703	4,455
50 and over	6.1	23.5	3,276	4,284

Source: U. S. Bureau of the Census, 1960 Census of Population, Women by Number of Children Ever Born, PC(2)-3A, Tables 23 and 24.

Stability of Marriage

About 82 percent of white women of childbearing age who had ever been married were living with their first husbands at the time of the 1960 census (Table 7.7). An additional 9 percent had remarried and were living with their current husband. The corresponding percentages for nonwhite women were 61 and 10, respectively.

Table 7.7   Percent distribution by marital characteristics of women 15-44 years old, by color and age: United States, 1960

Color and age	All women, percent ever married	Women ever married						
		Total	Husband present		Husband absent		Di-vorced	Wid-owed
			Women married once	Married more than once	Sepa-rated	Other		
WHITE								
Total	76.0	100.0	81.8	9.3	1.7	2.5	3.2	1.5
15-19	16.1	100.0	82.1	1.9	2.9	10.6	2.2	0.4
20-24	72.5	100.0	86.8	4.1	2.1	4.2	2.5	0.4
25-29	90.3	100.0	85.6	7.3	1.6	2.2	2.8	0.5
30-34	93.5	100.0	82.7	9.8	1.6	1.8	3.2	1.0
35-39	94.1	100.0	79.4	11.9	1.6	1.6	3.6	1.9
40-44	93.9	100.0	76.5	12.6	1.7	1.6	4.0	3.6
NONWHITE								
Total	71.7	100.0	61.4	10.3	13.3	5.8	4.9	4.4
15-19	16.2	100.0	71.2	1.3	10.3	14.8	1.5	0.9
20-24	64.4	100.0	70.9	3.3	12.1	9.7	2.7	1.2
25-29	84.2	100.0	66.4	7.3	13.9	6.1	4.2	2.1
30-34	90.4	100.0	61.0	11.0	14.4	4.9	5.2	3.5
35-39	92.5	100.0	56.3	14.3	13.7	4.0	6.0	5.7
40-44	93.6	100.0	52.7	15.5	12.4	3.6	6.4	9.4

Source: U. S. Bureau of the Census, 1960 Census of Population, Women by Number of Children Ever Born, PC(2)-3A, Tables 16 and 17.

At each age from 20-24 through 35-39, well over 90 percent of white women ever married had a husband present but this was true of less than 75 percent of nonwhite women. Women 15-19 had a smaller proportion with husband present than those of more mature age, for such reasons as husband being away in military service and some unwed mothers perhaps misreporting their marital status as separated, widowed, or divorced.

At each age relatively more nonwhite women than white women were separated.

Except at the earliest childbearing ages shown, the proportion of women who had remarried and were living with their current husbands considerably exceeded the proportion who were currently widowed or divorced. This indicates that many of the women who become widowed or divorced during the childbearing age remarry, often after a short time.

Other data, not shown in Table 7.7, indicate that above-average proportions of white women currently separated or divorced have been married more than once, which suggests that when a first marriage is not successful there is an increased chance that the second marriage also will not be successful, although most remarriages do remain intact. This is illustrated by the data in Table 7.8.

Table 7.8 Proportion of women married more than once, by marital status and color, for women 35-44 years old: United States, 1960

Marital status	White		Nonwhite	
	Percent distribution	Percent married more than once	Percent distribution	Percent married more than once
Total ever married	100.0	14.4	100.0	21.4
Married husband present	90.2	13.6	69.5	21.4
Separated	1.6	26.3	13.1	20.2
Other married husband present	1.6	20.9	3.8	21.9
Widowed	2.7	15.0	7.4	19.7
Divorced	3.8	25.4	6.2	24.6

Source: U. S. Bureau of the Census, 1960 Census of Population, Women by Number of Children Ever Born, PC(2)-3A, Tables 28 and 29.

The 1950 census obtained information on years in present marital status, by age at occurrence. These data provide some information on the distribution of women of childbearing age by age at divorce and age at remarriage, by number of children ever born (Tables 7.9 and 7.10). (Most remarriages of women of childbearing age involve women previously divorced, as the incidence of widowhood is low.) Women in remarriages for less than 2 years and women divorced less than 2 years have very similar patterns in respect to distribution by age at occurrence of remarriage or divorce and by number of children ever born. In both, more than half are below age 30-34, most often at age 20-24 and then at age 25-29. Large proportions of the women of each age are childless. The data for women in remarriages include births occurring up to 2 years after remarriage, so it is reasonable to suppose that the proportions who are childless at the time of remarriage are larger than those shown in Table 7.9.

Table 7.9   Distribution by number of children ever born, for women married more than once, husband present, in present marriage for less than 2 years, 15-44 years old at time of remarriage, by age at remarriage: United States, 1950

Age at current marriage	Women	Percent by children ever born			
		Total	None	1 and 2	3 or more
14-19	32,040	100.0	55.2	41.9	2.8
20-24	88,620	100.0	41.9	50.9	7.1
25-29	87,600	100.0	33.7	50.7	15.6
30-34	66,300	100.0	30.0	48.5	21.6
35-39	67,260	100.0	30.2	49.2	20.6
40-44	39,960	100.0	28.1	40.5	31.5

Source: U. S. Bureau of the Census, 1950 Census of Population, Duration of Current Marital Status, P-E, No. 2E, Table 8.

Table 7.10   Distribution of number of children ever born, for women divorced less than 2 years, 15-44 years old at time of divorce, by age at divorce: United States, 1950

Age at divorce	Women	Percent by children ever born			
		Total	None	1 and 2	3 or more
14-19	17,040	100.0	52.8	46.0	1.2
20-24	57,240	100.0	38.1	55.2	6.7
25-29	51,960	100.0	32.1	53.7	14.2
30-34	36,090	100.0	31.0	50.6	18.4
35-39	32,370	100.0	28.4	44.2	27.4
40-44	31,260	100.0	27.8	46.5	25.6

Source: U. S. Bureau of the Census, 1950 Census of Population, Duration of Current Marital Status, P-E, No. 2E, Table 23.

Tables 7.11 and 7.12 present data from the 1960 census on the distribution of women 35-44 years old, by age at first marriage and current marital status. These show clearly that among women of a given current age (35-44), those in interrupted first marriages are women who on the average first married at a younger age than women still in intact first marriages. This pattern reflects the combined effect of marriage stability by age at marriage and of varying intervals since

Table 7.11   Distribution of white women 35-44 years old ever married, by age at first marriage and by marital status: United States, 1960

Age at first marriage	Total ever married	Husband present		Husband absent		Di-vorced	Wid-owed
		Woman married once	Married more than once	Sepa-rated	Other		
Women (thousands)	10,356	8,075	1,269	169	167	396	280
			Percent by age at marriage				
Total	100.0	100.0	100.0	100.0	100.0	100.0	100.0
14-17	14.9	11.9	30.4	21.8	17.1	19.8	19.3
18-19	20.0	18.8	27.4	20.1	18.3	21.8	20.0
20-21	21.0	21.5	19.4	18.3	19.3	20.1	19.8
22-24	23.4	25.2	14.3	19.0	20.3	19.5	21.3
25-26	8.3	9.0	4.0	6.9	7.7	7.4	7.7
27-29	6.5	7.1	2.7	6.6	7.3	6.0	6.1
30-44	6.0	6.5	1.8	7.3	9.8	5.5	5.8
			Percent by marital status				
Total	100.0	78.0	12.3	1.6	1.6	3.8	2.7
14-17	100.0	62.2	25.0	2.4	1.9	5.1	3.5
18-19	100.0	73.2	16.8	1.6	1.5	4.2	2.7
20-21	100.0	79.6	11.3	1.4	1.5	3.6	2.5
22-24	100.0	84.1	7.5	1.3	1.4	3.2	2.5
25-26	100.0	85.3	5.9	1.4	1.5	3.4	2.5
27-29	100.0	85.4	5.1	1.7	1.8	3.6	2.6
30-44	100.0	85.4	3.8	2.0	2.7	3.6	2.6
Median age at marriage	21.4	21.8	19.4	20.8	21.5	20.4	21.1

Source: U. S. Bureau of the Census, 1960 Census of Population, **Women by Number of Children Ever Born**, PC(2)-3A, Table 18.

Table 7.12 Distribution of nonwhite women 35-44 years old ever married, by age at first marriage and by marital status: United States, 1960

Age at first marriage	Total ever married	Husband present		Husband absent		Di-vorced	Wid-owed
		Woman married once	Married more than once	Sepa-rated	Other		
Women (thousands)	1,231	672	183	161	47	76	91
				Percent by age at marriage			
Total	100.0	100.0	100.0	100.0	100.0	100.0	100.0
14-17	25.2	19.8	38.3	28.7	23.9	27.0	31.5
18-19	17.9	16.6	21.2	18.4	16.4	19.6	18.9
20-21	15.2	15.2	15.3	15.1	13.4	16.1	15.5
22-24	17.4	19.0	13.4	16.7	16.6	17.3	15.4
25-26	7.5	8.6	4.7	7.1	7.8	6.9	6.6
27-29	7.3	8.6	3.8	6.5	9.1	6.6	5.9
30-44	9.5	12.2	3.4	7.6	12.7	6.5	6.2
				Percent by marital status			
Total	100.0	54.6	14.9	13.1	3.8	6.2	7.4
14-17	100.0	42.9	22.6	14.9	3.6	6.6	9.3
18-19	100.0	50.7	17.7	13.5	3.5	6.7	7.9
20-21	100.0	54.5	15.0	13.0	3.4	6.5	7.6
22-24	100.0	59.6	11.5	12.5	3.7	6.1	6.6
25-26	100.0	62.3	9.3	12.2	4.0	5.6	6.5
27-29	100.0	64.4	7.7	11.7	4.8	5.6	6.0
30-44	100.0	70.1	5.3	10.5	5.1	4.2	4.9

Source: U. S. Bureau of the Census, 1960 Census of Population, Women by Number of Children Ever Born, PC(2)-3A, Table 19.

first marriage. That is, if intervals since first marriage were held constant (as is not the case in the data shown), the stability of marriages would still vary by age at marriage. Also, the women of current age 35-44 who first married at a young age were at risk of a marriage disruption for a longer time than the women who married at an advanced age. Youngest of all at first marriage in the data shown are the women who have remarried. Thus, 58 percent of white women 35-44 years old, married more than once and living with their current husband, first married before age 20 as compared with 31 percent of those still living with their first husband and 42 percent of separated and divorced white women. In part, that reflects the fact that women in remarriages must have had some intermediate time between marriages, so the data are more selective of women with long intervals since first marriage or early age at marriage than in the case of women presently separated or divorced.

Among white women 35-44 years old, the proportions currently separated, widowed, and divorced vary little in magnitude by age at first marriage. The proportions are largest among those age 14-17 at marriage, lowest among those 20-26 at marriage, and increase among those 27-29 and 30-44 at marriage.

If time since first marriage were the main cause of differences, those proportions should be largest for women aged 14-17 at first marriage and decline steadily thereafter. The data suggest, therefore, that after a certain age at marriage, an increased incidence of separation or divorce or widowhood more than offsets the effect of a generally shorter interval since first marriage.

Data for marriage cohorts hold constant the time since first marriage and provide further clues on the relation between age at first marriage and marriage stability. These data confirm that women who marry at age 22-24 generally have the most stable marriages, provided one does not go more than 40 or 50 years past the first marriage date. Eventually, the selective effect of mortality is such that only couples who married very young survive. For example, among white women first married in 1945-49 and in 1930-34, the following proportions of surviving women were still living with their first husbands as of August 1959:

Age at first marriage	Percent living with first husband, for women first married in specified period	
	1945-49	1930-34
14-17	72.7	60.5
18-19	85.5	69.5
20-21	87.5	71.0
22-24	90.5	76.8
25-29	85.8	72.4
30+	81.4	53.1

Source: U.S. Bureau of the Census, *Current Population Reports,* Series P-20, No. 108, Table 14.

The women first married in 1945-49 were 10 to 14 years past the date of first marriage as of 1959, or long enough to have had over three-fourths of their ultimate number of children, and those first married in 1930-34 were 25 to 29 years past the date of first marriage. Cohorts more recent than the one of 1945-49 had higher proportions living with first husband than that cohort. Those later than the one of 1930-34 had progressively smaller proportions than that cohort, with more decline among women of advanced ages of first marriage than of young ages.

Table 7.13 presents data on number of children ever born per 1,000 women 35-44 years old, in detail by current marital status and age at

Table 7.13   Children ever born per 1,000 women 35-44 years old, by age at first marriage and by marital status: United States, 1960

Age at first marriage	Total ever married	Husband present		Husband absent		Di-vorced	Wid-owed
		Woman married once	Married more than once	Sepa-rated	Other		
WHITE							
Total	2,572	2,634	2,456	2,540	2,494	1,878	2,357
14-17	3,280	3,485	2,914	3,395	3,261	2,656	3,107
18-19	2,868	2,989	2,548	2,844	2,853	2,164	2,711
20-21	2,641	2,741	2,267	2,598	2,635	1,855	2,333
22-24	2,441	2,530	1,993	2,198	2,391	1,553	2,066
25-26	2,203	2,281	1,828	1,948	2,156	1,259	1,892
27-29	1,939	2,008	1,686	1,667	1,760	1,108	1,593
30-44	1,285	1,292	1,614	1,258	1,233	865	1,225
NONWHITE							
Total	3,065	3,364	2,753	2,734	2,713	2,130	3,036
14-17	4,067	5,005	3,295	3,437	3,701	2,764	3,690
18-19	3,561	4,175	2,731	3,005	3,383	2,538	3,377
20-21	3,137	3,590	2,563	2,772	2,617	1,919	2,917
22-24	2,627	2,905	2,057	2,291	2,382	1,766	2,682
25-26	2,318	2,476	2,118	2,126	2,036	1,514	2,325
27-29	2,072	2,147	2,150	1,977	2,095	1,421	1,944
30-44	1,523	1,514	1,932	1,542	1,379	1,136	1,649

Source: U. S. Bureau of the Census, 1960 Census of Population, Women by Number of Children Ever Born, PC(2)-3A, Tables 18 and 19.

first marriage that matches that in Table 7.11 and 7.12. The data on children chiefly reflect fertility before a marital disruption in the case of women currently separated, widowed, or divorced.

Generally speaking, the women 35-44 years old still living with their first husbands are the most fertile, both overall and for each age of first marriage. Exceptions occur in some marital statuses among the women reported as first married at age 27-29 or 30-44. These exceptions may reflect misreporting of times married or of a date of remarriage instead of a date of first marriage, but could possibly also reflect some childbearing before marriage.

Among white women, the women currently separated have borne more children than women who are widowed, whereas the reverse situation applies to nonwhite women. In both color groups the separated and widowed women have borne more children than those who have remarried and are living with a current husband. Least fertile are the divorced women. For women of childbearing age, most remarriages involve women who previously were divorced, as may be seen from annual vital statistics on marriages by previous marital status of bride and groom. Probably women with few or no children have a better prospect for remarriage than women with many children, other things being equal.

It is not known how many children the women with disrupted first marriages would have had if their first marriage had remained intact. Certainly, some divorces occur because one spouse or the other wants children and none have been forthcoming. A probably overstated indication of the effect of marital disruptions on fertility can be obtained if it is assumed that the women would have had fertility as high as that for women living with first husband, for each age at marriage, and if the age at first marriage is weighted by distributions shown in Tables 7.11 and 7.12 for each marital status. (In the rare exceptions where the women of interrupted first marriage have higher fertility for a late age at first marriage than those still in first marriage, the higher fertility is used.) The results of the computations based on the procedure just mentioned are given in Table 7.14.

Because of their earlier age at first marriage, the women with disrupted first marriages would have had more children on the average had they been as fertile for each age at marriage as the women still living with their first husbands. Among white women 35-44 years old ever married, the actual rate of 2,572 children per 1,000 women was 96 percent of the rate of 2,682 that would have been obtained if the women of each age at first marriage had been as fertile as the women still living with their first husbands. This implies an overall fertility loss of about 4 percent from marriage interruptions. The corresponding overall loss for nonwhite women is about 14 percent. These figures probably overstate the extent of the overall loss, because it is unlikely that the women of some marital statuses would actually have been as fertile as women of intact first marriages had their marriage not been interrupted. Inability to have children is sometimes a factor in divorce, and widowhood is probably partly selective of women whose husbands had health problems or substandard fecundity while they were living.

Table 7.14   Children ever born per 1,000 women 35–44 years old, by color and marital status of woman: United States, 1960

Color and marital status	Actual (1)	Hypo- thetical (2)	(1) as percent of (2)	(1) as percent of rate for women married once husband present
WHITE				
Ever married	2,572	2,682	95.2	97.6
Married once, husband present	2,634	2,634	100.0	100.0
Married more than once, husband present	2,456	2,946	83.4	93.2
Separated	2,540	2,751	92.3	96.4
Other married, husband absent	2,494	2,666	93.5	94.7
Divorced	1,878	2,764	67.9	71.3
Widowed	2,357	2,744	85.9	89.5
NONWHITE				
Ever married	3,065	3,586	85.5	91.1
Married once, husband present	3,364	3,364	100.0	100.0
Married more than once husband present	2,753	4,004	68.8	81.8
Separated	2,734	3,694	74.0	81.3
Other married, husband absent	2,713	3,478	78.0	80.6
Divorced	2,130	3,689	57.7	63.3
Widowed	3,036	3,780	80.3	90.2

Source: Derived from Tables 7.11 and 7.12. See text for explanation of column (2).

Perhaps it should be noted that there is often a very short interval between divorce or widowhood and remarriage. According to data from the April 1953 Current Population Survey, 950,000 women remarried between January 1950 and April 1953. Of these, 660,000 were previously divorced and 284,000 were previously widowed, and 6,000 did not report previous marital status. The median interval between divorce and remarriage was 2.7 years and that between widowhood and remarriage was 3.5 years. These data involve women of all ages, not just those of childbearing age. Presumably, the intervals would be shorter if the data were limited to women of childbearing age.

Summary

A part of the baby boom that began after World War II was a result of increases in the proportion of women of childbearing age who had married. Data from the Current Population Survey indicate that the rise for women under age 25 reached a peak around 1956, and that declines have since occurred. Women born around 1935 appear to have a history of earlier marriages than prior or later cohorts and a slightly higher percentage of them may eventually marry than women of younger or older birth cohorts.

At each age from 20-24 through 35-39, well over 90 percent of ever-married white women, but less than 75 percent of ever-married nonwhite women, were living with their husbands at the time of the 1960 census. These proportions include women in remarriages as well as those in first marriages. Most remarriages of women of childbearing age involve women who were previously divorced. Among divorced and recently remarried women, the proportion who are childless is high. A rough indication of the overall loss of fertility from disrupted first marriages is provided by 1960 census data which indicate that the number of children ever born per 1,000 white women ever married, 35-44 years old, is 98 percent of the corresponding rate for white women in intact first marriages; for nonwhite women, the corresponding percentage is 91. The indication of loss is only approximate, because there is no way of knowing how many children divorced and widowed women would have had if their marriages had remained intact. The divorces, especially, may have involved some couples who did not want or could not have children.

An examination of data on children ever born by average age at marriage of women indicates that a 2-year shift upwards or downwards is likely to change the average number of children ever born by roughly 8 percent for white women and 24 percent for nonwhite women. Women who marry men either much younger or much older than themselves tend to have fewer children than women with husbands about 3 years older; this pattern possibly reflects an older average age at marriage and a shorter time for possible childbearing when the woman is much younger or older than the husband.

Great care is needed in describing and analyzing statistics on illegitimacy in the United States, partly because estimates of illegitimate births are subject to unknown biases and partly because various measures of illegitimacy can give quite different impressions of trends and variations in the incidence of illegitimate births. The purpose of this chapter is to examine a number of these statistical problems. First, problems in the registration of illegitimate births are examined. Later portions of the chapter deal with trends and differentials in three measures of illegitimacy and discuss their advantages and disadvantages. Finally, some of the factors that may be associated with variations in illegitimacy are taken up.

Definitions and Methods of Estimating

Estimates of the number of illegitimate births in the United States are based on information entered on birth certificates of states that require the reporting of the child's legitimacy. In some states a birth is defined as illegitimate if the mother reports herself as not currently married. The birth certificates in a few of these states ask only whether the mother is married. If she is married, the child is assumed to be legitimate. In other states, an illegitimate birth is a child conceived "out of wedlock" either to an unmarried woman or to a married women by a man other than her husband. In all states a child born to a widowed or divorced woman is considered legitimate if conception occurred while the mother and her husband were still living together.

The proportions of illegitimate births to single and to previously married women are not known, because the mother's previous marital status is not required on the birth certificate of any state. However, a pilot study recently carried out in the National Center for Health Statistics suggests that the overwhelming majority of illegitimate births occur to women who were never married. In this study the surname of the child and the mother's maiden name were compared on a sample of birth certificates from 10 states that report legitimacy. When the birth was illegitimate, the child's surname was the same as the mother's maiden name in 90 percent of the cases. In the remaining 10 percent the mother was evidently married previously.

Not all conceptions occurring before marriage terminate in illegitimate births. In many cases the couple marries before delivery and the child is registered as legitimate. Some inferential data on this pattern of behavior are presented in Chapter 13, Table 13.9. According to this table, among white women who first married in 1955-59, 12.7 percent had a first birth before the end of the seventh month of marriage. This proportion is twice as great as the comparable proportion among white women who first married in 1940-44, so it is evident that the proportion of legitimate births conceived before marriage has increased substantially.

Some unmarried mothers may be living in consensual, or common law, unions, but the proportion of illegitimate births occurring under such circumstances in the United States is not known. In Puerto Rico, however, some data on this topic are available. In 1965, 23.2 percent of all births in Puerto Rico were classified as illegitimate. However, only 4.4 percent of all births occurred to women who were not living in either a legal or consensual union. The remaining 18.8 percent were "illegitimate" births, but the mother and father were living together. In other words, 81 percent of the illegitimate children were born to parents who were living in consensual unions. It seems unlikely, however, that the comparable proportion is as high in the United States.

Not all states require the reporting of legitimacy status on the birth certificate. In 1965 reporting of legitimacy was required in 34 states and the District of Columbia. Approximately 7 out of 10 of all estimated illegitimate births occurred in these areas. The reporting situation was much better three decades ago. In 1938, for example, 44 states and the District of Columbia asked for legitimacy on the birth certificate. The only states that did not require reporting then were California, Massachusetts, New York, and Texas.

In making estimates of the number of illegitimate births in the entire United States, the states are grouped into nine geographic divisions. The ratio of illegitimate to total live births for the residents of the reporting states in each division is then applied to *all* live births for residents of that division. The sum of the estimates for the nine divisions is the estimate for the United States. These estimates are prepared for white and nonwhite births separately.

A crucial and unsolved problem in the investigation of statistics on illegitimacy is the extent of misreporting in the states that require the reporting of this item. Many women undoubtedly succeed in reporting their illegitimate children as legitimate, but the extent of such misreporting is unknown. It cannot be assumed that the relative degree of misreporting has been constant over time and for different segments of the population, and the direction of the biases can only be guessed. It seems likely that the reporting of illegitimacy has improved over time. One reason for believing this is that the reporting of all births has improved. Another reason is that the proportion of births occurring in hospitals has increased greatly, and it is probably more difficult to misreport an illegitimate birth in a hospital than at home.

Measures of Illegitimacy

This section describes trends and variations in three measures of illegitimacy. Two of these have been frequently used in the past: the illegitimacy ratio (illegitimate births per 1,000 total births) and the illegitimacy rate per 1,000 unmarried women 15-44 years old. The third is one that has not been used previously, but has certain advantages: the illegitimacy rate per 1,000 women 15-44 years old. These statistics will be shown separately for the white and nonwhite population groups, because the difference between them is large.

One measure relating to illegitimacy that cannot be shown is the number of unwed mothers who remain unmarried, by age. It seems probable that many unwed mothers eventually marry and raise their children in a normal pattern of family life. But we have no idea of the proportion of women involved in such an adjustment.

The Illegitimacy Ratio. This is the number of illegitimate births per 1,000 total births. For the United States as a whole, this ratio was 77.4 in 1965. In other words, 7.74 percent of all births were classified as illegitimate. Trends and color differentials in this ratio are shown for 1940-65 in Table 8.1. Over the entire 25-year period the ratio has risen by 104 percent. On the average, illegitimacy ratios for nonwhite births have been nine times higher than for white births. Factors associated with the white-nonwhite differential will be discussed in a later section of this chapter.

The advantage of the illegitimacy ratio is that it tells the proportion of children born in any year who are involved in the many social problems associated with illegitimacy. It is useful, therefore, as a measure of the relative need for services to unwed mothers and their children.

The illegitimacy ratio, however, is a poor measure to use in analyzing factors associated with illegitimacy. This is because the numerator

Table 8.1 Estimated number of illegitimate births and ratio
of illegitimate births to total births, by color:
United States, 1940-65

(Due to rounding estimates to the nearest hundred, figures by color
may not add to totals)

Year	Number			Ratio per 1,000 births		
	Total	White	Nonwhite	Total	White	Nonwhite
1965	291,200	123,700	167,500	77.4	39.6	263.2
1964	275,700	114,300	161,300	68.5	33.9	245.0
1963[a]	259,400	104,600	154,900	63.3	30.4	235.5
1962[a]	245,100	94,700	150,400	58.8	27.0	227.8
1961	240,200	91,100	149,100	56.3	25.3	223.4
1960	224,300	82,500	141,800	52.7	22.9	215.8
1959	220,600	79,600	141,100	52.0	22.1	218.0
1958	208,700	74,600	134,100	49.6	20.9	212.3
1957	201,700	70,800	130,900	47.4	19.6	206.7
1956	193,500	67,500	126,000	46.5	19.0	204.0
1955	183,300	64,200	119,200	45.3	18.6	202.4
1954	176,600	62,700	113,900	44.0	18.2	198.5
1953	160,800	56,600	104,200	41.2	16.9	191.1
1952	150,300	54,100	96,200	39.1	16.3	183.4
1951	146,500	52,600	93,900	39.1	16.3	182.8
1950	141,600	53,500	88,100	39.8	17.5	179.6
1949	133,200	53,500	79,700	37.4	17.3	167.5
1948	129,700	54,800	74,900	36.7	17.8	164.7
1947	131,900	60,500	71,500	35.7	18.5	168.0
1946	125,200	61,400	63,800	38.1	21.1	170.1
1945	117,400	56,400	60,900	42.9	23.6	179.3
1944	105,200	49,600	55,600	37.6	20.2	163.4
1943	98,100	42,800	55,400	33.4	16.5	162.8
1942	96,500	42,000	54,500	34.3	16.9	169.2
1941	95,700	41,900	53,800	38.1	19.0	174.5
1940	89,500	40,300	49,200	37.9	19.5	168.3

Source: National Center for Health Statistics, Vital Statistics of the United States, 1965, Vol. I, Natality, Table 1-25

[a]Figures for white and nonwhite births in 1962 and 1963 have
been adjusted to include estimates for New Jersey, and therefore differ
from originally published figures. The reporting of color was not required on birth certificates in that state for a major portion of these
two years.

and the denominator of the ratio may be subject to quite different influences. The numerator (illegitimate births) is subject to all the influences that determine the number of such births in a given year, but the denominator (total births) is subject predominantly to the influences that affect births within marriage (e.g., family size preferences, desired spacing of births, success in using contraception, etc.). Consequently, the illegitimacy ratio changes not only in response to those factors directly influencing illegitimate births but also in response to those factors directly influencing legitimate births. In the past several years, for example, there has been a decline in the number of legitimate births, which appears to be associated with certain shifts in the spacing of births within marriage, changes in desired family size, and changes in the effectiveness with which couples use contraception. A corresponding decline has not occurred among illegitimate births. As a consequence of the decline in the denominator, the illegitimacy ratio has increased more rapidly than the number of illegitimate births or than any other measure of illegitimacy. Between 1960 and 1965, for example, the illegitimacy ratio increased by 47 percent. The comparable percentage increases in other measures of illegitimacy are as follows:

Number of illegitimate births	30 percent
Illegitimate births per 1,000 women 15-44	21 percent
Illegitimate births per 1,000 unmarried women 15-44	9 percent

The same point can be made about certain differentials in the illegitimacy ratio. Table 8.2 shows, for example, that the illegitimacy ratio is higher at ages 15-19 than at any later age at childbirth. But, as Table 8.4 indicates, other measures show that the incidence of illegitimacy is often higher at ages 20-24 and 25-29. The reason that the illegitimacy ratio is so high at ages 15-19 is simply that the denominator of the ratio (total births, most of which are legitimate) is relatively lower at ages 15-19 than at ages 20-24 and 25-29.

Although the illegitimacy ratio has its uses as an index of relative needs for services, it is clearly a poor analytical measure of illegitimacy.

Illegitimate Births per 1,000 Women 15-44. Although this rate does not relate illegitimate births to the population at risk (i.e., to the number of unmarried women), it is useful (1) because it indicates the proportion of all women in the childbearing years of life who have an illegitimate birth in any given year, and (2) because it facilitates comparisons with the fertility rate (the total number of births per 1,000 women 15-44).

Table 8.2 Estimated number of illegitimate births and ratio of illegitimate births to total births, by color and age of mother: United States, 1940, 1950, 1960, and 1965

(Due to rounding estimates to the nearest hundred, figures by color may not add to totals)

Color and age of mother	Number of illegitimate births				Illegitimate births per 1,000 total births			
	1965	1960	1950	1940	1965	1960	1950	1940
Total	291,200	224,300	141,600	89,500	77.4	52.7	39.8	37.9
Under 15	6,100	4,600	3,200	2,100	785.3	678.5	637.3	644.8
15-19	123,100	87,100	56,000	40,500	208.3	148.4	133.5	134.7
20-24	90,700	68,000	43,100	27,200	67.8	47.7	38.1	36.8
25-29	36,800	32,100	20,900	10,500	39.8	29.4	20.5	16.3
30-34	19,600	18,900	10,800	5,200	37.0	27.5	18.1	13.0
35-39	11,400	10,600	6,000	3,000	40.3	29.5	20.4	14.9
40 and over	3,700	3,000	1,700	1,000	42.9	31.0	21.3	15.0
White	123,700	82,500	53,500	40,300	39.6	22.9	17.5	19.5
Under 15	1,400	1,200	700	500	572.8	475.4	419.4	443.7
15-19	50,700	32,800	19,900	16,000	114.3	71.6	62.4	69.7
20-24	43,400	26,700	17,800	14,700	38.4	21.9	18.3	22.7
25-29	14,900	10,700	7,900	5,200	18.8	11.4	8.7	8.9
30-34	7,200	6,000	4,200	2,200	16.1	10.2	7.9	6.0
35-39	4,500	3,900	2,300	1,300	19.0	12.7	9.0	7.3
40 and over	1,600	1,300	700	500	22.2	15.8	10.2	8.5
Nonwhite	167,500	141,800	88,100	49,200	263.2	215.8	179.6	168.2
Under 15	4,600	3,500	2,500	1,600	864.0	822.4	745.8	751.2
15-19	72,400	54,300	36,100	24,500	492.0	421.5	358.4	344.4
20-24	47,300	41,300	25,300	12,500	229.9	199.6	159.0	136.4
25-29	21,900	21,300	13,000	5,300	162.8	141.3	114.7	88.3
30-34	12,400	12,900	6,600	2,900	149.0	129.9	102.4	80.1
35-39	6,900	6,700	3,600	1,700	148.8	127.7	98.5	75.3
40 and over	2,000	1,700	1,000	600	140.1	116.8	92.9	77.4

Source: National Center for Health Statistics, Vital Statistics of the United States, 1965, Vol. I, Natality, Table 1-27, and comparable tables in reports for 1940, 1950, and 1960.

Table 8.3 shows that only a very small fraction of women of childbearing age deliver an illegitimate child in any given year. In 1965, for example, the proportion was 7.5 per 1,000 or 0.8 percent; in 1940 it was 0.3 percent. If anyone wanted to make the problem of illegitimacy appear minor, these statistics would be ideal for the purpose.

The most useful feature of the illegitimacy rate for all women is that it employs the same population base as the commonly used fertility rate, and the two measures can be compared easily. For example, in 1965 the fertility rate was 96.6 births per 1,000 women 15-44. This can be regarded as the sum of two components: the rate for legitimate births (89.1) and the rate for illegitimate births (7.5). Trends in these two components of the fertility rate since 1940 are shown in Fig. 8.1 for the white and nonwhite populations. Several observations can be made on the basis of these comparisons:

Table 8.3 Estimated number of illegitimate births per 1,000 women 15-44 and per 1,000 unmarried women 15-44, by color: United States, 1940-65

Year	Rate per 1,000 women 15-44[a]			Rate per 1,000 unmarried women 15-44[b]		
	Total	White	Nonwhite	Total	White[c]	Nonwhite[c]
1965	7.5	3.6	35.2	23.5	11.6	97.6
1964	7.2	3.4	34.7	23.0	11.0	97.2
1963	6.9	3.1	34.1	22.5	10.5	97.1
1962	6.6	2.9	33.9	21.9	9.8	97.5
1961	6.6	2.8	34.3	22.7	10.0	100.8
1960	6.2	2.6	33.1	21.6	9.2	98.3
1959	6.2	2.5	34.0	21.9	9.2	100.8
1958	5.9	2.4	32.8	21.2	8.8	97.8
1957	5.8	2.3	32.3	21.0	8.6	95.3
1956	5.6	2.2	31.4	20.4	—	—
1955	5.3	2.1	30.0	19.3	—	—
1954	5.1	2.1	28.9	18.7	—	—
1953	4.7	1.9	26.7	16.9	—	—
1952	4.4	1.8	24.8	15.8	—	—
1951	4.3	1.7	24.4	15.1	—	—
1950	4.1	1.8	23.1	14.1	6.1	71.2
1949	3.9	1.8	21.0	13.3	—	—
1948	3.8	1.8	19.9	12.5	—	—
1947	3.9	2.0	19.2	12.1	—	—
1946	3.7	2.1	17.3	10.9	—	—
1945	3.5	1.9	16.6	10.1	—	—
1944	3.2	1.7	15.3	9.0	—	—
1943	3.0	1.5	15.4	8.3	—	—
1942	3.0	1.4	15.3	8.0	—	—
1941	3.0	1.5	15.2	7.7	—	—
1940	2.8	1.4	14.0	7.1	3.6	35.6

Source: National Center for Health Statistics.

[a]Population enumerated as of April 1 for 1940, 1950, and 1960, and estimated as of July 1 for all other years.

[b]Population enumerated as of April 1 for 1940 and 1950, and estimated as of July 1 for all other years. The illegitimacy rates for unmarried women shown in this table differ from those published in various issues of Vital Statistics of the United States. The rates shown here are based on a smoothed series of population estimates for unmarried women, by color and age, which were not available when the rates previously published were computed.

[c]Estimates of the unmarried population by color are not available in inter-censal years until 1957.

1. The rate for illegitimate births has risen more rapidly than the rate for legitimate births.
2. The rate for white illegitimate births has risen more rapidly than for nonwhite illegitimate births since 1955; in the period since 1960 the nonwhite rate has leveled off, but the white rate has continued to rise rapidly.
3. If there were no illegitimate births, the fertility rates of white and nonwhite groups would be nearly equal. Another way of stating this is that most of the difference between white and nonwhite fertility rates can be attributed to the higher rate for illegitimate births among nonwhite women.

Insofar as illegitimate births represent unwanted children, the latter observation is consistent with findings reported elsewhere,[1] that nonwhite married women want no more children than white married women and would have fewer children if they were more successful in preventing unwanted births.

Illegitimate Births per 1,000 Unmarried Women 15-44. This rate, commonly known as the illegitimacy rate, relates illegitimate births

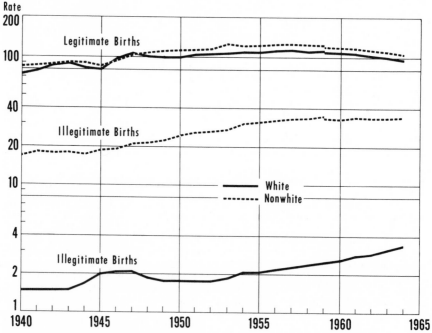

Fig. 8.1. Legitimate and illegitimate births per 1,000 women 15-44 years of age, by color: United States, 1940-64.

to the population subject to the risk of having an illegitimate birth: unmarried women in the childbearing years of life. Trends are shown for 1940-65 in Table 8.3. Rates by age and color are shown in Table 8.4.

Table 8.4 Estimated number of illegitimate births per 1,000 women 15-44 and per 1,000 unmarried women 15-44, by color and age of woman: United States, 1940, 1950, 1960, and 1965

Color and age of woman	Rate per 1,000 total women 15-44[a]				Rate per 1,000 unmarried women 15-44[b]			
	1965	1960	1950	1940	1965	1960	1950	1940
Total (15-44)[c]	7.5	6.2	4.1	2.8	23.5	21.6	14.1	7.1
15-19	14.7	13.2	10.6	6.6	16.7	15.3	12.6	7.4
20-24	13.4	12.3	7.3	4.6	39.9	39.7	21.3	9.5
25-29	6.5	5.8	3.3	1.9	49.3	45.1	19.9	7.2
30-34	3.5	3.1	1.8	1.0	37.5	27.8	13.3	5.1
35-39	1.9	1.7	1.1	0.6	17.4	14.1	7.2	3.4
40-44[d]	0.6	0.5	0.3	0.2	4.5	3.6	2.0	1.2
White (15-44)[c]	3.6	2.6	1.8	1.4	11.6	9.2	6.1	3.6
15-19	6.9	5.7	4.3	2.9	7.9	6.6	5.1	3.3
20-24	7.3	5.5	3.4	2.8	22.1	18.2	10.0	5.7
25-29	3.0	2.2	1.4	1.0	24.3	18.2	8.7	4.0
30-34	1.5	1.1	0.8	0.5	16.6	10.8	5.9	2.5
35-39	0.8	0.7	0.5	0.3	8.3	6.1	3.2	1.7
40-44[d]	0.3	0.2	0.2	0.1	2.3	1.8	0.9	0.7
Nonwhite (15-44)[c]	35.2	33.1	23.1	14.0	97.6	98.3	71.2	35.6
15-19	67.0	66.7	54.7	34.8	75.8	76.5	68.5	42.5
20-24	56.9	58.7	36.2	18.7	152.6	166.5	105.4	46.1
25-29	30.6	30.3	18.7	8.4	164.7	171.8	94.2	32.5
30-34	17.6	17.6	10.7	5.4	137.8	104.0	63.5	23.4
35-39	9.5	9.5	5.8	3.2	63.3	56.3	31.3	13.2
40-44[d]	2.9	2.8	1.9	1.4	16.8	14.5	8.7	5.0

Source: National Center for Health Statistics.

[a]Population enumerated as of April 1 for 1940, 1950, and 1960, and estimated as of July 1 for 1965.

[b]Population enumerated as of April 1 for 1940 and 1950, and estimated as of July 1 for 1960 and 1965. The illegitimacy rates for unmarried women shown in this table differ from those published in various issues of Vital Statistics of the United States. The rates shown here are based on a smoothed series of population estimates for unmarried women, by color and age, which were not available when the rates previously published were computed.

[c]Rates computed by relating total births, regardless of age of mother, to women 15-44.

[d]Rates computed by relating births to mothers aged 40 and over to women aged 40-44.

Although, as mentioned earlier, the illegitimacy rate has risen less rapidly than other measures of illegitimacy in the years since 1960, this has not always been the case. Between 1940 and 1960 the illegitimacy rate for unmarried women increased more rapidly than any other measure of illegitimacy. The percentage increases between 1940 and 1960 in various measures of illegitimacy are as follows:

Illegitimacy ratio	39 percent
Illegitimate births per 1,000 women 15-44	121 percent
Illegitimate births per 1,000 unmarried women 15-44	207 percent

The exceptionally rapid rise in the illegitimacy rate was brought about by an increase in the number of illegitimate births and a decline in the number of unmarried women. As Table 8.5 shows, the number of unmarried women declined between 1940 and 1960. Also, the proportion of women who were unmarried declined in this 20-year period. In spite of these changes, the number of illegitimate births increased substantially.

Table 8.5 Number and percentage of unmarried women 15-44, by color and age: United States, 1940, 1950, and 1960

Color and age	Number of unmarried women (in thousands)			Percent of all women who are unmarried		
	1960	1950	1940	1960	1950	1940
Total (15-44)	10,289	10,017	12,523	28.5	29.3	39.1
15-19	5,555	4,434	5,439	84.3	83.3	88.4
20-24	1,686	2,021	2,870	30.5	34.4	48.7
25-29	765	1,050	1,461	13.8	16.7	25.9
30-34	688	814	1,016	11.3	13.8	19.6
35-39	761	830	888	11.9	14.5	18.5
40-44	834	868	849	14.1	16.9	19.4
White (15-44)	8,802	8,779	11,142	27.7	28.9	39.1
15-19	4,868	3,907	4,863	84.3	83.9	89.3
20-24	1,422	1,781	2,599	29.5	34.4	49.7
25-29	618	911	1,298	12.8	16.3	25.9
30-34	559	711	892	10.4	13.5	19.3
35-39	631	715	759	11.1	14.1	17.8
40-44	704	753	730	13.3	16.3	18.5
Nonwhite (15-44)	1,486	1,238	1,381	34.8	32.4	39.3
15-19	687	527	576	84.2	79.4	81.7
20-24	264	240	271	37.8	34.3	40.4
25-29	147	138	163	21.1	19.8	25.7
30-34	129	104	124	17.6	16.9	23.0
35=39	130	115	129	18.3	18.3	24.0
40-44	130	115	119	21.0	22.1	27.9

Source: U. S. Bureau of the Census, 1960 Census of Population, Vol. I, Characteristics of the Population, Part 1, U. S. Summary, Table 176; and 1950 Census of Population, Vol. II, Characteristics of the Population, Part 1, U. S. Summary, Table 102.

Part of this rise in the illegitimacy rate may be due to selective factors. If one thinks of the unmarried population as being subdivided according to the risk of illegitimacy, and if the low-risk women are more likely to marry than the high-risk women, then a rise in the proportion married will eliminate the low-risk group from the population base of unmarried women and leave the women who are most likely to have an illegitimate birth. This is sheer speculation, however. To substantiate such a hypothesis one would have to show, through careful research, that there was an inverse relation between the probability of marriage and the probability of illegitimacy among unmarried women. This may not be the case.

Also, such a hypothesis could not explain all of the rise in illegitimacy, for even when the illegitimacy rate is based on all women, rather than only on the unmarried, one sees that a rise has occurred.

Factors Contributing to Color Differences
Every measure of illegitimacy discussed shows that the rate is much higher among nonwhite than among white women. Generally the difference is on the order of 9 to 1 (i.e., the ratio of the nonwhite to the white measure). What accounts for this large difference?

First of all, there may be differences in the reporting of illegitimate births that make it easier for white women to conceal their children's legitimacy status. However, there are also reporting biases that may work in the opposite direction (e.g., a higher proportion of births in hospitals for white women). On balance, there is no basis for guessing whether white or nonwhite illegitimate births are better reported.

One factor that helps to keep the ratio of nonwhite to white measures of illegitimacy high is the fact that a higher proportion of nonwhite women have two or more illegitimate births. Consequently, if the measure of illegitimacy is based on first births rather than births of all orders, the nonwhite-white differential is reduced. In 1960 the reduction in the differential for the illegitimacy ratio was from 9 to 1 for all births to 7 to 1 for first births. The smaller ratio is a better indicator of the relative tendency of women to have *any* illegitimate births.

To establish the extent to which differences in socioeconomic status are associated with color differences in the incidence of illegitimacy, one would have to classify births by the socioeconomic status of the mother (e.g., such variables as educational attainment, income, religion, etc.). Unfortunately, it is not possible to do this, because the relevant information is not collected on birth certificates. It seems probable that such an analysis would reveal that the color difference is small for certain groups—for example, the better educated—and that the high rates of illegitimacy are concentrated among the poor and less-educated members of both color groups.

Another factor that is probably associated with the higher nonwhite rate of illegitimacy is less use of contraception. Although there are no data relating to the use of contraception in premarital sexual behavior, it seems quite likely that more use of contraception is made by white couples engaged in such relations than by nonwhite couples. This conjecture is based on the greater and more successful use of contraception by white married couples.[2]

Another factor that has been shown to be associated with higher rates of illegitimacy among nonwhite couples is a lesser tendency to resort to marriage when a premarital conception occurs. William Pratt has shown that among single women in the Detroit Metropolitan Area who became pregnant, the white women were more likely to marry than the nonwhite women.[3]

Finally, there have been suggestions that color differences in the incidence of illegitimacy are associated with differences in values and attitudes—for example, the supposedly greater tolerance of unwed mothers among nonwhite groups. To the social scientist, however, such explanations have very low priority. In essence, they regard differences in behavior as expressions of differences in values on a one-to-one basis, without any attempt to establish whether or not there really are differences in values when other factors in the social and economic environment are held constant. In fact, values and behavior may vary independently. For example, nonwhite married couples have more children, on the average, than white married couples, but they do not *want* more children than white couples.[4] They tend to want fewer but are less successful than white couples in controlling their fertility. For such reasons, it is dangerous to ascribe color differences in the behavior leading to higher rates of illegitimacy among nonwhite women as due primarily to different values. This may or may not be the case, and only careful research can give an answer.

Factors Contributing to the Rising Illegitimacy Rate

Every measure studied indicates that the incidence of illegitimate births has risen since 1940. Different measures show different percentage increases, but all show increases. One factor that may account for some of this rise is a greater improvement in the registration of illegitimate births than in the registration of legitimate births. As noted earlier, the rise in the proportion of births in hospitals may make it more difficult to conceal an illegitimate birth than was formerly the case. However, it seems highly unlikely that the entire upward trend in illegitimacy is due solely to improved reporting.

One factor that may help to account for the rise in illegitimacy is the reduction of sterility associated with venereal disease. This cannot be demonstrated with certainty, but it appears to be a tenable hypothesis, particularly for the nonwhite population. We do know that among nonwhite married women, the prevalence of childlessness was once quite high. Among ever-married nonwhite women 50-54 years of age enumerated in the 1960 census, for example, 28 percent reported that they had never had any children. The proportion was much lower for younger women (14 percent for ever-married nonwhite women 25-29 years old). It seems likely that this trend toward fewer childless women represents an increase in fecundity, probably due to the reduced prevalence of venereal disease.[5] If there has been an increase in the fecundity of the nonwhite population, it would affect the unmarried as well as the married, and increase the likelihood that premarital intercourse would lead to pregnancy and childbirth.

Such a trend may also have affected illegitimacy rates among certain segments of the white population, particularly the poor and less educated, who generally have had less access to adequate medical care.

Again, it should be emphasized that these suggestions are speculative. There are no research findings directly linking an increase in fecundity with an increase in illegitimacy. But in an area in which speculation is much more common than research, the hypothesis of increased fecundity appears to have somewhat more merit than other inadequately supported explanations.

Another possible explanation for the rise in illegitimacy is that it is more difficult now than it was in the 1930's to obtain an illegal abortion. Unfortunately, there is even less information about illegal abortion in this country than about illegitimacy, so that no evidence is available tending either to support or refute this hypothesis.

In view of what has happened to age at marriage and patterns of family growth in the United States since 1940, the rise in illegitimacy is baffling. Throughout the late 1940's and the 1950's, couples married at progressively younger ages and had their first births relatively early in marriage. The proportion married increased substantially at ages 20-24 and 25-29, as the figures in Table 8.5 indicate. Economic conditions seemed to make it easier than ever for couples to marry and start their families at relatively young ages.[6] Under such circumstances, it would seem reasonable to believe that premarital pregnancies would more frequently lead to marriage before the birth of the child than was the case in the 1930's, and that the proportion of women having children before marriage would, therefore, decline. But this has not happened. We must conclude that the increase in illegitimacy has not been satisfactorily explained. Clearly, research is needed to explore more thoroughly the factors associated with trends and differentials in the incidence of illegitimacy.

Summary

Statistics on illegitimacy in the United States are of unknown quality. The number of states requesting information about legitimacy status on the birth certificate has declined over the past 30 years. However, the states that do require reporting of legitimacy may have improved the registration of illegitimate births.

Trends and differentials in three measures of illegitimacy are described. The ratio of illegitimate births to total births is the least useful measure for analytical purposes. The illegitimacy rate based on all women 15-44 years of age is useful because it is comparable to the commonly used fertility rate. The illegitimacy rate based on unmarried women 15-44 years of age is useful because it relates illegitimate births to the population at risk.

All of these measures show that illegitimacy is more common among nonwhite women than among white women. One important factor in this differential has been shown to be the greater likelihood that a white woman will marry after she becomes pregnant than will a nonwhite woman.

All measures also show that illegitimacy has become increasingly prevalent over the past quarter of a century. The reasons for this rise are unknown. Our lack of knowledge in this area emphasizes the need for research.

9 / Education and Fertility

Nature of Data
The last three censuses of the United States have included questions on last grade of school completed. In the 1960 census the question was divided into two parts and asked of persons of school age and older in the 25 percent sample: "What is the highest grade (or year) of regular school he has ever attended?" and "Did he finish this grade (or year)?" The monograph *The Fertility of American Women* contained a rather detailed analysis of the relation of fertility to educational attainment of women and ever-married women in 1940 and 1950.[1] Materials from that report will be drawn upon as needed for indications of trends in fertility by educational attainment since 1940. Chapter 10 includes a discussion of the relative merits of educational attainment of the woman and occupation group of the husband as indices of socioeconomic status in studies of differential fertility.

Briefly, this chapter considers recent trends in educational attainment of ever-married women in the United States; trends in proportions ever married by educational attainment; percent changes in fertility rates during the past decade by education; fertility rates by educational attainment of the wife and by education of the wife and husband jointly considered; and indices of trends in fertility differentials by education of the wife. Chapter 11 analyzes fertility by age, and age at marriage, of wife by occupation, education, and income of the husband.

Trends in Educational Attainment of Ever-Married Women
There has been improvement since 1950 in the educational attainment of ever-married women, both white and nonwhite, although the changes during the 1950-60 decade were not quite so sharp as those during the period 1940-50. In both decades the improvement was relatively greater for nonwhite than for white women. Nevertheless, in 1960 the educational attainment of ever-married white women was still considerably higher on the average than that of nonwhite women. For instance, the proportion of ever-married white women 25-29 years of age whose education was "none or elementary" was 35 percent in 1940, 20 percent in 1950, and 13 percent in 1960. Among the nonwhite women, the comparable percentages were 72, 51, and 28 (Tables 9.1 and 9.2).[2]

Marriage in Relation to Educational Attainment

During the years 1940-50 there was a marked trend toward earlier marriage; more women also married, especially among the college-educated. This trend was only slightly evident in the years 1950-60. For instance, in 1940 among native white women 20-24 years of age and reporting 4 or more years of college, the proportion ever married was 25 percent. The comparable proportions were 44 percent for white women in 1950 and 55 percent in 1960. Similarly, among white women 20-24 years of age reporting completion of high school but no further education, the proportion ever married was 40 percent in 1940 (for native white), 64 percent in 1950, and 76 percent in 1960.

As a consequence, there is now a much weaker inverse relation of educational attainment to proportions ever married, especially among women 25 years of age and over. Thus, among white women 30-34 years of age in 1960, the proportions ever married were 90 percent for those reporting 4 years of college, 94 percent for those reporting

Table 9.1   Percent distribution by years of school completed, for ever-married white women 15-49 years old, by age: United States, 1960 and 1950

Year and years of school completed	15-19	20-24	25-29	30-34	35-39	40-44	45-49
1960							
Total, education reported	100.0	100.0	100.0	100.0	100.0	100.0	100.0
College: 4 or more	0.1	4.0	7.1	7.0	5.9	6.0	5.7
1-3	2.8	11.4	11.3	10.9	10.8	9.6	9.6
High school: 4	30.9	47.8	45.5	42.6	42.7	36.7	28.8
1-3	48.5	25.8	22.7	23.2	21.5	22.6	22.7
None or elementary	17.7	11.0	13.4	16.2	19.1	25.0	33.1
1950							
Total, education reported	100.0	100.0	100.0	100.0	100.0	100.0	100.0
College: 4 or more	0.2	3.1	5.2	5.4	5.4	5.9	5.0
1-3	1.9	8.4	9.2	8.9	8.9	9.5	8.6
High school: 4	25.2	42.4	42.3	36.6	29.2	23.5	19.5
1-3	43.0	26.7	23.0	23.1	23.0	21.2	18.9
None or elementary	29.7	19.4	20.4	26.0	33.5	39.8	48.1

Source: Derived from U.S. Bureau of the Census, 1960 Census of Population, Women by Number of Children Ever Born, PC(2)-3A, Table 25; and Grabill, Kiser, and Whelpton, The Fertility of American Women, Table 69.

4 years of high school, and 95 percent for those reporting 8 years of elementary school.

As indicated in Table 9.3, the highest proportions ever married among both white and nonwhite women in most of the age groups shown are those for women reporting 1-3 years of high school. Some selective factors may be involved, in that many girls drop out of high school because of marriage. Among women whose education was restricted to elementary school, there tended to be a direct relation of specific grade attained to proportions ever married. White and nonwhite women in the two extreme educational groups, those reporting no schooling at all (or less than 1 year) and those reporting 5 or more years of college, were characterized by lowest proportions ever married. Again selective factors may be involved. Those reporting 5 or more years of college training may be composed largely of women electing to do graduate work because of lack of opportunity for, or interest in, marriage. The group of women reporting no schooling or

Table 9.2   Percent distribution by years of school completed, for ever-married nonwhite women 15-49 years old, by age: United States, 1960 and 1950

Year and years of school completed	15-19	20-24	25-29	30-34	35-39	40-44	45-49
1960							
Total, education reported	100.0	100.0	100.0	100.0	100.0	100.0	100.0
College: 4 or more	0.1	1.9	4.8	4.5	4.0	3.6	3.0
1-3	1.8	6.7	6.9	6.2	5.1	4.3	3.4
High school: 4	15.9	30.6	27.9	24.1	21.5	15.7	10.8
1-3	49.6	37.0	32.2	29.3	25.6	22.5	19.4
None or elementary	32.7	23.8	28.3	35.9	43.8	53.9	63.4
1950							
Total, education reported	100.0	100.0	100.0	100.0	100.0	100.0	100.0
College: 4 or more	0.1	1.2	2.8	2.8	2.5	2.9	1.7
1-3	0.9	4.4	4.1	3.6	3.7	3.0	2.6
High school: 4	7.9	17.8	17.5	12.9	9.8	7.1	6.0
1-3	36.5	30.5	24.3	20.6	17.0	14.3	10.8
None or elementary	54.6	46.1	51.4	60.1	67.0	72.7	79.0

Source: Derived from U.S. Bureau of the Census, 1960 Census of Population, Women by Number of Children Ever Born, PC(2)-3A, Table 25; and Grabill, Kiser, and Whelpton, The Fertility of American Women, Table 70.

less than 1 year is a select group in that it probably contains many with mental and physical defects severe enough to preclude school attendance and matrimony.

The pattern of the relation of educational attainment to percent ever married is much the same for white and nonwhite women. For most age groups and educational levels considered, the proportions ever married tend to be a little lower for nonwhite than for white women. The chief exception is the higher proportion married among nonwhite than among white women of lowest educational attainment (less than 1 year).

Table 9.3　Percent ever married among women of specified ages, by education and color:　United States, 1960

Years of school completed		White			Nonwhite		
		20–24	30–34	45–49	20–24	30–34	45–49
Total		72.5	93.5	93.5	64.4	90.4	94.3
College:	5 or more	47.3	74.6	72.7	34.5	78.8	88.7
	4	56.3	89.5	88.4	45.2	88.2	90.0
	1–3	47.8	92.4	92.7	42.2	90.1	94.0
High school:	4 years	75.9	94.2	93.3	62.4	89.7	92.5
	1–3	86.5	96.2	95.6	71.9	92.6	95.0
Elementary:	8	83.6	94.6	95.2	72.1	90.8	94.9
	5–7	78.6	93.5	94.9	70.9	91.3	95.1
	1–4	66.0	87.9	92.9	60.6	87.8	94.5
	Less than 1	26.2	56.0	75.2	48.4	73.7	88.9

Source:　Derived from U.S. Bureau of the Census, 1960 Census of Population, Women by Number of Children Ever Born, PC(2)-3A, Table 25.

Percent Changes in Fertility Rates by Educational Attainment of the Wife, 1950-60

The 1940-50 increase in age-specific fertility rates was restricted largely to women under 35 years of age. At older ages the 1950 fertility rates were lower than those for 1940. This reflected the fact that the postwar baby boom had its initial and greatest impact on the younger women, who were largely under 35 in 1950. The older women could not roll back the years and participate in the baby boom. However, by 1960 the women in the vanguard of the baby boom were nearing the end of the childbearing period, and the cumulative fertility rates for 1960 tended to be higher than those for 1950 at all ages.

Among the age groups of women experiencing increases in fertility during the 1940-50 period, the increases tended to be directly related to educational attainment and thus to bring about a diminution of the educational differentials in fertility.[3]

During the decade, 1950-60 there was some continuation of the tendency for percentage increases in fertility to be directly related to educational attainment, *but not for women under 25 years of age.* In fact, among ever-married white women 20-24 years of age there was a rather striking, although not complete, inverse relation of increases in fertility during 1950-60 to educational attainment. The increases extended from 27 percent for those reporting 4 or more years of college to 47 percent for those reporting 1-3 years of high school (Table 9.4 and Fig. 9.1). The increase was 36 percent for those reporting no schooling or only elementary education. Thus, the increases in fertility by age and education tended to diminish the educational differentials in fertility for women 25 years of age and over and to strengthen or enhance them for younger women.

By color, the increases in fertility during the years 1950-60 tended to be larger for nonwhite than for white women, especially in the 25-39 age ranges. As among white women, the increase in the fertility of nonwhite ever-married women tended to be directly related to educational attainment for ages 30-44 and inversely related to education for ages 20-24 (Table 9.5 and Fig. 9.1).

Fertility Differentials by Education, Color, and Type of Residence, 1940-60

Although there was a distinct trend toward a lessening of educational differentials in fertility during the decade 1950-60, these differentials still existed for white and nonwhite women in 1960. As indicated in Fig. 9.2 and in Tables 9.6 and 9.10, among both white and nonwhite women in the United States as a whole, fertility rates of all women and ever-married women at all age groups of the childbearing span were consistently lowest for those reporting 4 or more years of college and highest for those reporting only 8 years of elementary school or less. The intermediate classes tended to fall into positions consistent with the principle of inverse relation of fertility to educational attainment. For both white and nonwhite women, the differentials in fertility were sharper for all women than for ever-married women because of the previously described relation of proportions married to educational attainment.

As for the factor of residence, the range of the fertility rate
ever-married white women was narrower in urban than in rural a
It was narrower in urbanized areas than in other urban areas. I
also narrower in rural nonfarm than in rural farm areas (Tables 9
9.9). The foregoing statements appear to hold for nonwhite wc
as well, but the small number of rural-farm nonwhite women
college education precludes certainty on this point (Tables 9.1
9.12).

The variations in fertility by educational attainment in 1960
much wider among nonwhite than among white women. Amon
women and ever-married women under 25 years of age, the fert

Table 9.4 Percent change, 1950-60, in number of children ever born per 1,000 white women 15-49 year
old, by age, marital status, years of school completed, and urban and rural residence of t
woman: United States

Age and years of school completed	United States		Urban		Rural nonfarm		Rural farm	
	All marital classes	Ever married	All marital classes	Ever married	All marital classes	Ever married	All marital classes	Ever marri
15-19								
College: 1-3	126.3	49.6	131.3	50.6	87.8	a	404.8	a
High school: 4	86.2	47.3	100.0	50.7	74.5	45.0	45.8	54.3
1-3	27.2	36.3	41.7	40.1	10.6	30.9	-11.6	34.8
None or elementary	16.9	44.8	34.6	56.3	-1.0	34.1	-7.5	41.8
20-24								
College: 4 or more	55.0	26.8	66.1	37.2	39.2	5.9	3.5	-2.7
1-3	39.8	31.9	46.9	37.6	34.3	17.8	46.8	47.6
High school: 4	59.2	41.2	71.7	47.2	41.4	33.3	32.9	34.5
1-3	55.6	46.8	64.4	53.1	46.1	40.6	38.4	37.3
None or elementary	35.7	35.6	51.0	47.0	23.1	28.9	18.1	27.1
25-29								
College: 4 or more	42.4	30.4	43.5	30.8	48.0	35.5	24.6	17.0
1-3	54.3	46.6	57.6	48.8	52.0	46.0	47.3	40.5
High school: 4	53.9	45.9	59.3	49.7	44.7	41.0	35.7	33.7
1-3	39.9	37.3	47.9	44.2	30.4	29.4	24.6	25.5
None or elementary	25.1	25.0	39.0	36.7	20.2	21.4	10.8	15.5
30-34								
College: 4 or more	43.4	34.2	47.2	36.7	38.9	31.0	26.3	22.2
1-3	46.4	40.4	51.7	44.5	38.4	34.4	40.8	35.5
High school: 4	40.4	35.4	45.5	39.5	31.8	29.6	29.4	26.5
1-3	29.8	26.8	36.3	32.6	24.4	23.1	16.9	14.9
None or elementary	21.0	20.2	35.0	32.4	13.6	14.6	11.2	12.8
35-39								
College: 4 or more	52.0	39.0	52.9	38.3	56.3	46.4	47.1	35.0
1-3	40.1	34.5	45.2	38.3	37.4	33.0	33.7	28.8
High school: 4	37.5	32.4	44.0	37.7	30.1	26.9	23.0	20.2
1-3	25.0	22.9	30.3	27.8	25.4	23.9	15.3	14.1
None or elementary	13.4	13.0	24.2	23.2	8.9	9.3	0.7	0.6
40-44								
College: 4 or more	49.8	37.6	52.0	38.7	47.1	34.9	50.7	41.4
1-3	30.6	25.7	37.5	31.7	30.1	25.6	24.7	18.7
High school: 4	29.6	24.4	33.4	27.3	25.4	22.2	17.0	15.6
1-3	13.2	13.0	19.1	17.1	14.1	12.7	1.4	0.0
None or elementary	3.9	3.6	9.6	9.2	4.9	4.8	-4.8	-5.4
45-49								
College: 4 or more	40.8	27.2	46.1	30.9	35.4	18.8	17.4	11.7
1-3	20.6	16.0	26.0	19.9	19.0	14.6	16.9	16.1
High school: 4	14.4	10.7	16.5	12.3	9.8	8.5	4.6	3.5
1-3	3.7	1.8	5.0	3.1	15.7	13.1	-4.4	-4.3
None or elementary	-5.0	-5.2	-3.1	-3.4	0.5	0.5	-8.7	-9.2

Source: Derived from U.S. Bureau of the Census, 1960 Census of Population, Women by Number of
Children Ever Born, PC(2)-3A, Table 25; and 1950 Census of Population, Fertility, P-E, No. 5C, Table 2

a Percent change not shown where fewer than 4,000 women in 1950.

rates of the nonwhite tended to surpass those of the white at all educational levels. The relative excess tended to decrease with lowering of educational level (Table 9.13). At older ages the nonwhite women who finished college were characterized by conspicuously low fertility and those of elementary school status by conspicuously high fertility, in comparison with white women of similar age, education, and residence. At ages 30-49 the nonwhite women with 1-3 years of college had somewhat lower fertility than white women of comparable age and education.

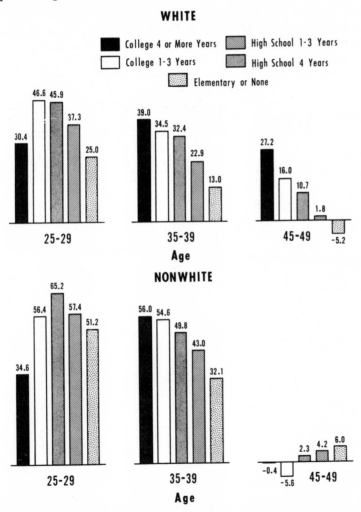

Fig. 9.1. Percent change, 1950-60, in number of children ever born per 1,000 ever-married women of selected ages, by color and years of school completed: United States.

For both white and nonwhite women, the differentials in fertility by educational attainment tended to be widest in the South and narrowest in the Northeast (Fig. 9.3 and 9.4).

Although not presented in the tables here, census tabulations were made regarding fertility by more detailed breakdown of the "none or elementary" group. Among the white ever-married women in the United States, the breakdown of this group exhibited a sharp and consistent inverse relation of fertility to years of school completed. Thus, at ages 35-39 the average number of children per ever-married woman was 4.1 for those never completing a year of school, 3.8 for those reporting 1-4 years, 3.3 for those reporting 5-7 years, and 2.4 for those reporting 8 years. Among the nonwhite ever-married women

Table 9.5 Percent change, 1950-60, in number of children ever born per 1,000 nonwhite women 15-49 years old, by age, marital status, years of school completed, and urban and rural residence of the woman: United States

Age and years of school completed	United States		Urban		Rural nonfarm		Rural farm	
	All marital classes	Ever married	All marital classes	Ever married	All marital classes	Ever married	All marital classes	Ever married
15-19								
College: 1-3	a	a	129.2	a	a	a	a	a
High school: 4	80.4	66.4	88.1	62.0	74.0	a	a	a
1-3	3.4	35.1	4.8	33.7	-10.2	37.3	-18.5	38.1
None or elementary	8.1	49.0	14.8	55.5	-18.6	32.3	10.3	54.6
20-24								
College: 4 or more	47.7	25.7	46.2	23.6	a	a	a	a
1-3	23.6	28.9	17.0	25.9	44.6	a	a	a
High school: 4	37.5	36.1	39.9	38.5	12.0	16.2	35.6	51.3
1-3	49.6	55.1	50.9	56.5	43.0	56.7	36.3	50.4
None or elementary	38.0	48.2	54.5	62.8	26.4	42.9	27.3	41.3
25-29								
College: 4 or more	39.1	34.6	44.3	42.0	a	a	a	a
1-3	67.3	56.4	68.8	59.7	a	a	a	a
High school: 4	66.9	65.2	69.9	68.7	47.2	34.6	29.5	47.8
1-3	56.2	57.4	62.3	63.3	51.3	52.9	27.7	33.8
None or elementary	44.4	51.2	64.1	70.1	37.3	46.5	26.8	34.5
30-34								
College: 4 or more	49.7	43.6	56.5	48.2	a	a	a	a
1-3	73.8	71.9	72.4	71.2	a	a	a	a
High school: 4	62.9	62.9	68.8	69.6	43.1	a	a	a
1-3	51.6	51.6	57.1	57.6	44.6	41.4	40.1	41.3
None or elementary	41.9	46.1	66.1	68.8	42.7	50.2	26.8	32.3
35-39								
College: 4 or more	57.9	56.0	63.1	62.3	a	a	a	a
1-3	54.7	54.6	68.6	69.7	a	a	a	a
High school: 4	50.5	49.8	59.4	58.8	a	a	a	a
1-3	42.6	43.0	55.3	55.3	48.2	47.7	9.8	14.0
None or elementary	29.8	32.1	47.1	49.4	36.0	37.4	28.1	29.9
40-44								
College: 4 or more	17.4	17.0	32.9	31.5	a	a	a	a
1-3	29.4	27.7	46.7	46.1	a	a	a	a
High school: 4	23.1	23.7	29.1	29.7	a	a	a	a
1-3	16.7	18.0	20.1	21.7	28.0	27.6	16.5	14.4
None or elementary	16.2	17.6	23.0	24.2	34.2	35.8	22.5	23.6
45-49								
College: 4 or more	3.5	-0.4	2.0	-2.7	a	a	a	a
1-3	-5.7	-5.6	-11.6	-10.7	a	a	a	a
High school: 4	1.1	2.3	2.0	3.4	a	a	a	a
1-3	5.1	4.2	3.8	3.4	36.8	a	14.1	a
None or elementary	4.8	6.0	5.7	7.2	32.4	32.1	10.5	10.7

Source: Derived from U.S. Bureau of the Census, 1960 Census of Population, Women by Number of Children Ever Born, PC(2)-3A, Table 25; and 1950 Census of Population, Fertility, P-E, No. 5C, Table 22.

aPercent change not shown where fewer than 4,000 women in 1950.

35-39 years old, the averages were respectively 4.1, 4.0, 3.8, and 3.3. At younger ages, however, the highest average number of children born to ever-married nonwhite women was consistently found not for those that never completed a year but for those reporting 1-4 years in school. It should also be mentioned that for both white and nonwhite total women (regardless of marital status), the women with less than 1 year of schooling were characterized by relatively low fertility. For instance, this general fertility rate for white women 35-39 years old was 2.7 per woman for those with no school year completed as compared with 3.5 for those with 1-4 years of schooling. Among the nonwhite, the two averages were 3.4 and 3.7. As already indicated, spinsterhood was relatively frequent among those who failed to complete a year of school.

The Current Population Survey of 1964 revealed a persistence of the inverse relation of fertility to educational attainment of ever-married women. The number of children ever born per 1,000 ever-married women 15-44 years old, standardized for age, extended from 1,848 for those with 4 years or more of college to 2,247 for those with 4 years of high school and 3,464 for those reporting less than 8 years of elementary school.[4]

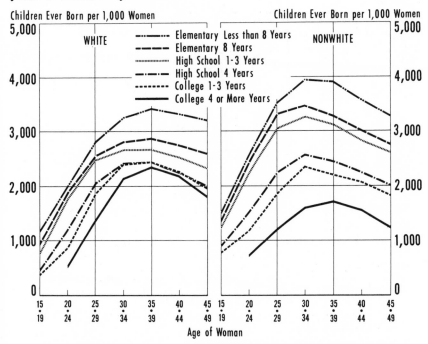

Fig. 9.2. Number of children ever born per 1,000 ever-married women 15-49 years old, by age, color, and years of school completed: United States, 1960.

Table 9.6   Number of children ever born per 1,000 white women, 15-49 years old, by age, marital status, and educational attainment of the woman: United States, 1960, 1950, and 1940

Age and years of school completed		Total white women			Ever-married white women		
		1960	1950	1940[a]	1960	1950	1940[a]
15-19							
College:	4 or more	b	89	b	b	b	b
	1-3	43	19	9	383	256	281
High school:	4	121	65	29	470	319	349
	1-3	103	81	40	799	586	591
None or elementary		180	154	106	1,024	707	732
20-24							
College:	4 or more	296	191	65	535	422	319
	1-3	425	304	122	890	675	493
High school:	4	912	573	280	1,202	851	698
	1-3	1,539	989	650	1,779	1,212	1,073
None or elementary		1,510	1,113	810	1,941	1,431	1,338
25-29							
College:	4 or more	1,091	766	313	1,376	1,055	642
	1-3	1,629	1,056	613	1,872	1,277	935
High school:	4	1,894	1,231	757	2,064	1,415	1,086
	1-3	2,327	1,663	1,234	2,479	1,805	1,503
None or elementary		2,394	1,913	1,571	2,687	2,150	1,942
30-34							
College:	4 or more	1,843	1,285	704	2,148	1,601	1,110
	1-3	2,223	1,518	1,050	2,405	1,713	1,347
High school:	4	2,294	1,634	1,164	2,435	1,798	1,456
	1-3	2,577	1,986	1,692	2,679	2,112	1,920
None or elementary		2,796	2,311	2,223	3,027	2,519	2,529
35-39							
College:	4 or more	2,028	1,334	918	2,353	1,693	1,381
	1-3	2,297	1,639	1,366	2,450	1,822	1,665
High school:	4	2,320	1,687	1,462	2,450	1,851	1,751
	1-3	2,582	2,066	2,009	2,685	2,184	2,238
None or elementary		2,928	2,582	2,725	3,132	2,772	3,002
40-44							
College:	4 or more	1,871	1,249	1,065	2,195	1,595	1,598
	1-3	2,126	1,628	1,598	2,279	1,813	1,911
High school:	4	2,148	1,657	1,671	2,275	1,829	1,962
	1-3	2,438	2,153	2,240	2,539	2,274	2,482
None or elementary		2,830	2,724	2,998	3,011	2,906	3,269
45-49							
College:	4 or more	1,519	1,079	1,231	1,828	1,437	1,831
	1-3	1,825	1,513	1,707	1,970	1,698	2,067
High school:	4	1,879	1,643	1,747	2,013	1,818	2,026
	1-3	2,228	2,148	2,370	2,332	2,290	2,607
None or elementary		2,708	2,852	3,134	2,868	3,025	3,400

Source: Derived from U.S. Bureau of the Census, 1960 Census of Population, Women by Number of Children Ever Born, PC(2)-3A, Table 25; and Grabill, Kiser, and Whelpton, The Fertility of American Women, Tables 75 and 76.

[a]Data for 1940 relate to native white women.

[b]Rate not shown where base is less than 1,000 in 1960, 4,000 in 1950, or 3,000 in 1940.

Table 9.7   Number of children ever born per 1,000 white women,
15-49 years old, by age, marital status, and educational
attainment of the woman: Urban, 1960, 1950, and 1940

Age and years of school completed		Total white women			Ever-married white women		
		1960	1950	1940[a]	1960	1950	1940[a]
15-19							
College:	4 or more	b	98	b	b	b	b
	1-3	37	16	9	369	245	273
High school:	4	104	52	22	452	300	306
	1-3	102	72	32	789	563	555
None or elementary		179	133	78	1,022	654	663
20-24							
College:	4 or more	274	165	61	509	371	285
	1-3	382	260	108	853	620	432
High school:	4	850	495	221	1,147	779	607
	1-3	1,450	882	520	1,712	1,118	941
None or elementary		1,460	967	610	1,877	1,277	1,125
25-29							
College:	4 or more	1,049	731	294	1,350	1,032	607
	1-3	1,554	986	541	1,823	1,225	846
High school:	4	1,797	1,128	611	1,986	1,327	930
	1-3	2,215	1,498	1,003	2,385	1,654	1,279
None or elementary		2,264	1,629	1,208	2,553	1,867	1,572
30-34							
College:	4 or more	1,799	1,222	664	2,131	1,559	1,070
	1-3	2,148	1,416	900	2,350	1,626	1,192
High school:	4	2,195	1,509	988	2,354	1,687	1,287
	1-3	2,449	1,797	1,404	2,564	1,933	1,639
None or elementary		2,605	1,929	1,755	2,826	2,134	2,046
35-39							
College:	4 or more	1,980	1,295	854	2,333	1,687	1,328
	1-3	2,209	1,521	1,198	2,379	1,720	1,502
High school:	4	2,214	1,538	1,275	2,359	1,713	1,579
	1-3	2,420	1,857	1,669	2,534	1,983	1,903
None or elementary		2,639	2,124	2,143	2,840	2,306	2,406
40-44							
College:	4 or more	1,813	1,193	979	2,169	1,564	1,528
	1-3	2,017	1,467	1,376	2,187	1,660	1,712
High school:	4	2,023	1,516	1,471	2,163	1,699	1,783
	1-3	2,279	1,914	1,870	2,389	2,040	2,125
None or elementary		2,487	2,269	2,372	2,666	2,441	2,631
45-49							
College:	4 or more	1,474	1,009	1,119	1,807	1,380	1,755
	1-3	1,719	1,364	1,492	1,875	1,564	1,865
High school:	4	1,754	1,505	1,554	1,896	1,689	1,845
	1-3	2,035	1,939	1,978	2,148	2,084	2,230
None or elementary		2,360	2,436	2,490	2,513	2,601	2,751

Source: Derived from U.S. Bureau of the Census, 1960 Census of
Population, Women by Number of Children Ever Born, PC(2)-3A, Table 25; and
Grabill, Kiser, and Whelpton, The Fertility of American Women, Tables 75
and 76.

[a]Data for 1940 relate to native white women.

[b]Rate not shown where base is less than 1,000 in 1960, 4,000 in
1950, or 3,000 in 1940.

Table 9.8   Number of children ever born per 1,000 white women 15-49 years old, by age, marital status, and educational attainment of the woman: Rural nonfarm, 1960, 1950, and 1940

Age and years of school completed		Total white women			Ever-married white women		
		1960	1950	1940[a]	1960	1950	1940[a]
15-19							
College:	1-3	77	41	6	399	b	b
High school:	4	185	106	49	506	349	400
	1-3	125	113	63	821	627	650
None or elementary		197	199	140	1,027	766	762
20-24							
College:	4 or more	437	314	74	667	630	384
	1-3	662	493	168	1,008	856	574
High school:	4	1,086	768	416	1,305	979	807
	1-3	1,756	1,202	914	1,913	1,361	1,238
None or elementary		1,628	1,322	1,024	2,044	1,586	1,456
25-29							
College:	4 or more	1,302	880	370	1,484	1,095	716
	1-3	1,865	1,227	705	1,997	1,368	982
High school:	4	2,105	1,455	1,024	2,206	1,565	1,279
	1-3	2,572	1,973	1,576	2,664	2,058	1,742
None or elementary		2,602	2,164	1,907	2,869	2,363	2,198
30-34							
College:	4 or more	2,031	1,462	782	2,196	1,676	1,144
	1-3	2,399	1,734	1,195	2,502	1,861	1,448
High school:	4	2,480	1,882	1,414	2,560	1,976	1,613
	1-3	2,857	2,297	2,030	2,916	2,369	2,173
None or elementary		3,060	2,694	2,576	3,292	2,873	2,819
35-39							
College:	4 or more	2,200	1,408	1,038	2,397	1,637	1,412
	1-3	2,505	1,823	1,556	2,591	1,948	1,800
High school:	4	2,543	1,954	1,696	2,620	2,065	1,887
	1-3	2,951	2,354	2,342	3,014	2,432	2,504
None or elementary		3,305	3,035	3,036	3,511	3,211	3,271
40-44							
College:	4 or more	2,055	1,397	1,223	2,245	1,664	1,649
	1-3	2,357	1,811	1,699	2,442	1,944	1,916
High school:	4	2,407	1,919	1,907	2,483	2,032	2,108
	1-3	2,824	2,476	2,496	2,891	2,565	2,667
None or elementary		3,298	3,143	3,304	3,484	3,325	3,543
45-49							
College:	4 or more	1,657	1,224	1,496	1,827	1,538	1,950
	1-3	2,003	1,683	1,873	2,095	1,828	2,167
High school:	4	2,110	1,922	2,030	2,206	2,034	2,261
	1-3	2,684	2,319	2,667	2,745	2,428	2,845
None or elementary		3,268	3,253	3,388	3,437	3,420	3,641

Source: Derived from U.S. Bureau of the Census, 1960 Census of Population, Women by Number of Children Ever Born, PC(2)-3A, Table 25; and Grabill, Kiser, and Whelpton, The Fertility of American Women, Tables 75 and 76.

[a]Data for 1940 relate to native white women.

[b]Rate not shown where base is less than 4,000 in 1950 or 3,000 in 1940.

Table 9.9   Number of children ever born per 1,000 white women,
15-49 years old, by age, marital status, and educational
attainment of the woman: Rural farm, 1960, 1950, and
1940

Age and years of school completed		Total white women			Ever-married white women		
		1960	1950	1940[a]	1960	1950	1940[a]
15-19							
College:	1-3	106	21	10	589	b	b
High school:	4	140	96	36	534	346	405
	1-3	61	69	40	806	598	599
None or elementary		135	146	115	1,025	723	767
20-24							
College:	4 or more	356	344	76	687	706	b
	1-3	665	453	128	1,156	783	719
High school:	4	1,046	787	402	1,428	1,062	928
	1-3	1,660	1,199	860	1,962	1,429	1,306
None or elementary		1,428	1,209	963	2,039	1,604	1,531
25-29							
College:	4 or more	1,286	1,032	346	1,540	1,316	830
	1-3	2,043	1,387	806	2,187	1,557	1,281
High school:	4	2,273	1,675	1,187	2,450	1,832	1,554
	1-3	2,614	2,098	1,796	2,786	2,220	2,054
None or elementary		2,563	2,314	2,012	2,974	2,574	2,402
30-34							
College:	4 or more	2,106	1,667	892	2,353	1,925	1,402
	1-3	2,757	1,958	1,461	2,875	2,121	1,797
High school:	4	2,832	2,188	1,855	2,940	2,324	2,145
	1-3	3,084	2,639	2,431	3,159	2,750	2,665
None or elementary		3,237	2,910	2,925	3,529	3,129	3,277
35-39							
College:	4 or more	2,435	1,655	1,219	2,614	1,936	1,797
	1-3	2,900	2,169	1,799	2,970	2,306	2,121
High school:	4	2,912	2,367	2,274	2,993	2,491	2,517
	1-3	3,255	2,822	2,933	3,327	2,917	3,158
None or elementary		3,541	3,517	3,666	3,734	3,710	3,959
40-44							
College:	4 or more	2,296	1,524	1,511	2,460	1,740	2,045
	1-3	2,856	2,290	2,476	2,925	2,465	2,727
High school:	4	2,853	2,439	2,640	2,937	2,540	2,806
	1-3	3,106	3,063	3,288	3,167	3,168	3,483
None or elementary		3,616	3,798	4,063	3,765	3,981	4,337
45-49							
College:	4 or more	1,868	1,591	1,766	2,020	1,809	2,189
	1-3	2,485	2,126	2,488	2,590	2,230	2,790
High school:	4	2,596	2,482	2,624	2,698	2,606	2,790
	1-3	2,982	3,119	3,411	3,052	3,257	3,573
None or elementary		3,567	3,905	4,203	3,713	4,088	4,437

Source: Derived from U.S. Bureau of the Census, 1960 Census of
Population, Women by Number of Children Ever Born, PC(2)-3A, Table 25; and
Grabill, Kiser, and Whelpton, The Fertility of American Women, Tables 75
and 76.

[a]Data for 1940 relate to native white women.

[b]Rate not shown where base is less than 4,000 in 1950 or 3,000 in
1940.

Table 9.10   Number of children ever born per 1,000 nonwhite women, 15-49 years old, by age, marital status, and educational attainment of the woman: United States, 1960, 1950, and 1940

Age and years of school completed		Total nonwhite women			Ever-married nonwhite women		
		1960	1950	1940[a]	1960	1950	1940[a]
15-19							
College:	1-3	105	b	22	790	b	b
High school:	4	193	107	56	917	551	505
	1-3	180	174	87	1,232	912	731
None or elementary		254	235	151	1,456	977	828
20-24							
College:	4 or more	322	218	126	739	588	b
	1-3	497	402	165	1,177	913	654
High school:	4	954	694	388	1,530	1,124	890
	1-3	1,622	1,084	699	2,257	1,455	1,184
None or elementary		1,752	1,270	917	2,535	1,711	1,409
25-29							
College:	4 or more	872	627	277	1,218	905	611
	1-3	1,526	912	544	1,883	1,204	926
High school:	4	1,904	1,141	803	2,249	1,361	1,154
	1-3	2,664	1,705	1,275	3,050	1,938	1,622
None or elementary		2,880	1,994	1,641	3,446	2,279	2,017
30-34							
College:	4 or more	1,371	916	567	1,607	1,119	858
	1-3	2,126	1,223	967	2,359	1,372	1,277
High school:	4	2,309	1,417	1,160	2,574	1,580	1,425
	1-3	3,014	1,988	1,616	3,256	2,148	1,912
None or elementary		3,410	2,403	2,199	3,795	2,598	2,513
35-39							
College:	4 or more	1,510	956	753	1,730	1,109	1,041
	1-3	2,045	1,322	1,333	2,204	1,426	1,636
High school:	4	2,280	1,515	1,546	2,457	1,640	1,788
	1-3	2,929	2,054	1,921	3,128	2,187	2,138
None or elementary		3,422	2,636	2,669	3,715	2,812	2,923
40-44							
College:	4 or more	1,387	1,181	1,161	1,552	1,327	1,358
	1-3	1,920	1,484	1,683	2,077	1,627	1,906
High school:	4	2,117	1,720	2,005	2,252	1,820	2,204
	1-3	2,688	2,304	2,372	2,842	2,409	2,532
None or elementary		3,198	2,753	3,019	3,424	2,912	3,248
45-49							
College:	4 or more	1,108	1,071	1,355	1,238	1,243	b
	1-3	1,724	1,828	1,862	1,833	1,942	2,009
High school:	4	1,870	1,850	2,032	2,021	1,976	2,227
	1-3	2,497	2,376	2,669	2,628	2,521	2,812
None or elementary		2,972	2,835	3,281	3,141	2,964	3,478

Source: U. S. Bureau of the Census, 1960 Census of Population, Women by Number of Children Ever Born, PC(2)-3A, Table 25; 1950 Census of Population, Fertility, P-E, No. 5C, Table 22; 1940 Census of Population, Differential Fertility, 1940 and 1910—Women by Number of Children Ever Born, Table 50; and Grabill, Kiser, and Whelpton, The Fertility of American Women, Table 77.

[a]Data for 1940 relate to Negro women.

[b]Rate not shown where base is less than 4,000 in 1950 or 3,000 in 1940.

Table 9.11   Number of children ever born per 1,000 nonwhite women,
15-49 years old, of any marital status, by age, urban-
rural residence, and educational attainment of the
woman: 1960 and 1950

Age and years of school completed		1960			1950		
		Urban	Rural nonfarm	Rural farm	Urban	Rural nonfarm	Rural farm
15-19							
College:	1-3	110	66	a	48	a	a
High school:	4	205	167	70	109	96	101
	1-3	198	158	97	189	176	119
None or elementary		271	237	224	236	291	203
20-24							
College:	4 or more	326	334	a	223	a	a
	1-3	502	415	656	429	287	a
High school:	4	964	946	746	689	845	550
	1-3	1,628	1,667	1,392	1,079	1,166	1,021
None or elementary		1,709	1,775	1,905	1,106	1,404	1,496
25-29							
College:	4 or more	867	1,248	a	601	a	a
	1-3	1,504	1,728	a	891	a	a
High school:	4	1,876	2,107	1,960	1,104	1,431	1,514
	1-3	2,567	3,140	3,025	1,582	2,075	2,368
None or elementary		2,660	3,221	3,473	1,621	2,346	2,738
30-34							
College:	4 or more	1,360	1,459	a	869	a	a
	1-3	2,059	2,733	a	1,194	a	a
High school:	4	2,222	2,892	3,207	1,316	2,021	a
	1-3	2,844	3,790	4,494	1,810	2,621	3,208
None or elementary		2,988	4,111	4,923	1,799	2,880	3,882
35-39							
College:	4 or more	1,484	1,691	a	910	a	a
	1-3	1,984	2,568	a	1,177	a	a
High school:	4	2,202	2,887	3,256	1,381	a	a
	1-3	2,707	4,016	4,952	1,743	2,709	4,510
None or elementary		2,860	4,344	5,555	1,944	3,193	4,338
40-44							
College:	4 or more	1,380	1,377	a	1,038	a	a
	1-3	1,849	2,851	a	1,260	a	a
High school:	4	2,009	2,902	3,609	1,556	a	a
	1-3	2,446	3,818	5,211	2,037	2,983	4,472
None or elementary		2,545	4,328	5,667	2,069	3,224	4,628
45-49							
College:	4 or more	1,087	1,156	a	1,066	a	a
	1-3	1,594	2,621	a	1,803	a	a
High school:	4	1,775	2,420	3,777	1,741	a	a
	1-3	2,230	3,825	4,750	2,148	2,796	4,163
None or elementary		2,359	4,079	5,289	2,232	3,081	4,786

Source: U.S. Bureau of the Census, 1960 Census of Population,
Women by Number of Children Ever Born, PC(2)-3A, Table 25; and 1950 Census
of Population, Fertility, P-E, No. 5C, Table 22.

[a]Rate not shown where base is less than 1,000 in 1960 or 4,000 in
1950.

Table 9.12 Number of children ever born per 1,000 ever-married
nonwhite women, 15-49 years old, by age, urban-rural
residence, and educational attainment of the woman:
1960 and 1950

Age and years of school completed		1960			1950		
		Urban	Rural nonfarm	Rural farm	Urban	Rural nonfarm	Rural farm
15-19							
College:	1-3	788	a	a	a	a	a
High school:	4	946	806	a	584	a	a
	1-3	1,235	1,230	1,196	924	896	866
None or elementary		1,490	1,383	1,466	958	1,045	948
20-24							
College:	4 or more	718	a	a	581	a	a
	1-3	1,167	1,168	a	927	a	a
High school:	4	1,510	1,626	1,806	1,090	1,399	1,194
	1-3	2,217	2,409	2,416	1,417	1,537	1,606
None or elementary		2,410	2,646	2,937	1,480	1,851	2,078
25-29							
College:	4 or more	1,213	1,248	a	854	a	a
	1-3	1,860	2,048	a	1,165	a	a
High school:	4	2,206	2,494	2,745	1,308	1,853	1,857
	1-3	2,937	3,560	3,684	1,798	2,328	2,753
None or elementary		3,169	3,892	4,173	1,863	2,656	3,103
30-34							
College:	4 or more	1,587	1,721	a	1,071	a	a
	1-3	2,286	2,934	a	1,335	a	a
High school:	4	2,479	3,213	3,548	1,462	a	a
	1-3	3,082	4,002	4,895	1,955	2,830	3,465
None or elementary		3,309	4,662	5,433	1,960	3,104	4,107
35-39							
College:	4 or more	1,698	1,973	a	1,046	a	a
	1-3	2,143	2,659	a	1,263	a	a
High school:	4	2,372	3,105	3,521	1,494	a	a
	1-3	2,894	4,248	5,300	1,864	2,877	4,648
None or elementary		3,108	4,738	5,912	2,080	3,448	4,552
40-44							
College:	4 or more	1,542	1,519	a	1,173	a	a
	1-3	2,002	3,058	a	1,370	a	a
High school:	4	2,134	3,164	3,738	1,645	a	a
	1-3	2,592	4,014	5,304	2,129	3,145	4,636
None or elementary		2,727	4,659	5,958	2,196	3,432	4,819
45-49							
College:	4 or more	1,206	1,339	a	1,239	a	a
	1-3	1,698	2,726	a	1,901	a	a
High school:	4	1,915	2,626	4,305	1,852	a	a
	1-3	2,352	3,982	4,908	2,274	a	a
None or elementary		2,502	4,300	5,470	2,335	3,256	4,941

Source: U.S. Bureau of the Census, 1960 Census of Population,
Women by Number of Children Ever Born, PC(2)-3A, Table 25; and 1950 Census
of Population, Fertility, P-E, No. 5C, Table 22.

aRate not shown where base is less than 1,000 in 1960 or 4,000 in
1950.

Fertility by Education of the Wife and Husband

The foregoing section was concerned with fertility according to the educational status of the wife alone. The present section relates to fertility according to educational attainment of the *wife and husband jointly considered.*

Table 9.14 presents fertility rates for white and nonwhite women (married and husband present) 35-44 years of age and of given educational attainment *by education of the husband.* It will be noted that among white women reporting 4 or more years of college, there was a direct relation of number of children to educational attainment of the husband. The highest rate was for women whose husbands were also college graduates and the lowest rate was for women whose husbands had less than 8 years of schooling. As one proceeds from high to low educational attainment of the wife, one finds a gradual transition from the direct to the inverse relation of fertility to educational attainment of the husband. This holds in less pronounced form for the nonwhite group.

Table 9.13   Percent excess of average number of children ever born to nonwhite women over that of white women, ever married, by age and educational attainment of woman: United States and urban areas, 1960

Area and educational attainment	15-19	20-24	25-29	30-34	35-39	40-44	45-49
UNITED STATES							
College: 4 or more	a	38.1	-11.5	-25.2	-26.5	-29.3	-32.3
1-3	106.3	32.2	0.6	-1.9	-10.1	-8.9	-7.0
High School: 4	95.1	27.3	9.0	5.7	0.3	-1.0	0.4
1-3	54.2	26.9	23.0	21.5	16.5	11.9	12.7
None or elementary	42.2	30.6	28.2	25.4	18.6	13.7	9.5
URBAN							
College: 4 or more	a	41.1	-10.2	-25.5	-27.2	-28.9	-33.3
1-3	113.6	36.8	2.0	-2.7	-9.9	-8.5	-9.4
High School: 4	109.3	31.6	11.1	5.3	0.6	-1.4	1.0
1-3	56.5	29.5	23.1	20.2	14.2	8.5	9.5
None or elementary	45.8	28.4	24.1	17.1	9.4	2.3	-0.4

Source: Derived from U. S. Bureau of the Census, 1960 Census of Population, Women by Number of Children Ever Born, PC(2)-3A, Table 25.

[a]Rate not shown where base is less than 1,000.

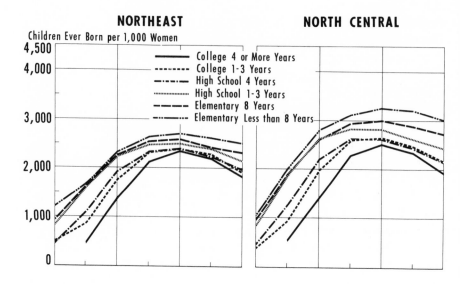

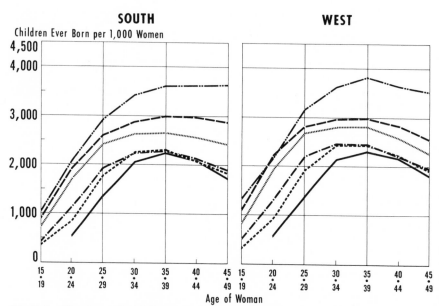

Fig. 9.3. Number of children ever born per 1,000 ever-married white women 15-49 years old, by age and years of school completed: Regions, 1960.

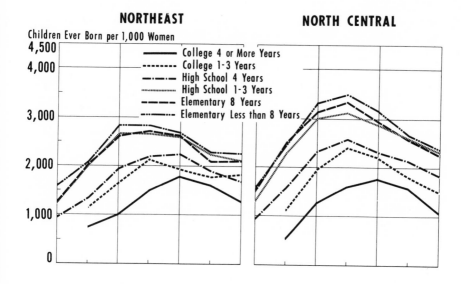

NORTHEAST

NORTH CENTRAL

Children Ever Born per 1,000 Women

——— College 4 or More Years
-------- College 1-3 Years
—·—·— High School 4 Years
··············· High School 1-3 Years
– – – Elementary 8 Years
··—··— Elementary Less than 8 Years

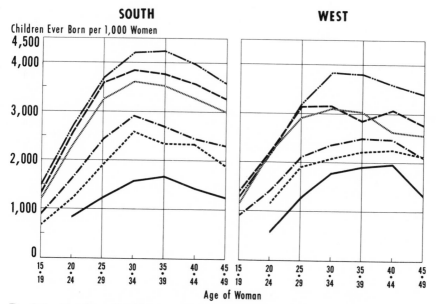

SOUTH

WEST

Children Ever Born per 1,000 Women

Age of Woman

Fig. 9.4. Number of children ever born per 1,000 ever-married nonwhite women 15-49 years old, by age and years of school completed: Regions, 1960.

Table 9.14   Number of children ever born per 1,000 women 35–44 years of age, married and husband present, by color and jointly considered education of the wife and husband: United States and urbanized areas, 1960

Color, residence and education of wife	Education of husband					
	College		High school		Elementary	
	4+	1–3	4	1–3	8	Under 8
UNITED STATES						
White						
College: 4 or more	2,461	2,275	2,175	2,000	1,964	1,853
1–3	2,572	2,381	2,388	2,291	2,492	2,317
High school: 4	2,409	2,354	2,386	2,417	2,542	2,532
1–3	2,362	2,457	2,530	2,590	2,805	2,911
Elementary: 8	2,290	2,550	2,529	2,711	2,910	3,219
Under 8	2,447	2,420	2,647	2,927	3,217	3,717
Nonwhite						
College: 4 or more	1,755	1,749	1,764	1,506	1,822	1,853
1–3	2,088	2,211	2,194	2,523	2,038	2,429
High school: 4	2,316	2,453	2,358	2,407	2,557	2,732
1–3	2,534	2,664	2,823	3,013	3,085	3,476
Elementary: 8	a	2,265	2,707	3,146	3,010	3,729
Under 8	a	2,655	2,815	3,320	3,632	4,219
URBANIZED AREAS						
White						
College: 4 or more	2,420	2,212	2,109	1,947	1,807	1,865
1–3	2,503	2,296	2,281	2,138	2,089	2,103
High school: 4	2,344	2,273	2,294	2,304	2,257	2,269
1–3	2,247	2,362	2,408	2,446	2,529	2,610
Elementary: 8	2,212	2,361	2,333	2,471	2,458	2,712
Under 8	2,384	2,277	2,476	2,631	2,779	3,145
Nonwhite						
College: 4 or more	1,770	1,781	1,688	1,508	1,516	1,951
1–3	2,034	2,141	2,115	2,282	1,906	2,157
High school: 4	2,234	2,345	2,242	2,269	2,424	2,472
1–3	2,169	2,564	2,687	2,733	2,713	2,886
Elementary: 8	a	2,081	2,496	2,650	2,670	2,943
Under 8	a	2,412	2,476	2,845	2,989	3,002

Source: U.S. Bureau of the Census, 1960 Census of Population, Women by Number of Children Ever Born, PC(2)-3A, Tables 26 and 27.

[a]Rate not shown where base is less than 1,000.

By making vertical comparisons within Table 9.14, one may analyze the relation of fertility to education of the wife within groups specific with reference to education of the husband. Here again the same situation holds, at least in part. Among women whose husbands were college graduates, there was at least an incomplete direct association of fertility to wife's education. Among wives of men who reported less than 8 years of elementary school, there was a strong inverse relation of fertility to wife's education. Again the occurrence of the direct relation is less pronounced among the nonwhite than among the white group.

Since amount of education is correlated with urban-rural residence, the above type of comparisons are also presented in Table 9.14 for white and nonwhite women 35-44 years old in urbanized areas (see also Fig. 9.5). The range of variation in fertility by educational attainment is reduced somewhat with this type of restriction, but the general principles stated above may be observed. Again, this also holds in less consistent form for the nonwhite. In urbanized areas the fertility rates tended to be lower for nonwhite than for white women (married and husband present) among couples with both wife and

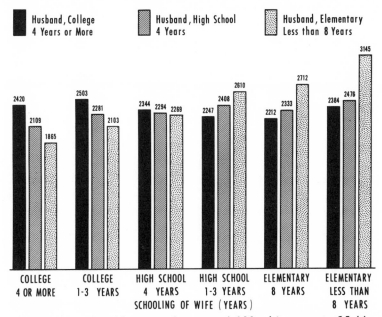

Fig. 9.5. Number of children ever born per 1,000 white women 35-44 years old, married and husband present, by years of school completed by wife and husband: Urbanized areas, 1960.

husband of college 4+, college 1-3, and high school 4 status. At lower educational levels the fertility of nonwhite women tended to surpass that of white women.

Among the possible explanations of the direct relation of fertility to education of one spouse when the other spouse is a college graduate is that in such a group one is dealing largely with families planned as to size. It will be recalled that the Indianpolis Fertility Study revealed a *direct* relation of fertility to socioeconomic status among native white couples of completely planned fertility. It is also possible that the low fertility of couples with widely different education is due in part to high proportions of late marriages, remarriages, and relatively wide differences in ages of the husband and wife. In this connection it may be noted that the pertinent data relate to women described as "married and husband present" regardless of number of times married or age of husband. Among white women 35-44 years old in urbanized areas and reporting 4 years or more of college, the proportions childless ranged from 10.8 percent for those whose husbands were also college graduates to 29.0 percent for those whose husbands had less than 8 years of elementary school.

The foregoing differentials in fertility by educational attainment of wife and husband are in harmony with the educational differentials in prevalence and effectiveness of family planning described in Chapter 3.

Indices of Trends in Fertility Differentials by Education of the Woman, 1940-60

Two indices have been used for indicating trends of fertility differentials by educational attainment during the period 1940-60. These are (1) the average percent deviation of the fertility rates of *specific educational classes* from the base rate for *all* women of given age, color, marital status, and type of residence (Tables 9.15 and 9.16), and (2) the relative spread of the fertility rates by educational attainment computed by expressing the fertility rate for each educational class as a percent of the base rate (Tables 9.17 and 9.18).

Both indices are derived by relating the fertility rates by education to the average or "base rate"[5] for all educational classes within a given group specific with reference to color, age, marital status, and residence. The former simply indicates the *average* of the percent differences of the fertility rates of all the educational classes from the base rate regardless of direction of the differences. The second portrays the complete range or spread of the fertility rates by education. It does this on a "relative" basis by interpreting the fertility rate of each educational class as a percent of the base rate. This is the method of "index numbers," in that it indicates the fertility of each class with the average expressed as 100. It facilitates analyses of trends and group comparisons of differential fertility by removing the factors of temporal changes and group differences in general magnitude of fertility rates.

Table 9.15 Measure of average interclass differences in cumulative fertility rates by years of school completed, white women by residence, age, and marital status: United States, 1940-60

Residence and age	Total white women			Ever-married white women		
	1960	1950	1940	1960	1950	1940
URBAN						
15-19	36.1	42.9	59.5	33.3	30.5	31.1
20-24	48.0	50.1	64.5	35.5	33.3	39.2
25-29	20.9	24.4	39.4	17.9	19.2	28.4
30-34	10.7	14.9	29.7	8.5	11.3	21.8
35-39	8.8	15.8	26.0	7.2	11.6	19.1
40-44	10.3	20.1	24.5	8.5	16.0	18.4
45-49	15.3	25.8	24.2	13.9	22.2	18.0
RURAL NONFARM						
15-19	29.6	38.1	57.4	29.5	a	a
20-24	39.3	41.0	63.9	32.5	28.2	38.3
25-29	19.1	27.0	42.2	18.7	24.4	32.7
30-34	12.6	19.2	33.6	12.5	17.6	27.8
35-39	13.1	21.7	29.7	12.9	21.0	25.5
40-44	15.0	24.0	27.9	15.3	22.9	25.1
45-49	21.9	29.5	25.8	22.1	27.8	23.0
RURAL FARM						
15-19	34.7	41.1	63.2	21.7	a	a
20-24	37.5	38.6	64.3	28.9	27.8	27.1
25-29	16.4	23.5	41.0	18.7	20.9	28.9
30-34	10.8	17.8	30.6	10.5	16.2	24.8
35-39	10.9	21.1	29.4	10.4	19.7	24.4
40-44	12.7	24.0	24.5	13.2	22.8	21.6
45-49	18.5	26.0	24.7	18.9	25.5	22.7

Source: Computed from U.S. Bureau of the Census, 1960 Census of Population, Women by Number of Children Ever Born, PC(2)-3A, Table 25; and Grabill, Kiser, and Whelpton, The Fertility of American Women, Table 92.

aMeasure not shown where fewer than 4,000 women in 1950 or 3,000 in 1940.

In general, both the average deviations and the indices of relative spread of the fertility rates indicate a strong trend since 1940 toward diminution of educational differentials in fertility of white women in the United States. This is shown by the decrease in the magnitude of the average deviations and by the narrowing of the relative spread of the fertility differentials by education. In most cases, however, the closing of the differentials was less marked during the 1950-60 decade than during the preceding decade. Thus, among urban ever-married white women 25-29 years of age, the average of the percent differences of the fertility rates of the several educational classes from the base rate was about 28 percent in 1940, 19 percent in 1950, and 18 percent in 1960 (Table 9.15).[6] As for relative spread of the rates by educational attainment among this same group, the indices for

Table 9.16 Measure of average interclass differences in cumulative fertility rates by years of school completed, for nonwhite women by age and marital status: United States and urban areas, 1940-60

Residence and age	Total nonwhite women			Ever-married nonwhite women		
	1960	1950	1940[a]	1960	1950	1940[a]
UNITED STATES						
15-19	23.5	38.5	46.9	24.0	22.4	15.8
20-24	42.2	40.4	47.5	41.4	28.0	22.7
25-29	29.8	32.2	40.7	29.8	28.0	32.8
30-34	24.8	30.1	37.1	24.9	28.3	32.6
35-39	25.8	32.5	35.2	25.8	31.6	31.5
40-44	26.7	28.9	29.5	26.8	28.1	28.1
45-49	29.6	27.8	29.8	29.7	26.3	27.8
URBAN						
15-19	23.3	36.4	----	22.5	21.2	----
20-24	41.7	37.8	----	31.6	24.4	----
25-29	28.2	28.4	----	25.8	23.9	----
30-34	21.4	22.7	----	20.3	20.5	----
35-39	19.2	23.7	----	19.0	16.6	----
40-44	18.0	22.6	----	17.5	21.3	----
45-49	21.8	18.1	----	21.2	16.6	----

Source: Computed from U.S. Bureau of the Census, 1960 Census of Population, Women by Number of Children Ever Born, PC(2)-3A, Table 25; 1950 Census of Population, Fertility, P-E, No. 5C, Table 22; and 1940 Census of Population, Differential Fertility, 1940 and 1910--Women by Number of Children Ever Born, Table 50.

[a]Data for 1940 relate to Negro women (not available by residence).

Table 9.17 Relative variation of cumulative fertility rates by years of school completed by white women 20-49 years old, by age and marital status: Urban, 1960, 1950, and 1940

(Base rate for each age group = 100)

Age and years of school completed	Total women			Ever-married women		
	1960	1950	1940	1960	1950	1940
20-24						
College: 4 or more	27	27	18	36	39	37
1-3	38	42	33	61	66	56
High school: 4	85	80	67	82	83	79
1-3	145	143	156	123	119	122
None or elementary	146	157	184	134	136	146
25-29						
College: 4 or more	55	58	37	63	69	54
1-3	81	78	69	85	82	76
High school: 4	94	89	77	92	89	83
1-3	116	118	127	111	111	114
None or elementary	118	128	153	119	125	141
30-34						
College: 4 or more	77	74	53	85	84	69
1-3	92	86	72	94	88	77
High school: 4	94	91	79	94	91	83
1-3	105	109	112	102	105	106
None or elementary	112	117	140	112	115	132
35-39						
College: 4 or more	83	72	53	91	86	70
1-3	93	85	74	93	87	79
High school: 4	93	86	79	92	87	83
1-3	101	104	103	99	101	100
None or elementary	111	119	133	111	117	126
40-44						
College: 4 or more	81	64	53	90	76	70
1-3	90	79	74	90	81	79
High school: 4	90	81	79	89	83	82
1-3	102	103	100	99	99	98
None or elementary	111	122	127	110	119	121
45-49						
College: 4 or more	71	51	55	80	63	75
1-3	83	69	73	83	72	79
High school: 4	85	76	76	84	78	78
1-3	98	98	97	95	96	95
None or elementary	114	123	122	112	119	117

Source: Computed from U.S. Bureau of the Census, 1960 Census of Population, Women by Number of Children Ever Born, PC(2)-3A, Table 25; and Grabill, Kiser, and Whelpton, The Fertility of American Women, Table 93.

See text for method of computing relative variations.

Table 9.18   Relative variation of cumulative fertility rates by years
of school completed by nonwhite women 20-49 years old, by
age and marital status: Urban, 1960 and 1950

(Base rate for each age group = 100)

Age and years of school completed	Total women		Women ever married	
	1960	1950	1960	1950
20-24				
College: 4 or more	23	23	34	43
1-3	35	45	55	68
High school: 4	68	72	71	80
1-3	114	114	105	105
None or elementary	120	116	114	109
25-29				
College: 4 or more	36	41	43	50
1-3	63	61	66	69
High school: 4	79	76	78	77
1-3	108	109	104	106
None or elementary	112	112	112	110
30-34				
College: 4 or more	49	52	52	58
1-3	74	71	74	72
High school: 4	80	78	81	79
1-3	103	107	100	106
None or elementary	108	107	108	106
35-39				
College: 4 or more	55	51	58	63
1-3	74	66	73	77
High school: 4	82	77	81	91
1-3	100	97	99	113
None or elementary	106	108	106	101
40-44				
College: 4 or more	57	53	59	56
1-3	76	64	77	65
High school: 4	82	79	82	79
1-3	100	103	99	102
None or elementary	104	105	105	105
45-49				
College: 4 or more	48	49	50	55
1-3	70	83	70	84
High school 4	78	81	79	82
1-3	98	99	98	100
None or elementary	104	103	104	103

Source: Computed from U.S. Bureau of the Census, 1960 Census of
Population, Women by Number of Children Ever Born, PC(2)-3A, Table 25;
1950 Census of Population, Fertility, P-E, No. 5C, Table 22.

See text for method of computing relative variations.

the three census dates may be compared as follows. With base rates expressed as 100, the range for 1940 extended from 54 for the college 4+ group to 141 for the none or elementary group. In 1950 the corresponding range was from 69 to 125 and in 1960 from 63 to 119 (Table 9.17).

For each census year considered, the interclass differences in fertility of white women by education were larger for total women than for ever-married women. This was true because the class differences in proportions married tended to run in the same direction as the class differences in marital fertility.[7]

Although educational differentials in fertility among white women tended to be greater in rural than in urban areas, there was not much difference by type of residence in the trends of the fertility differentials by educational attainment.

As for qualifications, note should first be taken of the maintenance, or even enlargement, since 1950 of the educational differentials in fertility among ever-married white women under 25 years of age. This is in contrast to the especially marked diminution of fertility differentials during the years 1950-60 among women 30-39 years of age.

It may also be noted that whereas the fertility differentials by education among ever-married white women 45-49 years of age were wider in 1950 than in 1940, they were narrower in 1960 than in both earlier years. The women of these older ages appeared to offer an exception to the 1940-50 trend toward convergence of fertility rates. As already indicated, however, women of these ages in 1950 had participated very little or not at all in the postwar baby boom. They were among the last cohorts to carry the torch of declining fertility. However, women 45-49 in 1960 *had* participated in the postwar baby boom. Furthermore, it has already been noted that the 1950-60 increases in fertility for women 40-49 tended to be directly related to educational attainment. Hence, women at the end of the childbearing period in 1960 provided no exception to the trend toward lessening of educational differentials in fertility.

In contrast to the situation among white women, there was little narrowing of educational differentials in fertility among nonwhite women during the decade 1950-60. In fact, for nonwhite ever-married women under 30, the interclass differences in fertility on the average were *larger* in 1960 than in 1950, and especially at ages 20-24. This held both for the United States as a whole and for urban areas. Among nonwhite women regardless of marital status, the interclass differences were lower in 1960 than in 1950 at all ages except 20-24 and 45-49. Among nonwhite women in urban areas, the educational differentials in fertility for ages 25-39 were virtually the same in 1960 as in 1950. Finally, it may be noted that some 63 percent of the ever-married white women 20-24 years old in 1960 had completed at least 4 years of high school, so the relatively high fertility of women of lower educational attainment affects only 37 percent. However, among the nonwhite women, the situation is virtually reversed because at these ages, 39 percent of the women had completed high school or attended college and 61 percent were below the high school 4 level.

Cohort Fertility by Educational Attainment

The foregoing discussion has related to intercohort comparisons of educational differentials in fertility among women and ever-married women of given ages. It is possible to arrange data from the past three censuses to compare fertility differentials at three successive ages *among the same cohorts of women.* Thus, it is possible to examine the fertility rates by educational attainment for all white and non-white women and ever-married women 20-24 years of age in 1940, 30-34 in 1950, and 40-44 in 1960. It is also possible to do the same for women 25-29 in 1940, 35-39 in 1950, and 45-49 in 1960. The former may be identified as a birth cohort of 1915-19 and the latter as a birth cohort of 1910-14. (Table 9.19 presents the data for all women and Table 9.20 for ever-married women.)

It is readily apparent that there are limitations to the data thus constructed, especially for the 1915-19 cohort of ever-married women who were 20-24 years of age in 1940 and 30-34 in 1950. One would expect a substantial number of recruits by ages 30-34 in 1950 from women marrying after ages 20-24. This limitation is less important for ever-married women 25-29, and it is nonexistent for women regardless of marital status. It is true, of course, that restriction of the data to native white women for 1940, as compared with white women for 1950 and 1960, yields some recruits from foreign-born white women at later ages. This, however, is believed to have no serious effect in view of the low proportion of foreign-born white women of childbearing age in the United States. The bearing on comparisons between the two older ages considered is believed to be especially small since both 1950 and 1960 fertility data relate to all white women. A corresponding limitation exists for nonwhite women in that the 1940 data relate to Negro women and those for 1950 and 1960 to nonwhite women. As already indicated, however, the great majority of nonwhite women in the United States are Negro.

Since the levels of cumulative fertility rates naturally increase sharply with age, especially during the first half of the childbearing period, the age-specific fertility rates for the two cohorts of white women were plotted on semilogarithmic scales, as shown in Fig. 9.6, in order to represent better the *relative* variations in fertility by education at successive ages.

Table 9.19   Children ever born per 1,000 women of specific birth cohorts at three points in their reproductive life, by color and education of the woman: United States

Color and birth cohort	Year	Age	College		High school		Elementary or none
			4+	1-3	4	1-3	none
WHITE							
1915-1919	1940[a]	20-24	65	122	280	650	810
"	1950	30-34	1,285	1,518	1,634	1,986	2,311
"	1960	40-44	1,871	2,126	2,148	2,438	2,830
1910-1914	1940[a]	25-29	313	613	757	1,234	1,571
"	1950	35-39	1,334	1,639	1,687	2,066	2,582
"	1960	45-49	1,519	1,825	1,879	2,228	2,708
NONWHITE							
1915-1919	1940[a]	20-24	126	165	388	699	807
"	1950	30-34	916	1,223	1,417	1,988	2,403
"	1960	40-44	1,387	1,920	2,117	2,688	3,198
1910-1914	1940[a]	25-29	277	544	803	1,275	1,425
"	1950	35-39	956	1,322	1,515	2,054	2,636
"	1960	45-49	1,108	1,724	1,870	2,497	2,972

Source: Derived from U.S. Bureau of the Census, 1960 Census of Population, Women by Number of Children Ever Born, PC(2)-3A, Table 25; 1940 Census of Population, Differential Fertility, 1940 and 1910-- Women by Number of Children Ever Born, Table 50; and Grabill, Kiser, and Whelpton, The Fertility of American Women, Table 75.

[a]Data for 1940 relate to native white and Negro women instead of white and nonwhite women.

Table 9.20   Children ever born per 1,000 ever-married women of specific birth cohorts at three points in their reproductive life, by color and education of the woman: United States

Color and birth cohort	Year	Age	College		High school		Elementary or none
			4+	1-3	4	1-3	
WHITE							
1915-1919	1940[a]	20-24	319	493	698	1,073	1,338
"	1950	30-34	1,601	1,713	1,798	2,112	2,519
"	1960	40-44	2,195	2,279	2,275	2,539	3,011
1910-1914	1940[a]	25-29	642	935	1,086	1,503	1,942
"	1950	35-39	1,693	1,822	1,851	2,184	2,772
"	1960	45-49	1,828	1,970	2,013	2,332	2,868
NONWHITE							
1915-1919	1940[a]	20-24	b	654	890	1,184	1,409
"	1950	30-34	1,119	1,372	1,580	2,148	2,598
"	1960	40-44	1,552	2,077	2,252	2,842	3,424
1910-1914	1940[a]	25-29	611	926	1,154	1,622	2,017
"	1950	35-39	1,109	1,426	1,640	2,187	2,812
"	1960	45-49	1,238	1,833	2,021	2,628	3,141

Source: Derived from U.S. Bureau of the Census, 1960 Census of Population, Women by Number of Children Ever Born, PC(2)-3A, Table 25; and Grabill, Kiser, and Whelpton, The Fertility of American Women, Tables 75 and 77.

[a] Data for 1940 relate to native white and Negro women instead of of to white and nonwhite women.

[b] Rate not shown where base is less than 3,000 in 1940.

It is apparent that among both the 1910-14 and 1915-19 cohorts of white women, total and ever married, the relative variations in fertility rates narrowed considerably as the women passed from their twenties (in 1940) to their thirties (in 1950). There was continued but relatively slight narrowing as the women advanced to their forties (in 1960). Even in the latter instance the diminution of the educational differentials in fertility was rather appreciable for women reporting at least 1 year of high school.

The age pattern of cohort fertility by education of nonwhite women was much the same as that described for white women. For the birth cohort of 1915-19, the fertility rates of nonwhite women exceeded those of white women at ages 20-24 at all educational levels. At later ages the fertility of nonwhite women of college attainment fell below that of white college-trained women, but at lower educational levels the fertility of nonwhite women was higher than that of white women.[8]

It should be emphasized that the described relations of cohort fertility to education, color, and age are based upon the experiences of the birth cohorts of 1910-14 and 1915-19. Whether results would be similar for later cohorts is unknown.

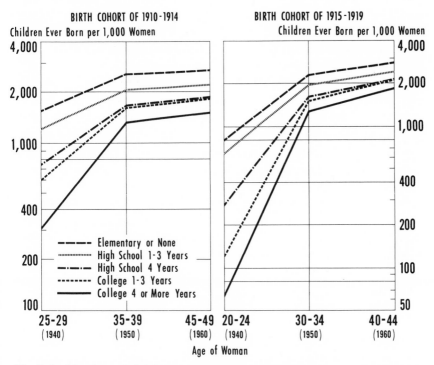

Fig. 9.6. Number of children ever born per 1,000 white women of the 1910-14 and 1915-19 birth cohorts at three points in their reproductive life, by education of the woman: United States. Data for 1940 relate to native white and Negro women instead of to white and nonwhite women.

Summary

Improvements in educational attainment were relatively greater for nonwhite than for white ever-married women during the years 1950-60. Nevertheless, the educational attainment was still considerably higher for white than for nonwhite women in 1960.

Since increases in proportions of women married by given ages had tended to be directly related with educational attainment during the two preceding decades, there was only a weak inverse relation of proportions married to educational attainment among women 25 years of age and over in 1960.

Because 1940-50 increases in fertility of white ever-married women 20-39 tended to be directly associated with educational attainment, the traditional inverse relation of fertility to educational attainment narrowed considerably.

The maintenance, or even enlargement, since 1950 of the educational differentials in fertility among white ever-married women under 25 years of age and among nonwhite women under 30 suggests that the phenomenon of educational differentials in fertility is not one that soon will disappear altogether.

Among women under 25 years old, the fertility of the nonwhite surpassed that of the white women at all educational levels. Among women 25 years of age and over and of college attainment, the fertility of nonwhite wives fell below that of white wives. At lower educational levels the nonwhite women tended to exceed the white women with respect to family size, and the percentage of this excess tended to increase with lowering of educational attainment.

The 1940, 1950, and 1960 census data were used to construct cohort fertility tables by color and educational attainment. Among birth cohorts of 1915-19 and 1910-14, the differentials in fertility by education became much smaller on a relative basis as the women passed from their twenties to their thirties and a little smaller as they progressed to their forties. Thus, the relatively strong differentials in fertility at young ages probably arise in part from differential age at marriage by education, and apparently the influence of this factor becomes less pronounced as the women in a cohort become older.

Nature of the Data

Brief consideration may first be given to some of the advantages and disadvantages of educational attainment of the woman and occupation group of the husband as indicators of socioeconomic status. Educational attainment is readily described in quantitative terms. It is a characteristic of virtual stability for persons 25 years of age and over and hence is amenable to use in analyses of cohort fertility. It has practically the same meaning for males and females and for ever-married and single persons.

Occupational class is less readily defined in quantitative terms. It is true that the broad occupational classes are commonly ranked in order from, say, the professional classes to the unskilled laborers. Nevertheless there is much heterogeneity of specific occupations and of the educational levels of people within a broad occupational class. For instance, teachers and ministers are conventionally assigned to the professional class although there are all grades of teachers and preachers. Furthermore, there are problems in the proper placement of certain broad occupational classes on any type of scale. The group of "service workers" in the census classification, for instance, is so heterogeneous that it is difficult to place it in any ranking. Similarly, the farm and nonfarm ways of life and work are commonly believed to be so different that the urban and rural categories are generally handled separately in studies of occupational differentials in fertility.

Unlike educational attainment, occupation does *not* remain virtually constant among adults as they pass through life. Although most of the changes in occupation may not involve the crossing of broad class lines, much interclass mobility does exist. Also unlike educational attainment, occupational group as a measure of socioeconomic status of families must relate to husbands only for the majority of families, that is, those in which the wife is not employed.

Despite the disadvantages of using occupational class as an indicator of socioeconomic status, it does have certain manifest strengths. The broad occupation groups are of heterogeneous composition, but they provide meaningful delineations of social status and style of life. Occupational class may change in time, but this provides an objective measure of social mobility.

A distinct advantage of occupational class in studies of differential fertility is the long series of existing data of this type. In contrast to questions on specific educational attainment, which were not asked until 1940, questions on occupation have been asked in censuses in the United States since 1820.

The question on total number of children ever born was first asked in the 1890 census. However, no advantage was taken of this first opportunity to analyze number of children ever born in relation to occupational class of the husband, and the original enumeration schedules were eventually lost by fire.[1] The question on children ever born was continued in the 1900 and 1910 censuses. It was dropped in 1920 and 1930 but was reintroduced in 1940. The question was asked of a 5 percent sample of ever-married women in 1940, of a 3 1/3 percent sample in 1950, and of a 25 percent sample in 1960. One hopes it will remain in the future enumerations. The question is occasionally asked also in the Current Population Survey.

Some of the 1900 census data on children ever born were utilized by Joseph A. Hill of the Census Bureau in his study, *Fecundity of Immigrant Women.*[2] However, the use of U.S. census data for study of occupational differentials in fertility was not begun until 1928, when the Milbank Memorial Fund assisted the Bureau of the Census in extracting relevant data from the original enumeration schedules of the 1910 census for a sample of about 100,000 native white couples from selected urban and rural areas of Northern and Western states. This resulted in the first fairly comprehensive inductive study of differential fertility according to occupational class in the United States.[3] It related to approximately the same period as an earlier pioneering study based upon the 1911 Census of England and Wales.[4]

By the early 1930's interest in trends and differentials in fertility in the United States was sufficient to stimulate the reintroduction of the question on children ever born in the 1940 census. This time the Bureau of the Census not only tabulated the 1940 fertility data in relation to occupation but also made parallel tabulations of the 1910 materials and published a series of reports relating to the two sets of data.[5]

Thus, except for 1920 and 1930, a series of census data on occupational differentials in fertility in the United States goes back to 1910. Some of the 1910 and 1940 materials are presented in this chapter, but the major part of the discussion relates to trends since 1950. Unless otherwise specified, the 1960 data presented in this chapter on fertility by occupation group of husband relate to women described as "married and husband present." Those for earlier census periods relate to women "married once and husband present."

Chapter 9 related fertility to educational attainment; this chapter relates it to occupation group; and Chapter 11 relates fertility to income, and considers the three variables jointly. Chapter 11 also discusses children ever born in connection with several other indices of socioeconomic status, including employment status of women, occupation of employed women, and characteristics of housing. It presents some special data on religious background in relation to fertility, including those based upon the Current Population Survey of 1957.

Percent Distribution of Married Women by Broad Occupation Group of the Husband in 1950 and 1960

The distribution of married women by occupational class of the husband in 1950 and 1960 (Tables 10.1 and 10.2) reflects a fairly substantial decline in proportions in agricultural and unskilled laboring jobs and increases in the proportions in white-collar and skilled worker jobs. On a relative basis the upgrading was somewhat sharper for nonwhite than for white husbands, but in 1960 the nonwhite men were

Table 10.1 Percent distribution by major occupation group of husband, for white women 15-49 years old, married and husband present, by age of woman: United States, 1960 and 1950

Year and occupation of husband	15-19	20-24	25-29	30-34	35-39	40-44	45-49
1960							
Total, occupation reported	100.0	100.0	100.0	100.0	100.0	100.0	100.0
Profess'l, techn'l, and kindred wkrs.	5.1	13.1	16.2	14.6	12.7	10.5	9.6
Mgrs., offs., and prop's., exc. farm	3.8	6.7	9.9	12.8	14.5	15.9	16.5
Clerical, sales, and kindred workers	13.5	15.5	14.5	14.3	13.9	13.4	13.1
Craftsmen, foremen, and kindred wkrs.	20.2	21.7	22.7	23.9	24.7	24.5	24.0
Operatives and kindred workers	36.6	27.6	22.9	20.7	20.1	20.1	19.1
Service workers, incl. private hshld.	3.4	3.7	3.8	3.9	4.1	4.4	5.1
Laborers, except farm and mine	10.8	6.6	4.7	4.2	4.1	4.2	4.4
Farmers and farm managers	2.6	3.2	4.0	4.4	5.1	6.1	7.1
Farm laborers and foremen	4.0	2.0	1.3	1.0	1.0	1.0	1.1
1950[a]							
Total, occupation reported	100.0	100.0	100.0	100.0	100.0	100.0	100.0
Profess'l, techn'l, and kindred wkrs.	2.4	7.1	9.9	9.3	9.2	9.0	8.0
Mgrs., offs., and prop's., exc. farm	3.1	6.3	9.5	13.0	15.7	17.3	17.2
Clerical, sales, and kindred workers	10.5	15.3	14.9	13.4	12.4	12.2	12.7
Craftsmen, foremen, and kindred wkrs.	17.2	20.1	22.1	22.7	22.5	22.6	22.3
Operatives and kindred workers	33.7	28.1	23.8	21.9	19.7	17.4	16.0
Service workers, incl. private hshld.	2.7	3.2	3.3	3.5	3.7	4.1	4.9
Laborers, except farm and mine	12.6	7.9	5.9	5.2	4.9	4.7	4.9
Farmers and farm managers	10.0	8.4	8.5	9.3	10.4	11.3	12.5
Farm laborers and foremen	8.0	3.5	2.2	1.7	1.6	1.4	1.5

Source: U. S. Bureau of the Census, 1960 Census of Population, Women by Number of Children Ever Born, PC(2)-3A, Table 31; Grabill, Kiser, and Whelpton, The Fertility of American Women, Table 47.

[a]The 1950 data relate to women married once and husband present.

on the average still considerably lower in occupational level than the white men. Thus, among white married women 25-29 years of age, the proportion with husbands in white-collar occupations was 34 percent in 1950 and 40 percent in 1960. Among the nonwhite women, the corresponding proportions were about 10 percent in 1950 and 17 percent in 1960.

Table 10.2 Percent distribution by major occupation group of husband, for nonwhite women 15-49 years old, married and husband present, by age of woman: United States, 1960 and 1950

Year and occupation of husband	15-19	20-24	25-29	30-34	35-39	40-44	45-49
1960							
Total, occupation reported	100.0	100.0	100.0	100.0	100.0	100.0	100.0
Profess'l, techn'l, and kindred wkrs.	1.9	3.8	6.3	5.7	4.6	3.9	3.4
Mgrs., offs., and prop's., exc. farm	0.5	1.4	2.2	2.9	3.2	3.6	3.6
Clerical, sales, and kindred workers	6.0	8.3	8.7	8.0	8.0	6.5	5.7
Craftsmen, foremen, and kindred workers	9.6	11.2	12.4	13.7	14.0	13.2	13.0
Operatives and kindred workers	30.4	31.3	31.2	29.9	28.5	27.6	25.3
Service workers, incl. private hshld.	15.2	13.4	11.5	11.6	11.8	13.0	14.9
Laborers, except farm and mine	23.1	21.9	19.9	19.8	20.2	20.7	20.8
Farmers and farm managers	2.8	2.4	2.7	3.8	5.0	6.1	7.2
Farm laborers and foremen	10.4	6.3	5.0	4.7	4.7	5.3	6.1
1950[a]							
Total, occupation reported	100.0	100.0	100.0	100.0	100.0	100.0	100.0
Profess'l, techn'l, and kindred wkrs.	0.5	1.5	2.7	3.1	2.8	3.1	1.9
Mgrs., offs., and prop's., exc. farm	0.8	1.3	1.8	2.8	3.0	3.2	3.6
Clerical, sales, and kindred workers	3.0	4.7	5.4	4.2	3.9	3.8	3.4
Craftsmen, foremen, and kindred workers	6.9	8.6	9.4	10.3	9.5	9.9	9.3
Operatives and kindred workers	24.8	26.6	26.2	23.9	22.2	20.0	17.4
Service workers, incl. private hshld.	8.8	10.7	11.6	12.2	12.2	13.5	14.0
Laborers, except farm and mine	26.3	26.0	24.5	23.9	24.8	23.4	23.4
Farmers and farm managers	14.6	12.9	12.2	14.2	17.2	18.7	21.6
Farm laborers and foremen	14.5	7.6	6.2	5.5	4.5	4.5	5.5

Source: U. S. Bureau of the Census, 1960 Census of Population, Women by Number of Children Ever Born, PC(2)-3A, Table 32, Grabill, Kiser, and Whelpton, The Fertility of American Women, Table 48.

[a]The 1950 data relate to women married once and husband present.

Percent Change in Fertility Rates 1950-60, by Occupation Group

During the decade of the 1950's, as during the preceding decade, the increases in fertility rates of white women tended to be relatively large in the occupational classes previously characterized by relatively low fertility. However, from 1940 to 1950 the *increases* in fertility were restricted largely to women under 35 years of age. The fertility rates of women of ages above 35 tended to be lower in 1950 than in 1940. From 1950 to 1960 the increases in fertility were observed for virtually all women under 45 years of age (Table 10.3).

In the classifications by occupation of husband the observed 1940-50 increases in fertility among white women under 35 years old tended to be largest for wives of professional men. The 1950-60 increases

Table 10.3 Percent change 1950-60 in number of children ever born per 1,000 women 15-49 years old, married and husband present, by age of wife and major occupation group of husband: United States, urban and rural

Age of wife and occupation of husband	White				Nonwhite			
	United States	Urban	Rural nonfarm	Rural farm	United States	Urban	Rural nonfarm	Rural farm
15-19								
Profess'l, techn'l, and kindred wkrs.	19.0	23.9	a	a	a	a	a	a
Mgrs., offs., and prop's., exc. farm	59.7	60.7	57.1	a	a	a	a	a
Clerical, sales, and kindred workers	41.5	39.4	55.4	a	a	a	a	a
Craftsmen, foremen, and kindred wkrs.	46.5	61.1	29.1	11.5	21.5	24.1	a	a
Operatives and kindred workers	29.3	35.4	19.5	38.5	36.8	38.0	38.0	a
Services workers, incl. private hshld.	41.8	57.3	a	a	59.0	62.7	a	a
Laborers, except farm and mine	25.2	20.9	37.4	4.8	37.5	31.8	43.5	a
Farmers and farm managers	30.6	a	17.0	36.8	14.1	a	a	19.0
Farm laborers and foremen	35.7	15.2	32.8	42.4	56.7	a	51.6	68.4
20-24								
Profess'l, techn'l, and kindred wkrs.	44.8	47.0	35.5	a	48.6	a	a	a
Mgrs., offs., and prop's., exc. farm	50.3	54.1	45.3	a	a	a	a	a
Clerical, sales, and kindred workers	49.8	50.8	45.4	61.0	35.9	33.8	a	a
Craftsmen, foremen, and kindred wkrs.	43.9	48.7	35.4	32.7	46.7	50.4	a	a
Operatives and kindred workers	40.0	47.1	30.8	25.5	50.9	53.5	52.8	a
Service workers, incl. private hshld.	39.3	42.5	29.1	a	35.9	35.7	a	a
Laborers, exc. farm and mine	31.6	39.7	25.5	13.7	41.4	42.9	37.7	a
Farmers and farm managers	24.3	79.4	43.6	23.3	32.2	a	a	35.2
Farm laborers and foremen	29.3	36.2	24.1	33.3	50.3	a	42.4	54.9
25-29								
Profess'l, techn'l, and kindred wkrs.	42.7	45.0	37.1	27.6	21.0	19.9	a	a
Mgrs., offs., and prop's., exc. farm	44.0	45.6	41.3	30.2	79.2	84.1	a	a
Clerical, sales, and kindred workers	52.0	53.5	44.6	31.9	42.5	40.3	a	a
Craftsmen, foremen, and kindred wkrs.	38.4	43.7	29.4	19.8	63.7	69.0	a	a
Operatives and kindred workers	37.6	44.5	28.0	15.4	47.2	54.4	35.8	a
Service workers, incl. private hshld.	39.2	40.4	35.0	a	74.9	77.0	a	a
Laborers, exc. farm and mine	30.8	40.2	23.5	12.5	52.3	63.2	30.4	a
Farmers and farm managers	18.0	- 4.3	25.5	19.2	24.4	a	a	31.1
Farm laborers and foremen	25.8	25.1	24.6	26.3	55.3	a	62.9	44.9
30-34								
Profess'l, techn'l, and kindred wkrs.	33.8	36.4	26.8	7.6	18.6	32.8	a	a
Mgrs., offs., and prop's., exc. farm	31.4	33.0	27.7	20.9	41.6	41.4	a	a
Clerical, sales, and kindred workers	41.3	43.7	34.4	11.1	42.8	56.1	a	a
Craftsmen, foremen, and kindred wkrs.	26.8	32.5	18.0	9.3	40.6	45.1	38.6	a
Operatives and kindred workers	24.9	30.6	18.1	6.5	39.1	48.6	31.3	a
Service workers, incl. private hshld.	31.8	33.5	25.7	a	68.8	68.9	a	a
Laborers, exc. farm and mine	19.2	29.2	10.8	7.1	58.0	71.3	39.9	a
Farmers and farm managers	11.3	-17.4	14.7	13.0	9.3	a	a	18.4
Farm laborers and foremen	21.8	22.6	13.8	28.9	54.9	a	37.1	69.0
35-39								
Profess'l, techn'l, and kindred wkrs.	35.9	36.8	35.2	27.4	33.2	52.9	a	a
Mgrs., offs., and prop's., exc. farm	29.1	30.5	28.1	13.4	42.0	44.9	a	a
Clerical, sales, and kindred workers	33.7	35.1	30.1	20.8	27.7	31.8	a	a
Craftsmen, foremen, and kindred wkrs.	18.8	23.7	13.9	3.0	23.6	27.6	a	a
Operatives and kindred workers	12.6	20.4	4.5	- 4.2	25.7	36.4	16.9	a
Service workers, incl. private hshld.	24.0	26.2	18.6	a	53.4	56.6	a	a
Laborers, exc. farm and mine	6.1	12.2	5.7	- 6.6	32.9	37.2	28.5	a
Farmers and farm managers	3.3	-21.6	18.9	3.8	9.4	a	a	14.6
Farm laborers and foremen	8.5	26.8	7.7	4.7	30.4	a	11.5	44.8
40-44								
Profess'l, techn'l, and kindred wkrs.	27.5	30.3	25.9	- 0.7	12.3	23.3	a	a
Mgrs., offs., and prop's., exc. farm	20.3	21.5	18.1	11.3	14.1	10.4	a	a
Clerical, sales, and kindred workers	20.3	21.5	20.3	- 5.8	22.7	30.1	a	a
Craftsmen, foremen, and kindred wkrs.	6.2	10.0	2.3	- 5.2	7.7	6.1	a	a
Operatives and kindred workers	3.0	7.0	- 0.4	- 8.0	8.4	5.6	33.7	a
Service workers, incl. private hshld.	12.1	12.2	10.0	a	25.4	22.7	a	a
Laborers, exc. farm and mine	- 6.1	- 5.5	0.1	- 8.4	13.4	18.6	9.1	a
Farmers and farm managers	- 5.3	-25.4	16.5	- 5.2	8.0	a	a	12.2
Farm laborers and foremen	0.9	13.7	- 2.7	0.7	38.5	a	37.6	a
45-49								
Profess'l, techn'l, and kindred wkrs.	15.5	18.2	15.7	-16.4	a	a	a	a
Mgrs., offs., and prop's., exc. farm	4.9	6.2	2.6	- 8.4	-12.0	- 0.2	a	a
Clerical, sales, and kindred workers	1.0	1.6	3.9	- 9.4	14.4	10.1	a	a
Craftsmen, foremen, and kindred wkrs.	- 3.7	- 3.5	- 2.4	- 6.0	2.1	- 3.4	a	a
Operatives and kindred workers	- 7.8	- 7.9	- 2.8	-18.0	- 3.6	- 8.1	15.9	a
Service workers, incl. private hshld.	- 5.2	- 5.9	- 6.3	- 7.7	- 1.9	- 4.6	a	a
Laborers, exc. farm and mine	-12.6	-14.4	- 5.2	-19.2	5.5	- 3.1	21.1	a
Farmers and farm managers	-12.8	-18.5	3.7	-13.0	- 1.2	a	a	2.3
Farm laborers and foremen	- 1.8	11.5	- 5.6	- 2.4	25.1	a	23.5	a

Source: Derived from U. S. Bureau of the Census, 1960 of Population, Women by Number of Children Ever Born, PC(2)-3A, Tables 31,32; and Grabill, Kiser, and Whelpton, The Fertility of American Women, Tables 54,55. Data for 1950 limited to women married once, husband present.

aRate not shown where fewer than 4,000 women in 1950.

among white women under 35 were higher in most cases for the proprietary and clerical than for the professional groups. They were relatively slight for women 35-39 and 40-44, but in these cases the wives
of professional men outranked the other occupational groups in
percent increase of number of children ever born. The smallest increases were almost invariably those for wives of unskilled laborers,
farmers, and farm laborers. Thus, the 1950-60 increases in fertility
for women aged 25-29 ranged from 18 percent for the wives of farmers to 52 percent for wives of clerical and sales workers (see Fig. 10.1).
This type of trend served to diminish the inverse relation of occupational class to fertility among white groups during the decade.

For the nonwhite group, there was no manifest tendency for the
increases in fertility to be largest among those of upper socioeconomic
status. On the contrary, the 1950-60 increases in fertility tended to
be relatively small for nonwhite wives of professional men. They
tended to be relatively large for nonwhite wives of service workers,
unskilled laborers, and farm laborers. This type of trend served to
sharpen the inverse relation of occupational class to fertility among
nonwhite groups during the decade.

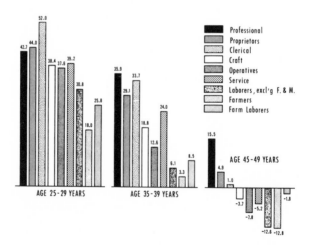

Fig. 10.1. Percent change 1950-60 in number of children ever born per 1,000
white women of specified ages, married and husband present, by major occupation group of husband: United States. Data for 1950 relate to women married
once and husband present.

Children Ever Born, by Major Occupation Group of the Husband

Age-specific fertility rates of white women, married and husband present, by occupation group of the husband, are shown by color and residence in Tables 10.4 to 10.7 for the censuses of 1910, 1940, 1950, and 1960.

A generally inverse relation of fertility to occupational rank of husband has existed throughout the period considered, that is, 1910-60. In 1960, as in 1910, the lowest fertility rates tended to be those for the wives of professional men and clerical and sales workers and the highest for the urban unskilled laborers and for the farmers and farm laborers.

According to the Current Population Survey of 1964 the number of children ever born per 1,000 women, married and husband present, 15-44 years old, standardized for age, ranged from 2,154 for wives of clerical and kindred workers and 2,176 for wives of professional, technical, and kindred workers to 3,320 for wives of unskilled laborers (except farm and mine) and 2,906 for wives of farmers and farm managers.[6]

Although the order of the broad occupational classes with respect to fertility has remained virtually unchanged since 1910, there has been a marked *reduction* in the fertility differentials by occupational class among the white married women. However, there has been a *widening* of the difference in fertility among nonwhite women under 35 years of age since 1950. As a consequence, whereas in 1950 the relative spread of the rates by occupational class was much the same for white and nonwhite women, in 1960 the interclass variations were sharper among the nonwhite than among the white women. The indices of fertility differentials by occupation group from 1910 to 1960 are discussed further later in this chapter.

Figure 10.2 presents the data for white and nonwhite women of specified ages in the United States. The high fertility of the wives of farmers and farm laborers stands out for both white and nonwhite women, and especially for the latter. In general, the range of the variations in fertility and the interclass differences in fertility tended to be wider among nonwhite than among white women—a possible reversal of the situation a generation ago. The differentials in fertility by occupation of husband also tended to be wider in "other urban" than in urbanized areas and wider in rural nonfarm than in urban areas. They were wider in the South than in the United States as a whole.

Table 10.4   Number of children ever born per 1,000 women 15-49 years old, married and husband present, by age and color of wife and major occupation group of husband: United States, 1960, 1950, 1940 and 1910

Age of wife and occupation of husband	White				Nonwhite			
	1960	1950[a]	1940[a]	1910[a]	1960	1950[a]	1940[a]	1910[a]
15-19								
Profess'l, techn'l, and kindred workers	546	459	326	501	1,122	b	b	b
Mgrs., offs., and prop's., exc. farm	725	454	401	585	b	b	b	b
Clerical, sales, and kindred workers	621	439	415	456	1,084	b	b	b
Craftsmen, foremen, and kindred workers	759	518	521	634	1,169	962	b	699
Operatives and kindred workers	755	584	551	669	1,241	907	537	750
Service workers, incl. private household	733	517	452	595	1,213	763	637	557
Laborers, except farm and mine	750	599	609	734	1,257	914	696	761
Farmers and farm managers	769	589	672	797	1,241	1,088	864	884
Farm laborers and foremen	787	580	610	683	1,340	855	698	825
20-24								
Profess'l, techn'l, and kindred workers	1,034	714	567	838	1,232	829	b	923
Mgrs., offs., and prop's., exc. farm	1,326	882	720	1,035	1,673	b	b	1,540
Clerical, sales, and kindred workers	1,188	793	625	886	1,634	1,202	778	1,219
Craftsmen, foremen, and kindred workers	1,498	1,041	898	1,218	2,011	1,371	1,052	1,353
Operatives and kindred workers	1,557	1,112	968	1,316	2,126	1,409	1,094	1,496
Service workers, incl. private household	1,407	1,010	809	1,121	1,851	1,362	875	1,067
Laborers, except farm and mine	1,573	1,195	1,093	1,491	2,248	1,590	1,167	1,523
Farmers and farm managers	1,609	1,294	1,306	1,629	2,753	2,083	1,766	2,063
Farm laborers and foremen	1,741	1,346	1,233	1,516	2,651	1,764	1,554	1,803
25-29								
Profess'l, techn'l, and kindred workers	1,826	1,280	880	1,232	1,547	1,278	1,049	1,903
Mgrs., offs., and prop's., exc. farm	2,106	1,462	1,101	1,607	2,220	1,239	b	1,911
Clerical, sales, and kindred workers	1,986	1,307	967	1,365	2,192	1,538	1,213	1,664
Craftsmen, foremen, and kindred workers	2,284	1,650	1,400	1,917	2,808	1,715	1,465	2,108
Operatives and kindred workers	2,388	1,736	1,500	2,017	2,984	2,027	1,619	2,198
Service workers, incl. private household	2,178	1,565	1,209	1,707	2,634	1,506	1,151	1,536
Laborers, except farm and mine	2,508	1,917	1,720	2,400	3,204	2,104	1,744	2,311
Farmers and farm managers	2,516	2,132	2,056	2,661	3,981	3,199	2,947	3,513
Farm laborers and foremen	2,892	2,298	2,004	2,518	3,912	2,519	2,437	2,964
30-34								
Profess'l, techn'l, and kindred workers	2,377	1,777	1,321	1,820	2,126	1,793	1,286	2,714
Mgrs., offs., and prop's., exc. farm	2,465	1,876	1,526	2,206	2,755	1,945	b	2,378
Clerical, sales, and kindred workers	2,387	1,689	1,365	1,906	2,475	1,733	1,272	2,452
Craftsmen, foremen, and kindred workers	2,631	2,075	1,920	2,605	3,168	2,254	2,150	2,887
Operatives and kindred workers	2,738	2,193	2,084	2,775	3,369	2,422	2,072	3,148
Service workers, incl. private household	2,478	1,880	1,690	2,325	2,947	1,746	1,586	1,909
Laborers, except farm and mine	2,929	2,457	2,448	3,248	3,643	2,305	2,212	3,080
Farmers and farm managers	3,020	2,713	2,805	3,706	4,818	4,408	4,028	4,837
Farm laborers and foremen	3,617	2,969	2,800	3,565	5,138	3,318	3,101	3,988
35-39								
Profess'l, techn'l, and kindred workers	2,495	1,836	1,673	2,364	2,233	1,676	1,613	3,511
Mgrs., offs., and prop's., exc. farm	2,525	1,956	1,861	2,788	2,630	1,852	b	3,290
Clerical, sales, and kindred workers	2,416	1,807	1,730	2,483	2,529	1,980	1,810	3,031
Craftsmen, foremen, and kindred workers	2,659	2,239	2,377	3,347	3,128	2,530	2,544	3,755
Operatives and kindred workers	2,765	2,456	2,604	3,614	3,287	2,615	2,573	3,936
Service workers, incl. private household	2,539	2,048	2,141	2,982	2,807	1,830	1,926	2,625
Laborers, except farm and mine	3,045	2,871	3,049	4,074	3,599	2,709	2,849	3,934
Farmers and farm managers	3,174	3,072	3,475	4,663	5,456	4,985	4,891	6,302
Farm laborers and foremen	3,962	3,652	3,596	4,432	5,039	3,863	3,791	5,125
40-44								
Profess'l, techn'l, and kindred workers	2,311	1,812	1,926	2,749	2,150	1,914	2,438	4,201
Mgrs., offs., and prop's., exc. farm	2,336	1,942	2,144	3,259	2,500	2,192	b	3,453
Clerical, sales, and kindred workers	2,230	1,853	1,978	2,858	2,207	1,798	b	b
Craftsmen, foremen, and kindred workers	2,548	2,399	2,666	3,854	2,845	2,641	2,862	4,994
Operatives and kindred workers	2,690	2,612	2,931	4,157	2,997	2,764	2,821	4,662
Service workers, incl. private household	2,426	2,164	2,564	3,596	2,591	2,066	2,305	3,365
Laborers, exc. farm and mine	2,968	3,162	3,403	4,633	3,296	2,907	2,894	4,952
Farmers and farm managers	3,166	3,344	3,914	5,292	5,684	5,262	5,131	7,538
Farm laborers and foremen	4,017	3,980	4,281	4,967	5,119	3,696	3,970	6,170
45-49								
Profess'l, techn'l, and kindred workers	2,022	1,751	2,069	3,079	2,020	b	2,269	5,436
Mgrs., offs., and prop's., exc. farm	2,074	1,978	2,283	3,493	2,355	2,676	b	5,352
Clerical, sales, and kindred workers	1,948	1,928	2,108	3,242	2,042	1,785	b	b
Craftsmen, foremen, and kindred workers	2,389	2,480	2,847	4,224	2,758	2,702	3,059	5,663
Operatives and kindred workers	2,539	2,753	3,037	4,496	2,723	2,823	3,311	5,777
Service workers, incl. private household	2,291	2,416	2,737	4,027	2,281	2,324	2,379	3,762
Laborers, exc. farm and mine	2,933	3,356	3,627	4,869	3,110	2,948	3,195	5,599
Farmers and farm managers	3,060	3,510	4,104	5,551	5,248	5,313	5,335	8,213
Farm laborers and foremen	4,146	4,222	4,270	5,176	4,750	3,796	4,970	6,832

Source: U. S. Bureau of the Census, 1960 Census of Population, *Women by Number of Children Ever Born*, PC(2)-3A, Tables 31,32; and Grabill, Kiser, and Whelpton, *The Fertility of American Women*, Tables 54, 55.

[a]Data for 1950, 1940, and 1910 are for women married once, husband present. Data for 1940 and 1910 relate to native white and Negro women.

[b]Rate not shown where base is less than 1,000 women in 1960, 4,000 in 1950, 3,000 in 1940, or 1,200 in 1910.

Table 10.5   Number of children ever born per 1,000 women 15-49 years old, married and husband present, by age and color of wife and major occupation group of husband: Urban areas, 1960, 1950, 1940, and 1910

Age of wife and occupation of husband	White				Nonwhite	
	1960	1950[a]	1940[a]	1910[a]	1960	1950[a]
15-19						
Profess'l, techn'l, and kindred workers	540	436	328	453	1,125	b
Mgrs., offs., and prop's., exc. farm	707	440	362	532	b	b
Clerical, sales, and kindred workers	605	434	423	417	1,079	b
Craftsmen, foremen, and kindred workers	749	465	459	585	1,157	932
Operatives and kindred workers	742	548	495	592	1,225	888
Service workers, incl. private household	730	464	432	560	1,201	738
Laborers, except farm and mine	735	608	533	656	1,255	952
Farmers and farm managers	b	b	b	b	b	b
Farm laborers and foremen	636	552	b	b	b	b
20-24						
Profess'l, techn'l, and kindred workers	985	670	513	721	1,200	b
Mgrs., offs., and prop's., exc. farm	1,282	832	628	907	1,697	b
Clerical, sales, and kindred workers	1,155	766	584	817	1,601	1,197
Craftsmen, foremen, and kindred workers	1,445	972	799	1,116	1,970	1,310
Operatives and kindred workers	1,499	1,019	848	1,159	2,011	1,310
Service workers, incl. private household	1,367	959	767	1,066	1,832	1,350
Laborers, except farm and mine	1,495	1,070	951	1,360	2,140	1,498
Farmers and farm managers	1,236	689	b	1,284	b	b
Farm laborers and foremen	1,585	1,164	1,188	1,276	2,309	b
25-29						
Profess'l, techn'l, and kindred workers	1,789	1,234	805	1,076	1,489	1,242
Mgrs., offs., and prop's., exc. farm	2,053	1,410	1,025	1,426	2,180	1,184
Clerical, sales, and kindred workers	1,937	1,262	913	1,242	2,155	1,536
Craftsmen, foremen, and kindred workers	2,217	1,543	1,274	1,738	2,675	1,583
Operatives and kindred workers	2,296	1,589	1,298	1,782	2,803	1,816
Service workers, incl. private household	2,131	1,518	1,158	1,589	2,592	1,464
Laborers, except farm and mine	2,408	1,717	1,446	2,177	3,027	1,855
Farmers and farm managers	2,133	2,228	b	2,191	b	b
Farm laborers and foremen	2,853	2,280	1,815	2,019	3,412	b
30-34						
Profess'l, techn'l, and kindred workers	2,351	1,724	1,271	1,575	2,071	1,560
Mgrs., offs., and prop's., exc. farm	2,426	1,824	1,434	1,965	2,674	1,891
Clerical, sales, and kindred workers	2,353	1,638	1,300	1,752	2,484	1,591
Craftsmen, foremen, and kindred workers	2,559	1,931	1,759	2,370	2,994	2,063
Operatives and kindred workers	2,611	2,000	1,823	2,452	3,130	2,106
Service workers, incl. private household	2,426	1,817	1,597	2,173	2,801	1,658
Laborers, exc. farm and mine	2,801	2,168	2,125	2,946	3,382	1,974
Farmers and farm managers	2,591	3,138	b	2,817	2,363	b
Farm laborers and foremen	3,663	2,988	2,418	2,865	3,477	b
35-39						
Profess'l, techn'l, and kindred workers	2,455	1,794	1,603	2,058	2,181	1,426
Mgrs., offs., and prop's., exc. farm	2,476	1,898	1,761	2,526	2,507	1,730
Clerical, sales, and kindred workers	2,378	1,760	1,645	2,285	2,448	1,857
Craftsmen, foremen, and kindred workers	2,553	2,064	2,178	3,070	2,925	2,292
Operatives and kindred workers	2,601	2,161	2,299	3,178	2,995	2,196
Service workers, incl. private household	2,468	1,956	2,028	2,849	2,687	1,716
Laborers, except farm and mine	2,820	2,514	2,663	3,775	3,189	2,324
Farmers and farm managers	2,561	3,265	2,384	3,627	2,969	b
Farm laborers and foremen	3,948	3,114	b	3,647	3,573	b
40-44						
Profess'l, techn'l, and kindred workers	2,277	1,747	1,858	2,435	2,077	1,685
Mgrs., offs., and prop's., exc. farm	2,273	1,871	2,021	2,987	2,373	2,150
Clerical, sales, and kindred workers	2,180	1,794	1,881	2,694	2,155	1,656
Craftsmen, foremen, and kindred workers	2,425	2,204	2,437	3,635	2,565	2,418
Operatives and kindred workers	2,484	2,321	2,583	3,746	2,625	2,485
Service workers, incl. private household	2,341	2,087	2,420	3,482	2,472	2,015
Laborers, except farm and mine	2,702	2,858	2,978	4,441	2,874	2,424
Farmers and farm managers	2,496	3,344	2,610	4,121	3,053	b
Farm laborers and foremen	4,015	3,532	b	3,838	3,386	b
45-49						
Profess'l, techn'l, and kindred workers	1,983	1,678	1,964	2,759	1,935	b
Mgrs., offs., and prop's., exc. farm	2,014	1,897	2,128	3,261	2,305	2,309
Clerical, sales, and kindred workers	1,895	1,866	1,999	3,094	1,893	1,719
Craftsmen, foremen, and kindred workers	2,239	2,320	2,630	4,008	2,473	2,561
Operatives and kindred workers	2,315	2,514	2,679	4,121	2,344	2,550
Service workers, incl. private household	2,149	2,283	2,507	3,883	2,162	2,266
Laborers, except farm and mine	2,677	3,127	3,230	4,794	2,588	2,670
Farmers and farm managers	2,527	3,100	2,701	4,176	4,044	b
Farm laborers and foremen	4,022	3,607	b	4,424	3,218	b

Source: U. S. Bureau of the Census, 1960 Census of Population, Women by Number of Children Ever Born, PC(2)-3A, Tables 31,32; and Grabill, Kiser, and Whelpton, The Fertility of American Women, Tables 54, 55.

[a]Data for 1950, 1940, and 1910 are for women married once, husband present. Data for 1940 and 1910 relate to native white women. Data for nonwhite or Negro women not available by urban-rural residence for 1940 and 1910.

[b]Rate not shown where base is less than 1,000 women in 1960, 4,000 in 1950, 3,000 in 1940, or 1,200 in 1910.

Table 10.6　Number of children ever born per 1,000 women 15-49 years old, married and husband present, by age and color of wife and major occupation group of husband:　Rural nonfarm areas, 1960, 1950, 1940, and 1910

Age of wife and occupation of husband	White				Nonwhite	
	1960	1950[a]	1940[a]	1910[a]	1960	1950[a]
15-19						
Profess'l, techn'l, and kindred workers	563	b	b	552	b	b
Mgrs., offs., and prop's., exc. farm	773	492	431	650	b	b
Clerical, sales, and kindred workers	682	439	366	529	b	b
Craftsmen, foremen, and kindred workers	786	609	611	727	1,202	b
Operatives and kindred workers	785	657	610	750	1,312	951
Service workers, incl. private household	725	b	b	677	b	b
Laborers, except farm and mine	783	570	651	796	1,306	910
Farmers and farm managers	646	552	b	703	b	b
Farm laborers and foremen	830	625	679	771	1,339	883
20-24						
Profess'l, techn'l, and kindred workers	1,237	913	660	996	b	b
Mgrs., offs., and prop's., exc. farm	1,482	1,020	906	1,208	b	b
Clerical, sales, and kindred workers	1,329	914	776	1,064	2,108	b
Craftsmen, foremen, and kindred workers	1,624	1,199	1,085	1,432	2,241	b
Operatives and kindred workers	1,668	1,275	1,158	1,565	2,508	1,641
Service workers, incl. private household	1,582	1,225	944	1,267	1,977	b
Laborers, except farm and mine	1,711	1,363	1,220	1,612	2,552	1,853
Farmers and farm managers	1,536	1,070	1,099	1,465	3,046	b
Farm laborers and foremen	1,762	1,420	1,188	1,644	2,633	1,849
25-29						
Profess'l, techn'l, and kindred workers	1,969	1,436	1,021	1,459	1,975	b
Mgrs., offs., and prop's., exc. farm	2,282	1,615	1,253	1,855	b	b
Clerical, sales, and kindred workers	2,197	1,519	1,169	1,721	2,776	b
Craftsmen, foremen, and kindred workers	2,427	1,875	1,614	2,295	3,503	b
Operatives and kindred workers	2,543	1,986	1,811	2,444	3,714	2,735
Service workers, incl. private household	2,394	1,773	1,372	2,046	3,077	b
Laborers, except farm and mine	2,664	2,157	1,976	2,630	3,719	2,851
Farmers and farm managers	2,364	1,884	1,699	2,457	3,968	b
Farm laborers and foremen	2,965	2,379	2,007	2,675	3,985	2,446
30-34						
Profess'l, techn'l, and kindred workers	2,480	1,956	1,432	2,166	2,400	b
Mgrs., offs., and prop's., exc. farm	2,578	2,019	1,706	2,543	3,554	b
Clerical, sales, and kindred workers	2,511	1,868	1,560	2,344	2,770	b
Craftsmen, foremen, and kindred workers	2,782	2,358	2,165	3,032	4,140	2,987
Operatives and kindred workers	2,965	2,511	2,461	3,367	4,354	3,317
Service workers, incl. private household	2,687	2,137	2,004	2,798	4,028	b
Laborers, except farm and mine	3,114	2,810	2,674	3,547	4,492	3,210
Farmers and farm managers	2,756	2,402	2,581	3,381	4,226	b
Farm laborers and foremen	3,567	3,134	2,651	3,733	5,251	3,829
35-39						
Profess'l, techn'l, and kindred workers	2,665	1,971	1,810	2,786	2,822	b
Mgrs., offs., and prop's., exc. farm	2,678	2,091	2,028	3,169	3,500	b
Clerical, sales, and kindred workers	2,549	1,959	1,969	3,026	3,801	b
Craftsmen, foremen, and kindred workers	2,891	2,539	2,646	3,824	4,134	b
Operatives and kindred workers	3,085	2,951	3,010	4,439	4,493	3,844
Service workers, incl. private household	2,791	2,353	2,384	3,448	3,816	b
Laborers, except farm and mine	3,409	3,224	3,303	4,395	4,808	3,742
Farmers and farm managers	3,067	2,580	2,993	4,219	5,669	b
Farm laborers and foremen	3,963	3,681	3,358	4,649	4,652	4,174
40-44						
Profess'l, techn'l, and kindred workers	2,435	1,934	2,065	3,119	2,737	b
Mgrs., offs., and prop's., exc. farm	2,530	2,143	2,348	3,668	3,374	b
Clerical, sales, and kindred workers	2,430	2,020	2,229	3,255	b	b
Craftsmen, foremen, and kindred workers	2,826	2,763	2,956	4,242	4,217	b
Operatives and kindred workers	3,126	3,139	3,427	5,034	4,398	3,290
Service workers, incl. private household	2,707	2,460	2,826	4,025	3,636	b
Laborers, except farm and mine	3,352	3,350	3,709	4,876	4,507	4,131
Farmers and farm managers	3,089	2,652	3,278	4,729	5,462	b
Farm laborers and foremen	4,028	4,140	3,999	5,212	5,022	3,649
45-49						
Profess'l, techn'l, and kindred workers	2,167	1,873	2,325	3,569	2,622	b
Mgrs., offs., and prop's., exc. farm	2,272	2,215	2,502	3,810	2,655	b
Clerical, sales, and kindred workers	2,161	2,079	2,443	3,627	3,449	b
Craftsmen, foremen, and kindred workers	2,727	2,793	3,182	4,600	3,984	b
Operatives and kindred workers	3,019	3,107	3,538	5,243	4,122	3,557
Service workers, incl. private household	2,733	2,915	3,445	4,512	3,094	b
Laborers, except farm and mine	3,331	3,515	3,922	4,916	4,643	3,833
Farmers and farm managers	2,949	2,843	3,506	5,068	4,483	b
Farm laborers and foremen	4,209	4,456	4,332	5,311	4,642	3,759

Source:　U. S. Bureau of the Census, 1960 Census of Population, Women by Number of Children Ever Born, PC(2)-3A, Tables 31,32; and Grabill, Kiser, and Whelpton, The Fertility of American Women, Tables 54, 55.

[a]Data for 1950, 1940, and 1910 are for women married once, husband present. Data for 1940 and 1910 relate to native white women. Data for nonwhite or Negro women not available by urban-rural residence for 1940 and 1910.

[b]Rate not shown where base is less than 1,000 women in 1960, 4,000 in 1950, 3,000 in 1940, or 1,200 in 1910.

Table 10.7 Number of children ever born per 1,000 women 15-49 years old, married and husband present, by age and color of wife and major occupation group of husband: Rural farm areas, 1960, 1950, 1940, and 1910

Age of wife and occupation of husband	White				Nonwhite	
	1960	1950[a]	1940[a]	1910[a]	1960	1950[a]
Clerical, sales, and kindred workers	654	b	b	b	b	b
Craftsmen, foremen, and kindred workers	739	663	b	b	b	b
Operatives and kindred workers	755	545	625	b	1,170	b
Service workers, incl. private household	b	b	b	b	b	b
Laborers, except farm and mine	692	660	724	762	b	b
Farmers and farm managers	821	600	674	801	1,297	1,090
Farm laborers and foremen	796	559	594	508	1,411	838
20-24						
Profess'l, techn'l, and kindred workers	1,361	b	b	1,204	b	b
Mgrs., offs., and prop's., exc. farm	1,576	b	1,004	1,349	b	b
Clerical, sales, and kindred workers	1,496	929	919	1,218	b	b
Craftsmen, foremen, and kindred workers	1,694	1,277	1,234	1,432	b	b
Operatives and kindred workers	1,684	1,342	1,249	1,554	2,765	b
Service workers, incl. private household	1,552	b	b	b	b	b
Laborers, except farm and mine	1,711	1,505	1,360	1,634	2,655	b
Farmers and farm managers	1,641	1,331	1,319	1,636	2,812	2,080
Farm laborers and foremen	1,777	1,333	1,250	1,202	2,766	1,786
25-29						
Profess'l, techn'l, and kindred workers	2,300	1,803	1,434	1,913	b	b
Mgrs., offs., and prop's., exc. farm	2,413	1,853	1,554	2,259	b	b
Clerical, sales, and kindred workers	2,251	1,706	1,646	2,132	b	b
Craftsmen, foremen, and kindred workers	2,629	2,195	2,012	2,332	b	b
Operatives and kindred workers	2,728	2,363	2,091	2,660	3,765	b
Service workers, incl. private household	2,616	b	b	b	b	b
Laborers, except farm and mine	2,742	2,438	2,227	2,606	3,834	b
Farmers and farm managers	2,559	2,146	2,074	2,672	4,243	3,237
Farm laborers and foremen	2,835	2,245	2,022	2,087	3,969	2,740
30-34						
Profess'l, techn'l, and kindred workers	2,683	2,494	1,626	2,916	b	b
Mgrs., offs., and prop's., exc. farm	2,881	2,383	1,995	3,241	b	b
Clerical, sales, and kindred workers	2,813	2,532	2,235	2,840	b	b
Craftsmen, foremen, and kindred workers	3,084	2,822	2,615	3,441	b	b
Operatives and kindred workers	3,160	2,968	2,919	3,757	5,259	b
Service workers, incl. private household	3,139	b	b	b	b	b
Laborers, except farm and mine	3,335	3,114	3,132	4,025	5,006	b
Farmers and farm managers	3,076	2,721	2,817	3,726	5,287	4,464
Farm laborers and foremen	3,647	2,829	2,898	3,159	5,552	3,286
35-39						
Profess'l, techn'l, and kindred workers	2,911	2,285	2,289	3,872	b	b
Mgrs., offs., and prop's., exc. farm	3,009	2,654	2,582	3,976	b	b
Clerical, sales, and kindred workers	2,942	2,434	2,692	3,940	b	b
Craftsmen, foremen, and kindred workers	3,263	3,168	3,319	4,419	b	b
Operatives and kindred workers	3,405	3,554	3,698	4,595	5,759	b
Service workers, incl. private household	3,303	b	3,297	b	b	b
Laborers, except farm and mine	3,552	3,802	3,946	4,925	5,933	b
Farmers and farm managers	3,216	3,098	3,501	4,694	5,809	5,070
Farm laborers and foremen	3,968	3,790	3,720	3,863	5,900	4,074
40-44						
Profess'l, techn'l, and kindred workers	2,879	2,900	2,801	4,598	b	b
Mgrs., offs., and prop's., exc. farm	2,864	2,573	2,957	4,565	b	b
Clerical, sales, and kindred workers	2,806	2,977	2,981	4,349	b	b
Craftsmen, foremen, and kindred workers	3,239	3,417	3,884	4,759	b	b
Operatives and kindred workers	3,466	3,768	4,135	5,232	5,756	b
Service workers, incl. private household	3,414	b	4,012	b	b	b
Laborers, except farm and mine	3,868	4,224	4,329	5,107	5,292	b
Farmers and farm managers	3,211	3,388	3,950	5,332	6,041	5,382
Farm laborers and foremen	4,006	3,980	4,435	4,738	5,785	b
45-49						
Profess'l, techn'l, and kindred workers	2,503	2,994	2,906	4,282	b	b
Mgrs., offs., and prof's., exc. farm	2,496	2,726	3,444	4,772	b	b
Clerical, sales, and kindred workers	2,519	2,781	2,991	4,699	b	b
Craftsmen, foremen, and kindred workers	3,254	3,461	3,976	5,182	b	b
Operatives and kindred workers	3,409	4,158	4,399	5,621	5,426	b
Service workers, incl. private household	3,214	3,482	b	b	b	b
Laborers, except farm and mine	3,568	4,414	4,431	5,531	5,928	b
Farmers and farm managers	3,103	3,568	4,144	5,603	5,536	5,413
Farm laborers and foremen	4,134	4,235	4,385	5,130	5,396	b

Source: U. S. Bureau of the Census, 1960 Census of Population, Women by Number of Children Ever Born, PC(2)-3A, Tables 31,32; and Grabill, Kiser, and Whelpton, The Fertility of American Women, Tables 54, 55.

[a]Data for 1950, 1940, and 1910 are for women married once, husband present. Data for 1940 and 1910 relate to native white women. Data for nonwhite or Negro women not available for urban-rural residence for 1940 and 1910.

[b]Rate not shown where base is less than 1,000 women in 1960, 4,000 in 1950, 3,000 in 1940, or 1,200 in 1910.

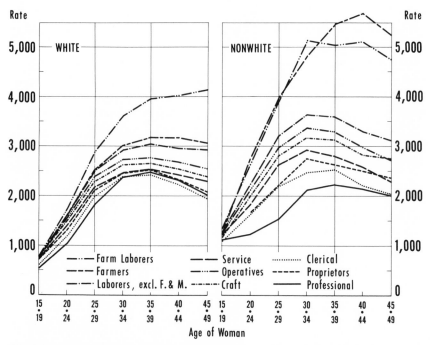

Fig. 10.2. Number of children ever born per 1,000 women 15-49 years old, married and husband present, by age and color of wife and major occupation group of husband: United States, 1960.

Although relatively few white or nonwhite couples now reside in rural farm areas, it is of interest to note that among the rural farm white residents, the 1960 occupational differentials in fertility were much the same as those in rural nonfarm areas. In both types of areas the fertility rates of professional and clerical workers tended to fall below those of managers and officials. However, although the white-collar classes fell below the laboring and farm classes with respect to fertility, they were not internally sharply differentiated. The farm laborers tended to exhibit highest fertility wherever they were found. However, they constitute a diminishing proportion of the population even at youngest ages.

A conspicuous feature of the nonwhite group is the relatively low fertility of the wives of professional men. Throughout ages 25-39 the fertility rates of nonwhite wives of professional men were 10-15 percent lower than those of white wives of professional men. At other occupational levels the fertility of nonwhite women tended to be higher than that of white women and the percent excess of nonwhite fertility over white fertility tended to be highest for farmers and farm laborers, intermediate for nonfarm manual workers, and lowest for proprietors and clerks. Among wives under 25 the fertility of the non-white group tended to surpass that of the white group at all occupational levels (Table 10.8). These situations tended to hold within urban areas alone as well as within the United States as a whole. They had their counterparts in the extremely low fertility levels in 1960 of nonwhite women who finished 1 year or more of college and especially those reporting 4 or more years of college. At lower educational levels the fertility rates of nonwhite women 25 years of age and over tended to surpass those of white women of comparable age and education. Among wives under 25, the fertility of nonwhite women exceeded that of their white counterparts at all educational levels (see Chapter 9).[7]

Table 10.8   Percent excess of average number of children ever born to nonwhite women over that of white women, married and husband present, by age of woman and major occupation group of husband: United States and urban areas, 1960

Area and occupation group	15-19	20-24	25-29	30-34	35-39	40-44	45-49
UNITED STATES							
Profess'l, techn'l, and kindred workers	105.5	19.1	-15.3	-10.6	-10.5	- 7.0	- 0.1
Mgrs., offs., and prop's., exc. farm	a	26.2	5.4	11.8	4.2	7.0	13.5
Clerical, sales, and kindred workers	74.6	37.5	10.4	3.7	4.7	- 1.0	4.8
Craftsmen, foremen, and kindred workers	54.0	34.2	22.9	20.4	17.6	11.7	15.4
Operatives and kindred workers	64.4	36.5	25.0	23.0	18.9	11.4	7.2
Service workers, incl. private household	65.5	31.6	20.9	18.9	10.6	6.8	- 0.4
Laborers, except farm and mine	67.6	42.9	27.8	24.4	18.2	11.1	6.0
Farmers and farm managers	61.4	71.1	58.2	59.5	71.9	79.5	71.5
Farm laborers and foremen	70.3	52.3	35.3	42.1	27.2	27.4	14.6
URBAN							
Profess'l, techn'l, and kindred workers	108.3	21.8	-16.8	-11.9	-11.2	- 8.8	- 2.4
Mgrs., offs., and prop's., exc. farm	a	32.4	6.2	10.2	1.3	4.4	14.4
Clerical, sales, and kindred workers	78.3	38.6	11.3	5.6	2.9	- 1.2	- 0.1
Craftsmen, foremen, and kindred workers	54.5	36.3	20.7	17.0	14.6	5.8	10.5
Operatives and kindred workers	65.1	34.2	22.1	19.9	15.1	5.7	1.3
Service workers, incl. private household	64.5	34.0	21.6	15.5	8.9	5.6	0.6
Laborers, except farm and mine	70.7	43.1	25.7	20.7	13.1	6.4	- 3.3
Farmers and farm managers	a	a	a	- 8.8	15.9	22.3	60.0
Farm laborers and foremen	a	45.7	19.6	- 5.1	- 9.5	-15.7	-20.0

Source: Derived from U.S. Bureau of the Census, 1960 Census of Population, Women by Number of Children Ever Born, PC(2)-3A, tables 31 and 32.

[a]Percent excess not shown where fewer than 1,000 women.

Children Ever Born, by Specific Occupation of Husband

There are a few interesting exceptions to the inverse relation of occupational class to fertility. These apparently are of long-standing duration and doubtless are due in part to the failure of the occupational categories to yield a continuum with respect to socioeconomic status. One case in point is the relatively low fertility rates of the wives of clerical and sales workers. Without exception, the age-specific fertility rates for this group are lower than those for the "managers, officials, and proprietors, except farm" group for white married women aged 20-24 through 45-49. This held for the United States as a whole and for the urban and rural nonfarm groups considered separately. In fact, in 1960, among the white wives 30-49 years of age in the United States, the age-specific fertility rates for the wives of clerical and sales workers were as low as or lower than those for wives of professional men.

Although the 1960 rates are given for the combined "clerical and sales" group for the sake of comparability with the rates for the earlier years, they are available separately for the two constituent classes. The fertility of the "clerical and kindred workers" was consistently lower than that of the "sales workers" in 1960. However, the fertility rates for even the "sales workers" tended to fall below those of the "managers, officials and proprietors, except farm" throughout ages 35-49 in the United States as a whole and in urban areas. Thus, among wives 35-39 in the United States, there were 2,525 children ever born per 1,000 wives of "managers, officials, and proprietors, except farm." The rate was 2,378 for wives of "clerical and kindred workers" and 2,447 for wives of "sales workers."

In their analysis of 1910 census data Sydenstricker and Notestein observed that the "selected clerks" in their sample (salesmen and clerks in stores and "other clerks," a group presumably analogous to the "clerical and sales" group) exhibited lower fertility than proprietors. They commented, "It is possibly worth noting that this lowest fertility group of the Business Class is also the lowest income group of the class."[8]

Low income per se, of course, would hardly be a reasonable interpretation as the sole cause of lower fertility, and the authors did not state that it was. They implied instead that the clerical group may be one with the aspirations of the upper classes and the income of the lower classes. It is possible that this class in particular strives to maintain given levels of living by such devices as employment of women and family planning.

The array of husbands' specific occupations within broad classes according to fertility levels points up several interesting situations. The immediately following class-by-class description relates to white women 35-44 years old, married and husband present, and living in urbanized areas (see Table 10.9). Among such women whose husbands were of the professional class, the lowest fertility levels were those of wives of medical and dental technicians; wives of authors, editors, and reporters; and wives of artists and art teachers, musicians and music teachers, and social scientists. At the other extreme, wives of college presidents, professors, and instructors, and those of clergymen and physicians and surgeons stood out with highest fertility.

Within the group of "managers, officials, and proprietors" there was little variation in the fertility of the specific occupation groups shown. The lowest rate was that for the officials and inspectors in state and local administrations and the highest for self-employed managers, officials, and proprietors.

Concerning the relatively low fertility of the "clerical and kindred workers" in 1960, it may be noted that a subdivision of this rate for white married women 35-44 years of age in the United States revealed a higher rate for mail carriers than for bookkeepers. It is possible that the mail carriers are of lower educational status, on the average, than the bookkeepers. It is also possible that since mail carriers are generally in civil service, they have a greater sense of security than the bookkeepers. Competition with peers may be keen insofar as the civil service entrance examination is concerned, but it may virtually end with accession to the job. A mail carrier knows the requirements for advancement. The goals with respect to modest increases in salary are known, and these are influenced largely by length of service and not by special effort on the part of the individual. For the bookkeeper in private industry, competition with others and the struggle for advancement perhaps is considerably keener than in the case of the mail carrier or other petty civil service workers. There was not much variation among the "sales workers." The lowest rate was for salesmen and sales clerks (NEC) and the highest was for insurance agents, brokers, and underwriters.

Among the craftsmen, relatively low fertility was found for tailors and furriers, compositors and type setters, shoemakers and repairers, and airplane mechanics and repairmen. Relatively high fertility was found for blacksmiths, cranemen, carpenters, metal molders, and plasterers and cement finishers.

Among the operatives or semi-skilled workers, the wives of laundry and dry-cleaning operatives, "checkers, examiners and inspectors in manufacturing," sailors and deck hands, and textile spinners and weavers exhibited relatively low fertility, and wives of welders and flame cutters, painters, truck drivers, furnace men, mine operatives and laborers (NEC), and sawyers exhibited high fertility.

Table 10. 9 Number of children ever born per 1,000 women 35-44 years old, married and husband present, by specific occupations of employed husbands, by color and residence: United States and urbanized areas, 1960

(Specified occupations within a broad group are listed in order of magnitude of the fertility rates for white women in the United States)

Specific occupation of the husband	White		Nonwhite	
	United States	Urbanized areas	United States	Urbanized areas
Professional, technical and kindred workers	2,417	2,347	2,198	2,081
Technicians: medical and dental	2,121	2,017	a	a
Authors, editors and reporters	2,144	2,038	a	a
Artists and art teachers	2,161	2,088	a	a
Social scientists	2,169	2,102	a	a
Musicians and music teachers	2,170	2,101	a	a
Accountants and auditors	2,182	2,165	a	a
Pharmacists	2,238	2,183	1,937	1,913
Designers and draftsmen	2,266	2,216	a	a
Engineers: aeronautical	2,306	2,280	a	a
Teachers (NEC)	2,337	2,192	a	a
Technicians: electrical and electronic	2,357	2,318	a	a
Engineers: civil	2,382	2,348	a	a
Teachers: elementary school	2,382	2,271	1,980	1,759
Social, welfare and recreation workers	2,398	2,310	2,169	1,896
Chemists	2,411	2,394	a	a
Architects	2,416	2,313	a	a
Teachers: secondary school	2,422	2,352	1,951	1,764
Other profess'l., technical and kindred workers	2,424	2,337	2,208	2,243
Engineers: mechanical	2,427	2,356	a	a
Other technical engineers	2,428	2,376	a	a
Natural scientists (NEC)	2,460	2,426	a	a
College presidents, professors, instr's. (NEC)	2,462	2,487	1,760	a
Lawyers and judges	2,466	2,449	a	a
Dentists	2,503	2,437	a	a
Engineers: electrical	2,511	2,457	a	a
Clergymen	2,790	2,693	2,780	2,403
Physicians and surgeons	2,922	2,826	2,044	2,009
Managers, officials and proprietors, exc. farm	2,431	2,353	2,567	2,379
Officials and insp's., state and local admin.	2,342	2,267	a	a
Other specified managers and officials	2,364	2,280	2,498	2,289
Mgrs., off'ls., and propr's., (NEC) - salaried	2,417	2,358	2,459	2,370
Mgrs., off'ls., and propr's., (NEC) - self-empl.	2,479	2,382	2,657	2,414
Clerical and kindred workers	2,302	2,233	2,340	2,236
Bookkeepers	2,196	2,090	a	a
Other clerical and kindred workers	2,292	2,229	2,384	2,269
Mail carriers	2,433	2,341	2,098	2,087
Sales workers	2,354	2,285	2,613	2,399
Salesmen and sales clerks (NEC)	2,333	2,256	2,784	2,500
Real estate agents and brokers	2,368	2,341	a	a
Insurance agents, brokers and underwriters	2,448	2,419	1,993	a
Other specified sales workers	2,462	2,367	a	a
Craftsmen, foremen and kindred workers	2,607	2,454	3,001	2,667
Tailors and furriers	2,034	1,927	a	a
Compositors and typesetters	2,243	2,213	a	a
Shoemakers and repairers, except factory	2,249	2,062	a	a
Printing craft., exc. compos., and typesetters	2,322	2,310	a	a
Mechanics and repairmen: airplane	2,370	2,214	2,335	a
Bakers	2,424	2,337	3,230	3,278
Toolmakers and die makers and setters	2,479	2,391	a	a
Linemen, servicemen, teleph., telegr., and power	2,488	2,419	3,179	a
Foremen (NEC)	2,500	2,416	2,645	2,624
Machinists and job setters	2,509	2,388	2,453	2,369
Locomotive engineers	2,512	2,429	a	a
Mechanics and repairmen: radio and TV	2,536	2,402	3,165	a
Stationary engineers	2,544	2,443	2,879	2,499
Cabinetmakers and patternmakers	2,572	2,526	a	a
Electricians	2,572	2,441	2,877	2,794
Tinsmiths, coppersmiths and sheet metal workers	2,591	2,480	a	a
Other mechanics, repairmen and loom fixers	2,603	2,425	2,784	2,469
Millwrights	2,624	2,397	a	a
Locomotive firemen	2,634	2,605	a	a
Plumbers and pipe fitters	2,637	2,563	3,386	2,770
Structural metal workers	2,639	2,604	a	a

(Continued)

Table 10.9
(continued)

Number of children ever born per 1,000 women 35-44 years old, married and husband present, by specific occupations of employed husbands, by color and residence: United States and urbanized areas, 1960

(Specified occupations within a broad group are listed in order of magnitude of the fertility rates for white women in the United States)

Specific occupation of the husband	White		Nonwhite	
	United States	Urbanized areas	United States	Urbanized areas
Other craftsmen and kindred workers	2,664	2,436	3,132	2,715
Mechanics and repairmen: automobile	2,704	2,499	3,105	2,722
Boilermakers	2,718	2,779	a	a
Painters (const.), paper hangers and glaziers	2,722	2,577	2,925	2,757
Masons, tile setters and stone cutters	2,748	2,599	3,313	3,061
Blacksmiths, forgemen and hammermen	2,798	2,681	a	a
Cranemen, derrickmen and hoistmen	2,800	2,557	2,900	2,591
Carpenters	2,877	2,623	3,640	2,963
Molders, metal	2,920	2,723	3,076	2,907
Plasterers and cement finishers	2,969	2,850	2,848	2,709
Operatives and kindred workers	2,730	2,484	3,156	2,712
Laundry and dry cleaning operatives	2,294	2,218	2,455	2,268
Checkers, examiners and inspectors, mfg.	2,370	2,236	2,816	2,730
Assemblers	2,490	2,320	2,559	2,443
Meat cutters, exc. slaughter and packing house	2,500	2,402	3,221	2,890
Taxicab drivers and chauffeurs	2,520	2,405	2,311	2,241
Filers, grinders and polishers, metal	2,655	2,474	2,876	2,780
Spinners and weavers, textile	2,660	2,292	a	a
Apprentices	2,667	2,489	a	a
Sailors and deckhands	2,673	2,237	a	a
Operatives and kindred workers (NEC)	2,678	2,462	3,100	2,712
Attendants, auto service and parking	2,679	2,448	3,134	2,718
Brakemen and switchmen, railroad	2,683	2,619	2,872	a
Bus drivers	2,686	2,454	3,204	2,099
Power station operatives	2,712	2,477	a	a
Other spec. operatives and kindred workers	2,754	2,400	3,165	2,682
Stationary firemen	2,755	2,473	3,369	2,854
Packers and wrappers (NEC)	2,761	2,574	3,028	2,593
Welders and flame-cutters	2,770	2,614	2,901	2,775
Painters, exc. construction and maintenance	2,811	2,649	3,171	2,747
Truck drivers and deliverymen	2,819	2,577	3,405	2,846
Furnacemen, smeltermen and heaters	2,849	2,578	3,165	3,166
Mine operatives and laborers (NEC)	3,391	2,755	4,422	a
Sawyers	3,412	2,980	4,591	a
Private household workers	2,290	a	2,188	1,663
Service workers, exc. private household	2,484	2,365	2,719	2,501
Elevator operators	2,177	2,085	2,368	2,158
Waiters, bartenders and counter workers	2,192	2,049	2,310	2,248
Barbers	2,334	2,211	2,416	2,211
Other service workers, exc. private household	2,366	2,232	2,703	2,485
Cooks, exc. private household	2,450	2,294	2,527	2,317
Policemen, sheriffs and marshals	2,468	2,473	2,385	2,256
Firemen, fire protection	2,521	2,522	a	a
Guards and watchmen	2,585	2,322	2,689	2,511
Charwomen, janitors and porters	2,817	2,628	2,877	2,639
Laborers, exc. farm and mine	3,008	2,665	3,458	2,879
Longshoremen and stevedores	2,603	2,586	3,137	3,003
Other specified laborers	2,747	2,486	3,153	2,635
Laborers (NEC)	3,011	2,708	3,435	2,907
Fishermen and oystermen	3,139	2,548	a	a
Lumbermen, raftsmen and wood choppers	3,998	a	5,092	a
Farmers and farm managers	3,170	2,499	5,572	2,837
Farm laborers and foremen	3,988	3,487	5,078	2,790
Unpaid family workers	3,161	a	a	a
Exc. unpaid and farm foremen	4,002	3,496	5,063	2,842

Source: U. S. Bureau of the Census, 1960 Census of Population, Women by Number of Children Ever Born, PC(2)-3A, Tables 33,34.

aRate not shown where base is less than 1,000.

Among service workers, the range was from low fertility of wives of elevator operators, waiters, and barbers to high fertility of wives of policemen, firemen, guards and watchmen, and janitors.

Among the "unskilled laborers, except farm," the fertility rates were relatively low for wives of longshoremen and "other specified laborers," in intermediate position for wives of fishermen and oystermen, and highest for wives of lumberers, raftsmen, and woodchoppers.

As for the nonwhite group, the lower fertility for nonwhite than for white wives of professional men held for each specific professional occupation for which data in Table 10.9 are available for wives 35-44 years old. However, the discrepancies were relatively large for wives of physicians and college teachers and for wives of teachers in elementary and secondary schools residing in urbanized areas.

The fertility of nonwhite wives tended to surpass that of white wives of husbands in specific occupations below the professional level. Exceptions found in the United States as a whole and in urbanized areas were the lower fertility rates of nonwhite wives of mail carriers, insurance agents, taxi drivers, and chauffeurs, and plasterers and cement finishers. In urbanized areas alone lower nonwhite than white fertility rates were found for wives of bus drivers and policemen. White and nonwhite wives of barbers in urbanized areas exhibited equal fertility rates. As already indicated, the greatest relative *excess* of nonwhite fertility rates over white rates was that among wives of unskilled laborers, farmers, and farm laborers.

The fertility rates of ever-married employed *women* by broad occupation group, by specific occupations, and by age and color are discussed in Chapter 11 in the section on Labor Force Status of Women.

Distribution of Women by Number of Children Ever Born, by Major Occupation Group of the Husband

The trends in the distribution of women by number of children ever born were discussed in Chapter 4. These indicated that the increases since 1940 in the average numbers of children ever born have arisen not from increases in proportions of very large families but from increases in the proportions of families of moderate size and from corresponding decreases in proportions of childless and one-child families. In this section the distributions of women by number of children ever born will be examined according to broad occupation group of the husband.

It was noted earlier that the narrowing of occupational differentials in average number of children ever born has been due to sharper rises in fertility rates of groups previously characterized by relatively low fertility rates. How do the occupational classes differ by distributions of families according to number of children ever born for given ages of the mother?

Also, it was previously noted that whereas differentials in fertility of white women by husband's occupation have diminished, those of nonwhite women have widened. The enhancement of the fertility differentials among nonwhite occupation groups has resulted from the sharper rise in fertility among the laboring classes than among the white-collar groups. What are the white-nonwhite differences in distributions of women by number of children within given occupation groups, and what are the white-nonwhite differences in trends of such distributions?

The data indicate strongly that the relatively high increase in average number of children born to white wives of professional men has been due mainly to relatively large increases in proportions having families of moderate size (2-4 children) and not to increase in proportions having five or more children. Thus, among urban white women 25-29 years of age (married and husband present) married to men of professional status, the proportion reporting 2-4 children ever born was 38 percent in 1950 and 57 percent in 1960. The proportion reporting 5 or more children was only 0.3 percent in 1950 and 2.0 percent in 1960. The proportion reporting no children or only one child dropped from 62 percent in 1950 to 41 percent in 1960. In 1950, 26 percent of the women of this class reported no children at all; in 1960 this proportion was 17 percent. To some extent earlier marriage was responsible for these trends, as was earlier childbirth.[9]

An interesting contrast is afforded by the white wives of unskilled laborers of similar age and residence. The fertility rate for urban white women 25-29 years old and married to laborers was about 40 percent higher in 1960 than in 1950. This too was achieved mainly by increase in proportion of families with 2-4 children, but the increase in proportion of large families was also noteworthy. Thus in 1950, 49 percent of the wives of this class reported 0-1 child, 47 percent reported 2-4 children, and 4 percent reported 5 or more. In 1960 only 27 percent reported 0-1 child, 62 percent reported 2-4 children, and 10 percent reported 5 or more.

The relative importance of the large family, of course, was higher among women of older ages. Figure 10.3 shows a few comparisons for married women at ages 35-39; women of these ages are sufficiently

young to reflect the postwar trends in fertility and are sufficien
old to have virtually completed their families.

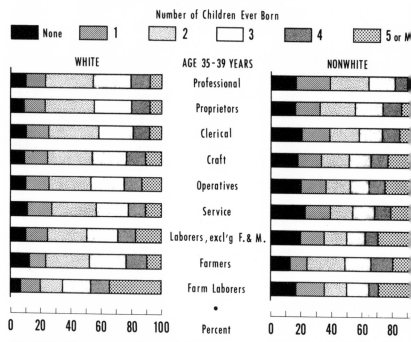

Fig. 10.3. Percent distribution by number of children ever born, for women
39 years old, married and husband present, by color of wife and major occu
tion group of husband: Urban areas, 1960.

Among urban white women 35-39 in 1960, the proportions chi
less varied little by occupation group of the husband. The range v
from 9 percent to 11 percent for the nonfarm occupations. In fa
the range was also narrow with respect to proportions reporting a
other specific number of children in the 0-4 category. The proporti
reporting 0-1 child was in the 23-28 percent range for the nonfa
occupational classes. The proportion reporting 2-4 children rang
from 58 percent for the unskilled laborers to 69 percent for t
professional and proprietary classes. The proportion reporting 5
more children extended from 8 percent for each of the three whi
collar classes to 17 percent for wives of unskilled laborers.

For each occupational class, the proportion of white women 35-
years old reporting 0-1 child declined with decreasing urbanization
residence and the proportion reporting 5 or more children increase

Thus, the proportions of wives of clerical workers 35-39 years old reporting 0-1 child in 1960 were 26 percent for urban areas, 24 percent for rural-nonfarm areas, and 19 percent for rural-farm areas. The proportions reporting 5 or more children were 8, 11, and 16 percent, respectively, in the three types of residence.

The data for nonwhite couples point up several situations and trends of interest. As already indicated in Chapter 4, the relatively large increase in fertility rates of nonwhite women has been due to declines in childlessness, declines in proportions with one child, and increases in proportions with 2-4 and 5 or more children. The sharper reductions in childlessness and the sharper increases in proportions with 5 or more children are important factors in the greater increase in nonwhite fertility than white fertility since World War II. They are important factors in the widening of the fertility differentials by color and by major occupation group of the husband among the nonwhite population.

In 1950 the proportion childless among urban nonwhite married women 25-29 years old was 31 percent for wives of unskilled laborers and 39 percent for wives of professional men. In 1960 the respective proportions were 12 percent and 25 percent. Among urban white women of comparable age the proportion childless in 1950 was 19 percent for wives of unskilled laborers and 26 percent for wives of professional men. In 1960 the respective figures were 11 and 17 percent. It was previously noted that at ages 20-24 the proportions childless were even lower among nonwhite than among white women in 1960. By occupation, this held for all except the professional class. Among urban wives of unskilled laborers 20-24 years old in 1960, the proportion childless was 15 percent for the nonwhite women and 23 percent for the white women.

In the 35-39 age group one may note the much lower proportions childless among nonwhite women in 1960 than in 1950. In 1960 the proportions childless among urban nonwhite married women 35-39 years old were 17 percent for wives of professional men and 20 percent for wives of unskilled laborers. In 1950 the percentage was over twice as high (41 percent) for nonwhite wives of professional men. It was considerably higher (33 percent) in 1950 than in 1960 for nonwhite wives of unskilled laborers. The proportions childless among nonwhite wives 35-39 in 1960 were higher than those of white wives at each occupational level (Fig. 10.3).

Like white women, nonwhite wives have exhibited declines in proportions reporting 0-1 child and increases in the proportion reporting 2-4 children. Unlike white wives, they have exhibited rather marked increases in the proportions reporting large families. They tend to exceed white wives in proportions childless and in proportions with 5 or more children. This holds for each age group 25 years of age and over and for each type of residence. It holds for each occupation group except the instances represented by few numbers, such as farmers in urban areas. In urban areas the proportion of nonwhite wives 35-39 years old in 1960 reporting 5 or more children extended from 9 percent for wives of professional men to 29 percent for wives of unskilled laborers. In rural nonfarm areas the proportions extended from 17 percent for wives of professional men to 51 percent for wives of unskilled laborers insofar as nonagricultural occupations were concerned. About 60 percent of the nonwhite wives of farmers and 45 percent of the nonwhite wives of farm laborers in rural nonfarm areas reported 5 or more children. In rural farm areas 60 percent of the nonwhite wives (35-39 years old) of farmers and 62 percent of the nonwhite wives of farm laborers reported 5 or more children. As already indicated, the rural farm population, white or nonwhite, is a small and diminishing proportion of the total.

The reduction of sterility from venereal infection may have been a factor in the decrease in childlessness among nonwhite women. Whatever the importance of this factor, the increase in average size of the nonwhite family has come about despite the presence of factors commonly regarded as deterrents to fertility. These are increasing urbanization, high rates of marital dissolution, and high rates of employment of women outside the home. On the other hand, the nonwhite women are of low economic status, and rates of illegitimacy have been high among them.

Parity Progression Ratios, by Occupational Class of the Husband and Age of Wife

As the term implies, the parity progression ratio is intended to indicate the extent to which women of a specific parity have progressed to the next parity. The ratios are computed from distributions of women of given age by number of children they have ever borne. The index is not strictly a ratio but a percentage. The parity progression ratio is the percentage of women ever married of parity N who had ever progressed to parity N + 1 (see Appendix A).

It will be noted that parity progression ratios are not "probabilities of birth," in that no specific time period such as 1 year is imposed. The birth probability is more refined, because it indicates the chances that a woman of N parity will proceed to N + 1 parity *within a given period of time,* commonly 1 year. In this section the parity progression ratios are presented by age of woman, but the progressions may have occurred at any prior time. However, the analysis by age introduces some control over time. Since the median age at marriage is about 20, the approximate average duration of marriage for each age group may be judged.

As expected, parity progression ratios tended to decline with increasing parity. The steepest drop is noted, however, in the comparison of the 2-to-3 ratio with the preceding 1-to-2 progression ratio. This means that the one-child family is no longer popular but the two-child family *is* one of the popular sizes.

Table 10.10 presents comparisons of the ratios among urban white married women by occupational class of the husband. Among wives 20-24 years of age, an inverse relation of the magnitude of the parity progression ratio to occupational class of the husband was apparent for each progression considered. Thus, the white wives of professional men exhibit the lowest ratios of progression and wives of unskilled and semi-skilled laborers (operatives) the highest. However, the differential by occupation in the ratios of progression from 0-to-1 and 1-to-2 parities is restricted only to the 20-24 age group and probably simply reflects the fact that women under 25 who are married to professional men have much shorter durations of marriage than do wives of unskilled laborers.

At older ages the disadvantage of late age at marriage is eliminated or greatly reduced insofar as 0-to-1 and 1-to-2 parity progressions are concerned. Among women 30 years of age and over, there was little in the way of occupational differentials in proportions of zero parity women having one child and in proportions of the one-child couples that have a second child by a given age. However, the inverse relation of occupational class to parity progression ratios became increasingly stronger in the 2-to-3, 3-to-4, and 4-to-5 progressions. In general, the data point up the fact that among women 30 years of age and over the inverse relation of family size to husband's occupational class was not appreciably accounted for by differences in proportions progressing to second parity but to variations in the progression to higher parities.

Table 10.10 Parity progression ratios—percent of women ever of given parity (N) who ever progressed to the next parity (N+1), for white women 20-49 years old, married and husband present, by age of woman and major occupation group of husband: Urban areas, 1960

Age of woman and parity progression	Total	Professional	Proprietors	Clerical	Craftsmen	Operatives	Service workers	Laborers exc. farm
20-24 years								
0 to 1	72.7	63.4	72.9	69.9	78.3	79.3	75.7	77.4
1 to 2	53.3	42.3	52.9	47.8	57.2	58.4	54.8	58.7
2 to 3	34.6	24.5	32.6	28.5	35.3	37.8	35.4	39.7
3 to 4	27.4	19.8	25.3	22.1	27.4	28.6	25.6	32.6
4 to 5	24.2	a	a	22.4	20.2	25.0	28.2	30.4
25-29 years								
0 to 1	86.8	82.9	87.6	85.5	89.4	89.8	87.5	89.0
1 to 2	76.6	71.0	77.7	74.1	79.4	79.5	77.5	80.3
2 to 3	51.9	44.9	49.1	47.4	53.8	56.1	53.0	59.0
3 to 4	39.9	30.4	35.1	35.3	40.5	44.7	39.7	51.3
4 to 5	34.6	24.6	27.8	28.8	34.0	38.8	34.7	44.3
30-34 years								
0 to 1	90.2	89.4	91.1	89.5	91.7	91.2	89.4	90.2
1 to 2	83.8	84.4	84.8	83.1	84.7	83.6	82.0	84.7
2 to 3	60.6	57.4	57.7	56.5	60.7	62.8	59.3	66.4
3 to 4	47.3	40.9	42.6	43.3	48.4	51.6	47.1	57.8
4 to 5	42.1	33.9	36.1	37.9	41.8	46.9	42.7	53.5
35-39 years								
0 to 1	89.7	89.7	91.0	89.0	90.7	90.0	88.8	89.6
1 to 2	83.4	85.5	84.7	83.2	83.1	82.8	81.2	83.8
2 to 3	59.9	59.3	58.4	56.0	60.6	61.6	59.7	64.9
3 to 4	49.9	45.1	45.5	46.1	50.9	52.8	51.4	58.7
4 to 5	46.1	38.6	39.9	42.5	45.8	51.0	49.3	58.8
40-44 years								
0 to 1	86.8	87.0	87.9	85.8	88.3	87.6	85.1	86.4
1 to 2	79.9	81.5	80.6	78.8	80.1	80.1	78.3	81.4
2 to 3	56.9	55.0	53.4	52.1	58.1	59.4	58.6	64.1
3 to 4	50.5	45.2	44.8	45.8	51.3	54.3	52.2	60.3
4 to 5	51.1	41.5	42.2	43.7	49.3	52.0	52.2	56.8
45-49 years								
0 to 1	82.3	82.5	83.2	80.4	84.0	83.8	80.4	83.5
1 to 2	75.6	76.4	75.8	72.8	76.1	76.7	74.9	79.9
2 to 3	54.5	49.0	49.2	47.9	56.2	58.7	56.0	65.7
3 to 4	50.5	41.6	43.4	43.1	51.8	54.5	53.3	62.2
4 to 5	50.6	40.5	41.4	43.2	51.7	53.0	53.0	61.9

Source: Computed from U.S. Bureau of the Census, 1960 Census of Population, Women by Number of Children Ever Born, PC(2)-3A, Table 31.

a Rate not shown where there are fewer than 4,000 women.

The proportions of women having experienced a progression from one parity to the next tended to rise with age, at least to a given age. The classifications by age, of course, are those of different women. Had they represented a cohort passing through life, the ratios would have been expected to decline with age. One would also expect a decline with age if one were dealing with *probabilities of birth* within a specific time such as 1 year. The fact that the ratios *increased* with age up to a given point simply means that women of an older age have had a longer time on the average to experience a given order of birth of a child. The fact that the 0-to-1 and 1-to-2 parity progression ratios reached a peak at about age 35 and declined at later ages probably means simply that women of older ages reflect the higher proportions of childless and one-child families that previously prevailed.

Finally, a word may be said about the trend of the fertility progression ratios during the past decade. Comparisons of those computed for urban white married women by major occupation group of the husband from the 1950 and 1960 census data appear to warrant the following generalizations:

1. For white women under 40 years of age (married and husband present) in urban and rural nonfarm areas and of given age and occupational class of husband, the 0-to-1, 1-to-2, 2-to-3, and 3-to-4 parity progression ratios tended to increase from 1950 to 1960. These increases occurred with but few exceptions, and they were substantial at young ages and low parities. The 4-to-5 parity progression ratio was rather consistently lower in 1960 than in 1950.

2. For women of the above descriptions 40-49 years of age, the 0-to-1, 1-to-2, and 2-to-3 parity progression ratios increased from 1950 to 1960. For the most part, the progression ratios of higher parities were lower in 1960 than in 1950, especially for women 45-49 years old.

Thus, although increases dominate the 1950-60 comparisons of most of the parity progression ratios, the decrease in the 4-to-5 ratio may serve to emphasize the lack of much desire for more than four children. It may also reflect the declines in fertility since 1957 and serve as an omen that these declines have been more basic than period declines in fertility.[10]

Indices of Trends of Fertility Differentials by Broad Occupational Class of the Husband, 1910-1960

As with educational attainment of the wife, two methods have been used to show trends in the fertility differentials by broad occupational class of the husband. These are (1) the *average* of the percentage deviations of the fertility rates of the seven nonagricultural occupational classes within a given age group from the base rate for the total age group, regardless of the direction of that deviation, and (2) the *relative spread* of the cumulative fertility rates by occupational class within each age group. This was obtained by expressing the fertility rate for each occupational class as a percent of the base rate for the total age group (see Chapter 9, pages 203-207).

The average deviations described under (1) above are presented for the urban and rural nonfarm white women (married and husband present) in Table 10.11. For the urban women the occupational differentials in fertility were about the same on the average in 1940 as in 1910. Probably it would be erroneous to infer from this similarity that no change occurred in the pattern of fertility differentials within the 30-year period. Indeed, it is quite possible that occupational differentials in fertility *increased* during the early part of the 1910-40 span, and decreased during the latter part of it.[11]

Table 10.11   Measure of average interclass differences in cumulative
fertility rates by major occupation group of husband for
white women, married and husband present, by residence and
age of woman: United States, 1960, 1950, 1940, and 1910

Residence and age	1960	1950[a]	1940[a]	1910[a]
URBAN				
15-19	7.7	12.8	13.3	11.1
20-24	10.6	12.7	16.8	16.3
25-29	7.7	9.6	16.0	17.7
30-34	5.3	7.4	15.2	16.3
35-39	4.1	9.5	15.2	16.2
40-44	5.5	13.5	15.0	16.7
45-49	8.9	17.1	15.1	15.7
RURAL NONFARM				
15-19	7.4	11.3	18.8	11.6
20-24	9.1	13.9	16.8	15.0
25-29	7.0	11.7	19.9	16.2
30-34	6.5	12.4	18.5	14.7
35-39	7.8	16.3	18.8	15.2
40-44	10.1	18.2	18.1	14.6
45-49	14.5	19.7	18.4	13.0

Source: Computed from U.S. Bureau of the Census, 1960 Census of
Population, Women by Number of Children Ever Born, PC(2)-3A, Table 31;
and Grabill, Kiser, and Whelpton, The Fertility of American Women,
Table 65.

[a]Data for 1950, 1940, and 1910 relate to women married once and
husband present.

Whatever may have been the trend during the 30 years from 1910 to 1940, there is no doubt that occupational differentials in fertility have narrowed sharply since 1940. Among urban white women, the 1940-50 reductions were especially marked at ages 25-39 and the 1950-60 reductions were especially marked at ages 15-19 and 35-49. For urban white women 35-39 years old the average interclass difference in fertility rate by occupational class was about 15 percent in 1940 and about 4 percent in 1960.

In 1940 and 1950 the occupational differentials in fertility tended to be wider on the average in rural nonfarm than in urban areas. In 1960 this type of difference was conspicuous only for women 40-49 years old. For women 15-29 the average fertility differentials by occupation were somewhat smaller in rural nonfarm than in urban areas.

It will be noted that the average of the percent deviations in fertility rates by occupational class of the husband ran lower than those by educational attainment of the wife. This holds true when the comparison is made for either urban or rural nonfarm areas. The average deviation, of course, is partly a function of the number of subgroups. However, the original data attest to the sharper differentials in fertility by education of the wife than by major occupation group of the husband. Possibly relevant are the previously mentioned attributes of education, that is, its amenability to quantitative expression, its stability over time, and the fact that in the present comparison education relates to the woman, who bears the children. It is also pertinent to point out that the relatively few agricultural workers residing in urban and rural nonfarm areas were eliminated in the classification by occupation but not in the classification by education of the woman. This has relevance in that agricultural workers probably are weighted by persons of relatively high fertility and low educational attainment.

The previously mentioned tendency for fertility differentials by socioeconomic status to be more pronounced among nonwhite than among white couples in 1960 is borne out by comparison of the average deviations for urban married women with husband present. In contrast to the decrease in the measures of average interclass differences in fertility for urban white women from 1950 to 1960 was the increase in these measures for urban nonwhite women at ages 25-34.

The *relative variations* in fertility rates by occupational class of the husband are shown in Figure 10.4 for urban and rural nonfarm white women. These indicate the changes in the pattern of relative variation of the seven specific nonagricultural classes in 1910, 1940, 1950, and 1960. As was the case with the average deviations, these data point up the lack of substantial change in the pattern and range of relative variations in fertility in 1940 as compared with 1910. They also point up the marked tendency toward narrowing of the range of variation after 1940. This holds for white wives in urban and rural nonfarm areas. Thus, if the fertility rate for all urban white married women 35-39 years old is expressed as 100, the range of the extreme rates for specific occupational classes is as follows: in 1940 the variation was from 80 for the professional class to 132 for the unskilled laborers, a range of 52 points. In 1950 the corresponding indices were 90 and 125, a range of 35 points. In 1960 the comparable figures were 97 and 112, a range of only 15 points.

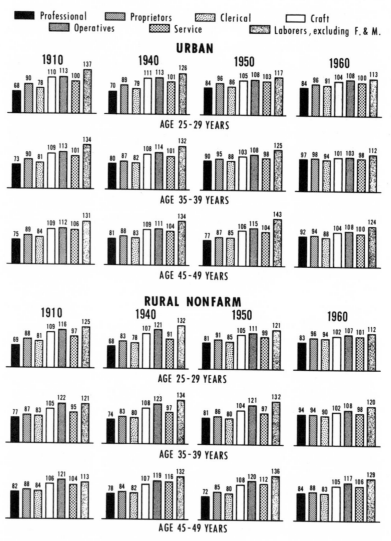

Fig. 10.4. Relative spread of cumulative fertility rates by major occupation group of husband, for white women, married and husband present, by age of woman: Urban and rural nonfarm areas, 1910, 1940, 1950, and 1960. Data for 1910 and 1940 relate to native white women. Data for 1910, 1940, and 1950 relate to women married once and husband present.

The pattern of the relative variations in fertility by occupational class was about the same in rural nonfarm as in urban areas, but in 1960 the spread of the rates tended to be a little wider in rural non-farm areas than in urban areas, especially at ages above 30.

Among urban nonwhite married women 25-34 years old, the relative variations in fertility by occupation group of the husband were somewhat wider in 1960 than in 1950.

Summary

The changes in the distribution of married women by occupational class of the husband during the decade 1950-60 reflect a continuation of the long-standing declines in proportions of unskilled laborers and agricultural workers and increases in the proportion of professional, business, and clerical workers. These changes were proportionately larger for nonwhite than for white couples during the years 1950-60, but nonwhite persons are still characterized by relatively low occupational status.

Among both white and nonwhite women, married and husband present, the average number of children ever born tended to be inversely related to occupational status of the husband. This held true for the white group despite continuation of a trend toward narrowing of occupational differentials in fertility. Among nonwhite women, in contrast, the differentials in fertility by occupation group of the husband widened during the 1950-60 decade, and this resulted in sharper differentials in fertility by occupation group among nonwhite than among white couples in 1960.

Stated in another manner, the fertility of nonwhite women as compared with that of white women was conspicuously high among wives of unskilled laborers, farmers, and farm laborers, and conspicuously low among wives of professional men. The fertility rates of nonwhite wives of school and college teachers, and of physicians, were particularly low.

The distribution of women by number of children ever born, and also the parity progression ratios by age of women, point up the popularity of the family size of 2-4 children and suggest the influence of trends and differentials in age at marriage on fertility trends and differentials. The impact of the declines in the birth rate since 1957 on trends and differentials in fertility is yet to be determined. In principle, however, it seems safe to predict a long-term trend toward further diminution of occupational differentials in fertility among white persons and an eventual similar trend among the nonwhite.

11 / Income and Other Social and Economic Factors

The two preceding chapters have dealt respectively with the relation of educational attainment of the woman and occupation group of the husband to average number of children born to women of specific age, color, residence, and so forth. The present chapter begins with a similar but briefer analysis of the relation of income of the husband during 1959 to cumulative fertility rates revealed by the 1960 census. It continues with discussion of fertility in relation to education, occupation, and income of the husband simultaneously considered, and then considers fertility in relation to employment status of women and occupation of employed women, housing conditions, and tenure and rental value of home. It concludes with a brief analysis of religion in relation to fertility, including some data from the 1957 Current Population Survey.

Husband's Income in Relation to Fertility

The relation of husband's income to number of children ever born is especially interesting. The data relate to income of the husband during 1959, the year preceding the 1960 census, and to children ever born, by age, color, and residence of women reported as "married and husband present." In the United States as a whole there tended to be a direct relation of children ever born to husband's income among white married women under 25 years old and an inverse relation among those 30 years of age and over (Table 11.1). There was virtual equality of average number of children by income of husband among women 25-29 years of age.

The inverse relation of number of children to husband's income existing among white wives 30 years of age and over tended to strengthen with increasing age of white women. It was stronger in the South as a whole than in the total United States. By type of residence, the above-described transition from direct to inverse relation of fertility of white married women to husband's income was most marked among the rural nonfarm women. The nearest approach to consistent uniformity of number of offspring by husband's income was among the white rural farm population. In the urbanized areas and the total urban areas the spread of the fertility rates by income was relatively slight for women 45-49 years of age.

Nevertheless, there was a well-defined transition from direct relation of husband's income to average number of children among the white

Table 11.1 Children ever born per 1,000 white wives with husband present by income of husband in 1959, by age of wife, and by type of residence: United States and the South, 1960

Age of wife and income of husband	United States	Urban	Rural nonfarm	Rural farm	South
20-24					
$15,000 and over	1,366	1,272	1,532	1,842	1,362
10,000 - 14,999	1,448	1,379	1,642	1,807	1,386
7,000 - 9,999	1,532	1,478	1,712	1,860	1,455
5,000 - 6,999	1,498	1,441	1,688	1,764	1,495
4,000 - 4,999	1,401	1,325	1,588	1,690	1,429
3,000 - 3,999	1,359	1,259	1,531	1,703	1,393
2,000 - 2,999	1,299	1,175	1,471	1,631	1,384
1.- 1,999 or loss	1,157	940	1,443	1,583	1,276
None	1,171	1,039	1,352	1,436	1,171
25-29					
$15,000 and over	2,191	2,116	2,392	2,801	2,182
10,000 - 14,999	2,178	2,116	2,373	2,630	2,120
7,000 - 9,999	2,226	2,183	2,376	2,614	2,131
5,000 - 6,999	2,191	2,113	2,410	2,666	2,133
4,000 - 4,999	2,150	2,031	2,371	2,653	2,110
3,000 - 3,999	2,182	2,038	2,345	2,638	2,168
2,000 - 2,999	2,212	2,014	2,401	2,554	2,288
1. - 1,999 or loss	2,247	1,921	2,562	2,527	2,443
None	2,090	1,765	2,370	2,617	2,230
30-34					
$15,000 and over	2,651	2,624	2,710	3,022	2,532
10,000 - 14,999	2,579	2,549	2,652	3,082	2,450
7,000 - 9,999	2,571	2,532	2,691	3,074	2,427
5,000 - 6,999	2,531	2,451	2,725	3,123	2,424
4,000 - 4,999	2,554	2,409	2,766	3,200	2,501
3,000 - 3,999	2,643	2,475	2,799	3,081	2,648
2,000 - 2,999	2,773	2,548	2,923	3,109	2,835
1.- 1,999 or loss	2,928	2,564	3,237	3,153	3,144
None	2,631	2,252	3,004	3,081	2,840
35-39					
$15,000 and over	2,733	2,680	2,898	3,414	2,664
10,000 - 14,999	2,601	2,559	2,721	3,088	2,496
7,000 - 9,999	2,583	2,529	2,755	3,166	2,450
5,000 - 6,999	2,576	2,473	2,833	3,270	2,499
4,000 - 4,999	2,619	2,455	2,863	3,295	2,579
3,000 - 3,999	2,755	2,512	3,002	3,286	2,804
2,000 - 2,999	2,947	2,620	3,207	3,277	3,070
1.- 1,999 or loss	3,097	2,671	3,486	3,281	3,367
None	2,905	2,368	3,434	3,450	3,166

Source: U.S. Bureau of the Census, 1960 Census of Population, Women by Number of Children Ever Born, PC(2)-3A, Table 37.

married women under 25 years old to inverse relation among those 30-49 years old. This transition from direct to inverse relation was generally more prominent for white than for nonwhite couples. The inverse relation of fertility to husband's income is the outstanding one among nonwhite wives, even at ages 20-24 and 25-29 (Table 11.2). However, among nonwhite as well as white wives, the differentials in fertility by husband's income were wider in the South as a whole than in the United States as a whole. Among the nonwhite women as among the white women, the differentials in fertility by income were also wider in the rural nonfarm than in the rural farm or urban areas.

It is not possible to give a good interpretation of the dual relation of fertility to income among white couples. It is well to keep in mind, however, that the above-described transition with age related to different cohorts—not to a single cohort passing through time.

It is possible that the direct relation observed for the younger cohorts is a harbinger of the same type of relation for the future even at older ages. If this is the case, the inverse relation observed at the older ages might be interpreted as the passing vestige of a former era. A closely related possibility is that current fertility of young women is more likely to be positively related with current income than is the total past fertility of long duration of marriage.

The direct relation of fertility to income or other measures of socioeconomic status has been found under various sets of conditions. It was found among completely planned families in the Indianapolis Study.[1] In the Princeton Fertility Study the proportion of two-child families having a third child or pregnancy within 3 years after the birth of the second child was directly associated with socioeconomic status among Catholic and Jewish couples but not among Protestant couples.[2] Deborah Freedman found that "An income which is above the average for one's status [that is, above the average income for the husband's occupational status and age] is associated with more children, but being in a higher absolute income means fewer children if the higher income is only what is usual for the husband's age and occupational status."[3]

It may well be, however, that the direct relation of fertility to income in the younger ages may simply reflect a greater tendency for the high-income than for the low-income people to concentrate their childbearing within the first decade of married life. If this is the case, it could account for much of the transition with age from direct to inverse relation of fertility to income.

Table 11.2   Children ever born per 1,000 nonwhite wives with husband
present, by income of husband in 1959, by age of wife, and
by type of residence: United States and the South, 1960

Age of wife and income of husband	United States	Urban	Rural nonfarm	Rural farm	South
20-24					
$15,000 and over	a	a	a	a	a
10,000 - 14,999	a	a	a	a	a
7,000 - 9,999	1,691	1,643	a	a	a
5,000 - 6,999	1,925	1,876	2,677	a	2,056
4,000 - 4,999	1,919	1,893	2,201	a	2,129
3,000 - 3,999	1,962	1,907	2,366	a	2,203
2,000 - 2,999	2,054	1,983	2,310	2,551	2,213
1. - 1,999 or loss	2,162	1,890	2,415	2,790	2,305
None	1,754	1,526	2,618	a	1,910
25-29					
$15,000 and over	a	a	a	a	a
10,000 - 14,999	2,155	2,038	a	a	a
7,000 - 9,999	2,251	2,222	2,659	a	2,479
5,000 - 6,999	2,426	2,395	2,812	a	2,558
4,000 - 4,999	2,623	2,581	2,981	a	2,849
3,000 - 3,999	2,691	2,626	3,062	3,450	2,855
2,000 - 2,999	2,995	2,827	3,521	3,606	3,214
1. - 1,999 or loss	3,250	2,746	3,719	4,052	3,451
None	2,785	2,268	3,579	3,918	3,228
30-34					
$15,000 and over	2,741	2,823	a	a	a
10,000 - 14,999	2,599	2,561	a	a	a
7,000 - 9,999	2,767	2,713	3,216	a	2,935
5,000 - 6,999	2,823	2,765	3,540	a	2,974
4,000 - 4,999	2,950	2,897	3,448	a	3,147
3,000 - 3,999	3,078	2,947	3,750	4,555	3,394
2,000 - 2,999	3,442	3,162	4,274	4,896	3,705
1. - 1,999 or loss	4,044	3,175	4,680	5,404	4,364
None	3,469	2,656	4,514	5,817	4,197
35-39					
$15,000 and over	2,673	2,446	a	a	a
10,000 - 14,999	2,425	2,272	a	a	a
7,000 - 9,999	2,830	2,760	3,608	a	3,214
5,000 - 6,999	2,803	2,727	3,600	a	3,065
4,000 - 4,999	2,846	2,733	3,964	a	3,128
3,000 - 3,999	3,099	2,928	3,968	5,172	3,462
2,000 - 2,999	3,408	3,044	4,489	4,967	3,728
1. - 1,999 or loss	4,195	2,989	4,843	5,995	4,527
None	3,472	2,476	4,765	5,737	4,247

Source: U.S. Bureau of the Census, 1960 Census of Population,
Women by Number of Children Ever Born, PC(2)-3A, Table 37.

[a]Rate not shown where base is less than 1,000.

According to the Current Population Survey of 1964, there was a rather marked inverse relation of the number of children ever born per 1,000 women 15-44 years old standardized for age, married and husband present, to family income during the 12 months preceding the survey. The rates extended from 2,075 for families reporting $10,000 and over to 3,323 for those reporting under $2,000.[4]

Fertility According to Multiple Indices of Socioeconomic Status

The special fertility tabulations of 1960 census data included one on number of children ever born among married women (married once and husband present) according to color, age, and age at marriage of the wife and three simultaneously considered socioeconomic attributes of the husband (occupational class, educational attainment, and his income during 1959). Some of those data are presented in Table 11.3. These women are divided into two age groups (35-44 and 45-54), and in each case into two age-at-marriage groups (14-21 and 22 and over).

First may be noted the nature of the *variations in fertility by income of the husband within groups of specific occupational and educational status.* It was stated in the previous section that the relation of fertility to husband's income tended to be direct, or positive, for white women under 25 years of age, virtually absent for those 25-29, and indirect, or inverse, for those aged 30 and over. However, Table 11.3 is not concerned with women under 35 years of age but only with those 35-44 and 45-54. Thus the present analysis is concerned with age groups in which there were rather strong *inverse* relations of fertility to husband's income considered alone. Nevertheless, the *analysis within groups of specific occupational and educational classes of the husbands and specific age at marriage of the wife* frequently yielded the direct relation of fertility of wife to income of the husband.

The most critical factor appeared to be age at marriage. Among women marrying at ages 22 or over and whose husbands were of given occupational and educational attainment, the relation of number of children ever born to husband's income was predominantly positive. This held within urbanized, other urban, rural nonfarm, and rural farm areas. It held for women 35-44 and 45-54 years of age (Table 11.3). For women marrying at ages 14-21, the relatively few cases of positive relation were mainly those of women whose husbands were of college attainment, in white-collar occupations, and residing in

Table 11.3 Multiple social and economic characteristics in relation to children ever born per 1,000 white women, married once, husband present, of specified age and age at marriage of the woman and by occupation, education, and 1959 income of the husband: Urbanized areas, 1960

Occupation, education and income in 1959 of the husband	Wives aged 35-44		Wives aged 45-54	
	Married at 14-21	Married at 22+	Married at 14-21	Married at 22+
Professional, technical, and kindred workers				
College: 1+				
$10,000+	2,694	2,551	2,140	2,018
7,000 - 9,999	2,645	2,239	2,064	1,658
4,000 - 6,999	2,469	2,031	2,125	1,639
2,000 - 3,999	2,412	1,925	2,135	1,594
Under 2,000	2,571	1,753	a	1,668
High school: 1-4				
$10,000+	2,530	2,180	2,133	1,814
7,000 - 9,999	2,583	2,232	2,170	1,633
4,000 - 6,999	2,531	1,951	2,290	1,526
2,000 - 3,999	2,688	1,763	2,294	1,299
Under 2,000	a	2,029	a	1,172
No high school				
$10,000+	a	a	2,373	1,856
7,000 - 9,999	2,598	2,008	2,270	1,551
4,000 - 6,999	2,700	2,104	2,434	1,696
Managers, officials, and proprietors, exc. farm				
College: 1+				
$10,000+	2,702	2,468	2,185	1,976
7,000 - 9,999	2,602	2,269	2,143	1,769
4,000 - 6,999	2,457	2,088	2,214	1,640
2,000 - 3,999	2,603	1,962	2,046	1,561
Under 2,000	2,593	2,061	2,229	1,604
High school: 1-4				
$10,000+	2,642	2,292	2,118	1,771
7,000 - 9,999	2,597	2,232	2,155	1,729
4,000 - 6,999	2,554	2,036	2,278	1,571
2,000 - 3,999	2,448	1,734	2,299	1,528
Under 2,000	2,472	1,804	2,134	1,638
No high school				
$10,000+	2,590	2,121	2,492	1,888
7,000 - 9,999	2,749	2,066	2,512	1,853
4,000 - 6,999	2,697	2,017	2,528	1,764
2,000 - 3,999	2,370	2,116	2,600	1,602
Under 2,000	2,770	1,820	2,879	1,311

(Continued)

Table 11.3 Multiple social and economic characteristics in
(continued) relation to children ever born per 1,000 white women,
married once, husband present, of specified age and
age at marriage of the woman and by occupation,
education, and 1959 income of the husband: Urbanized
areas, 1960

Occupation, education and income in 1959 of the husband	Wives aged 35-44		Wives aged 45-54	
	Married at 14-21	Married at 22+	Married at 14-21	Married at 22+
Clerical, sales, and kindred workers				
College : 1+				
$10,000+	2,761	2,469	2,205	1,882
7,000 - 9,999	2,580	2,304	2,083	1,683
4,000 - 6,999	2,512	2,054	2,087	1,560
2,000 - 3,999	2,206	1,740	2,075	1,245
Under 2,000	2,365	1,810	a	1,496
High school: 1-4				
$10,000+	2,519	2,298	2,161	1,662
7,000 - 9,999	2,540	2,269	2,045	1,679
4,000 - 6,999	2,504	2,003	2,253	1,585
2,000 - 3,999	2,514	1,660	2,308	1,397
Under 2,000	2,553	1,699	2,114	1,333
No high school				
$10,000+	2,944	2,341	2,114	1,668
7,000 - 9,999	2,642	2,043	2,391	1,644
4,000 - 6,999	2,553	2,028	2,394	1,616
2,000 - 3,999	2,665	1,853	2,565	1,478
Under 2,000	2,960	1,595	2,641	1,352
Craftsmen, foremen, and kindred workers				
College : 1+				
$10,000+	2,858	2,524	2,069	2,050
7,000 - 9,999	2,520	2,298	2,395	1,812
4,000 - 6,999	2,598	2,072	2,363	1,644
2,000 - 3,999	2,501	1,843	2,560	1,309
High school: 1-4				
$10,000+	2,732	2,311	2,251	1,817
7,000 - 9,999	2,711	2,324	2,443	1,820
4,000 - 6,999	2,682	2,108	2,588	1,747
2,000 - 3,999	2,764	1,841	2,850	1,615
Under 2,000	2,646	1,673	2,442	1,471
No high school				
$10,000+	2,839	2,418	2,587	1,861
7,000 - 9,999	2,793	2,223	2,703	1,865
4,000 - 6,999	2,891	2,083	2,771	1,785
2,000 - 3,999	3,308	2,061	3,144	1,809
Under 2,000	3,468	2,015	3,289	1,826

(Continued)

Table 11.3   Multiple social and economic characteristics in
(continued)   relation to children ever born per 1,000 white women,
married once, husband present, of specified age and
age at marriage of the woman and by occupation,
education, and 1959 income of the husband: Urbanized
areas, 1960

Occupation, education and income in 1959 of the husband	Wives aged 35-44		Wives aged 45-54	
	Married at 14-21	Married at 22+	Married at 14-21	Married at 22+
Operatives and kindred workers				
College : 1+				
$10,000+	2,475	2,339	a	2,091
7,000 - 9,999	2,885	2,307	2,825	1,838
4,000 - 6,999	2,766	2,115	2,559	1,776
2,000 - 3,999	2,839	1,351	a	1,388
High school: 1-4				
$10,000+	2,841	2,380	2,535	1,924
7,000 - 9,999	2,823	2,286	2,626	1,900
4,000 - 6,999	2,705	2,085	2,568	1,753
2,000 - 3,999	2,827	1,823	2,687	1,553
Under 2,000	3,153	1,373	2,889	1,800
No high school				
$10,000+	2,982	2,284	2,639	1,616
7,000 - 9,999	2,910	2,273	2,624	1,929
4,000 - 6,999	2,990	2,049	2,843	1,829
2,000 - 3,999	3,275	2,058	3,108	1,812
Under 2,000	3,627	2,079	3,313	1,838
Laborers, except farm and mine				
College: 1+				
$4,000 - 6,999	a	2,122	a	1,808
High school: 1-4				
$7,000 - 9,999	3,098	2,418	2,469	1,619
4,000 - 6,999	2,837	2,077	2,713	1,727
2,000 - 3,999	3,172	1,995	3,183	1,794
Under 2,000	3,326	a	a	a
No high school				
$7,000 - 9,999	2,860	2,551	3,201	2,209
4,000 - 6,999	3,363	2,117	3,282	1,932
2,000 - 3,999	3,631	2,315	3,731	2,277
Under 2,000	4,248	2,499	4,699	2,447

Source: U.S. Bureau of the Census, 1960 Census of Population,
Women by Number of Children Ever Born, PC(2)-3A, Table 39.

[a] Rate not shown where base is less than 1,000.

urban areas. Among women marrying at ages 22 and over, the direct relation of wife's fertility to husband's income tended to hold within each type of residence, but it was sharpest and most consistent in the urbanized and other urban areas and least common in the rural farm areas.

As for *the relation of education to fertility within groups of similar occupational and income status,* much again depends upon age at marriage of the wife. Among wives marrying at ages 14-21 the relation of education to fertility tended to be inverse. The few cases of direct relation of education to fertility were mainly those involving the higher occupational and income groups within urbanized and other urban areas.

Cases of direct or mixed relation of education to fertility were considerably more in evidence for women marrying at ages 22 or older than for those marrying at younger ages. The direct relation of education to fertility was predominant within the professional, proprietary, and clerical classes at either of the two top income classes. It tended to be more frequent in the urbanized and other urban areas than in the rural areas.

The *relation of occupational class to fertility within groups of specific educational and income levels* similarly was much influenced by age at marriage. Among women who had married at ages 14-21, the inverse relation of fertility to occupational class was predominant. However, this inverse relation tended to be slight or incomplete within urbanized and other urban areas. It tended to be sharp in rural nonfarm areas. Among women who married at ages 22 and older, there were suggestions of slight positive relations of fertility to occupational class of husbands within groups of upper educational and income status. In other urban areas the relation of occupational class to fertility tended to be mixed.

In summary, the analysis of fertility rates among white married women 35-54 years of age according to their age at marriage and according to the three simultaneously considered indicators of socioeconomic status of the husband appears to warrant the following statements: The direct relation of fertility to one indicator of socioeconomic status within groups specific with reference to the two other indicators of socioeconomic status was more frequently found among women of late than of early age at marriage, more frequently found among urban than among rural women, and more frequently found when the groups considered were of high than of low socioeconomic status according to the other two indicators. The ranking of the three indicators of socioeconomic status according to frequency with which it was directly associated with fertility when the remaining two indicators were controlled is as follows: income, education, and occupation.

The findings above are consistent with some mentioned earlier. In the preceding chapter it was noted that the relation of wife's fertility to husband's education was *direct* among women who completed college and *inverse* among women whose formal education was limited to elementary school or lower. Women college graduates perforce tend to marry rather late and doubtless also tend to be adept at family planning. This is mentioned because various studies have indicated a direct relation of fertility to socioeconomic status among completely planned families.

Finally, it may be noted that two of the earliest studies of differential fertility, one relating to the English census of 1911 and one relating to 1910 census of the United States, indicated a direct relation of fertility to socioeconomic status among women who married late.[5]

It should also be noted that age at marriage is an important determinant of differentials in fertility by color among women of given age, married once and husband present, and whose husbands were of given occupation group. Thus, among women 35-44 years of age whose husbands were in one of the three broad white-collar classes (professional, proprietary, clerical) or in the "service worker" class, the average number of children ever born *was larger for nonwhite than for white women if the wife was under 22 at marriage. The fertility rate was smaller for nonwhite than for white women if the wife was 22 or over at the time of marriage.* Within the other occupation groups (craft, operatives, laborers, and farmers and farm laborers) the fertility rate for nonwhite women exceeded that for white women regardless of the wife's age at marriage. However, the percent excess was consistently much lower for the wives marrying relatively late. Also among the relatively few cases of high income and high education, but of manual worker or agricultural status, the fertility of the nonwhite women tended to fall below that of white women of corresponding status if the wife was 22 or over at marriage, but not if she married at a younger age (see Table 11.4).

Table 11.4 Percent excess of average number of children ever born to nonwhite women over that of white women, married once and husband present, by age at marriage of woman and by occupation group, education, and income (1959) of the husband, for women 35-44: United States and urban areas, 1960

Area, education and income of the husband	Wives married at age 14-21								Wives married at age 22 and over							
	Profes-sionals	Propri-etors	Cleri-cals	Crafts-men	Opera-tives	Service workers	Laborers except farm & mine	Farmers and farm laborers	Profes-sionals	Propri-etors	Cleri-cals	Crafts-men	Opera-tives	Service workers	Laborers except farm & mine	Farmers and farm laborers
UNITED STATES																
Total	12.2	25.5	22.2	32.5	29.3	24.2	27.3	79.1	-18.0	-10.0	-7.0	0.9	8.5	-6.0	13.1	32.4
College: 1+	0.4	-1.5	5.2	18.7	19.0	10.6	a	a	-20.3	-13.4	-16.9	-10.1	-15.0	-4.9	-1.4	a
$10,000+	a	a	a	a	a	a	a	a	-17.8	a	a	a	a	a	a	a
7,000 - 9,999	-9.3	a	a	a	a	a	a	a	-7.1	a	a	a	a	a	a	a
4,000 - 6,999	5.3	a	11.5	a	20.5	a	a	a	-21.1	0.2	-16.2	-3.4	-12.5	-6.3	a	a
2,000 - 3,999	a	a	a	a	a	a	a	a	-12.3	a	a	a	a	a	a	a
High school: 1-4	27.0	22.0	16.5	24.8	23.9	19.8	31.0	61.6	-13.4	-9.8	-5.8	-2.7	-4.5	-10.0	0.2	9.7
$7,000 - 9,999	a	a	a	10.2	28.3	a	a	a	a	a	a	-13.1	-2.0	a	a	a
4,000 - 6,999	a	16.6	10.6	25.4	21.4	10.2	18.6	a	-10.9	-1.6	-3.7	0.4	-6.4	-5.4	-1.5	a
2,000 - 3,999	a	a	21.9	20.9	21.4	25.0	37.4	a	a	a	12.2	8.2	3.5	-2.3	-7.0	a
1- 1,999 or loss	a	a	a	42.0	26.3	11.8	35.4	96.9	a	a	a	a	12.8	22.3	54.2	13.5
No high school	a	35.7	38.6	31.2	26.1	22.2	21.9	67.5	a	-1.7	8.3	6.3	16.6	-1.1	15.5	41.5
$7,000 - 9,999	a	a	a	a	24.9	a	a	a	a	a	a	a	-15.1	a	a	a
4,000 - 6,999	a	a	38.9	21.5	14.5	36.2	17.6	49.1	a	a	-8.9	1.6	6.2	-1.6	9.6	33.5
2,000 - 3,999	a	51.7	34.3	22.3	20.9	15.4	11.6	63.2	a	-11.8	30.5	5.5	17.1	1.1	10.1	10.1
1- 1,999 or loss	a	a	a	28.6	21.3	4.0	22.1	66.4	a	a	a	25.5	30.0	5.9	12.4	45.7
URBAN																
Total	11.8	19.2	19.0	26.4	24.3	21.5	21.9	14.0	-18.6	-9.7	-6.8	-2.3	4.1	-8.5	4.8	-0.8
College: 1+	0.0	-2.6	6.6	18.5	21.3	12.2	a	a	-20.1	-11.9	-17.7	-7.7	-12.8	-7.7	-1.8	a
$10,000+	a	a	a	a	a	a	a	a	-18.1	a	a	a	a	a	a	a
7,000 - 9,999	-7.3	a	a	a	a	a	a	a	-6.3	a	a	a	a	a	a	a
4,000 - 6,999	4.3	a	13.3	a	21.3	a	a	a	-19.7	2.8	-17.1	0.0	-10.4	-7.8	a	a
2,000 - 3,999	a	a	a	a	a	a	a	a	-13.2	a	a	a	a	a	a	a
High school: 1-4	21.9	21.2	14.9	22.6	22.5	19.3	29.9	19.0	-19.4	-10.1	-4.9	-4.8	-4.9	-11.2	-3.9	10.6
$7,000 - 9,999	a	a	a	16.1	28.9	a	a	a	a	a	a	-10.8	-4.5	a	a	a
4,000 - 6,999	a	20.2	13.7	26.7	21.6	10.9	22.2	a	-15.5	0.7	-2.3	0.7	-5.8	-7.4	1.1	a
2,000 - 3,999	a	a	16.8	17.7	21.9	25.3	35.3	a	a	a	14.7	5.8	6.8	-0.4	-12.7	a
1- 1,999 or loss	a	a	a	24.4	15.9	22.9	24.6	a	a	a	a	a	35.8	41.5	41.5	a
No high school	a	26.5	34.7	24.4	21.1	20.9	15.3	1.7	a	0.4	9.9	2.0	11.8	-4.2	6.7	-16.3
$7,000 - 9,999	a	a	a	a	29.3	a	a	a	a	a	a	a	-19.9	a	a	a
4,000 - 6,999	a	a	40.4	24.2	18.7	38.6	18.3	a	a	a	-9.0	1.4	8.5	-1.9	8.7	a
2,000 - 3,999	a	a	26.7	10.5	17.2	17.5	7.1	-9.7	a	a	38.9	6.0	17.6	-2.1	3.7	a
1- 1,999 or loss	a	a	a	12.3	7.2	-15.1	9.7	-2.5	a	a	a	23.3	12.6	1.6	-5.5	a

Source: Computed from U. S. Bureau of the Census, 1960 Census of Population, Women by Number of Children Ever Born, PC(2)-3A, Tables 39, 40.

aPercent excess not shown where there are fewer than 1,000 nonwhite women.

Labor Force Status of Women and Occupation of Employed Women
According to definitions used in the 1960 census, the labor force consists of employed and unemployed civilians 14 years of age and over and members of the Armed Forces. The employed persons are those reporting that they were at work or with a job but not at work during the week preceding enumeration. The latter had a job or business from which they were temporarily absent because of bad weather, industrial dispute, vacation, illness or other personal reasons. The unemployed were persons not at work but looking for work. Persons who were neither employed nor unemployed (not at work, not with a job or business, and not looking for work) were classified as not in labor force.

There were notable increases from 1950 to 1960 in the proportion of white women in the labor force, particularly among the ever-married women in the latter half of the childbearing ages. Thus, among white ever-married women 45-49 years old, the proportion in the labor force was 29 percent in 1950 and 44 percent in 1960 (Table 11.5). The proportion of nonwhite women in the labor force was higher than that for white women of comparable age and marital status in both 1950 and 1960, but the increases during the decade were much smaller for nonwhite than for white women.

Table 11.5 Percentage of women in the labor force, by age, color, and marital status: United States, 1960 and 1950

| Age of woman | White | | | | Nonwhite | | | |
| | All marital classes | | Ever married | | All marital classes | | Ever married | |
	1960	1950	1960	1950	1960	1950	1960	1950
15-19	28.7	27.1	28.2	22.0	19.8	20.9	25.4	20.8
20-24	44.8	42.8	33.1	27.6	45.7	38.9	37.8	30.7
25-29	33.3	30.6	28.1	23.0	46.7	42.7	42.9	38.8
30-34	33.5	28.2	30.2	23.1	50.4	46.6	48.5	44.6
35-39	38.4	31.2	35.8	27.0	54.1	47.8	52.9	46.4
40-44	43.9	33.9	41.7	30.0	57.2	47.6	56.5	46.6
45-49	46.4	32.5	44.2	28.8	56.5	45.2	55.8	44.5

Source: Derived from U. S. Bureau of the Census, 1960 Census of Population, Women by Number of Children Ever Born, PC(2)-3A, Table 30, and Grabill, Kiser, and Whelpton, The Fertility of American Women, Table 94.

The tabulations of children ever born to women in the 1960 census according to labor force status of the women are provided in some detail. The employed women are subdivided into full-time workers and part-time workers on the basis of number of hours they worked during the week preceding enumeration. Those working 35 hours or more were considered as full-time and those working less than 35 hours were considered as part-time. The unemployed constituted a third group of women in the labor force for whom the tabulations were made.

The women not in the labor force were divided into four groups on the basis of year of last employment: 1959-60, 1955-58, 1954 or earlier, and "never worked."

Be it selective or determinative or both, the relation of labor force status to the fertility of ever-married women is very strong. Johnson reported labor force status to be one of the chief factors related to fertility in Europe.[6]

When the comparisons are made for the simple dichotomy it may be categorically stated that fertility rates were consistently lower for women in the labor force than for those not in the labor force. This held for white and nonwhite women and for total and ever-married women of all ages and in each type of residence in the United States in 1960. Similar relations have been reported for earlier census data and from other studies for the United States and other countries. The excess fertility of the women not in the labor force over that of women in the labor force tended to be greater for the white than for the nonwhite women. For both white and nonwhite women it tended to be larger for all women than for ever-married women because single women are more likely to be in the labor force than married women. The foregoing statement holds despite the fact that widowed and divorced women of working age are also more likely to be in the labor force than currently married women of similar age.

The relation of fertility to the more detailed subdivisions of labor force status differs somewhat by age of woman. However, the following statements may be made. The women reported as full-time workers were sharply and with almost complete consistency characterized by lowest average number of children ever born and by highest proportions childless. Also, the women 30 years of age and over who were not in the labor force and had never worked were rather sharply and consistently characterized by highest average number of children ever born and by relatively low proportions childless. However, at ages under 30 the highest fertility rates tended to be those for the women who were not in the labor force but had worked in 1954 or earlier (Table 11.6 and Fig. 11.1). Probably a selective factor is involved. Among women under 30 who had not worked for 6 years or more, many undoubtedly dropped out of the labor force *because* of the coming of children.

Table 11.6   Children ever born per 1,000 women and ever-married women and percent childless among ever-married women, of selected ages, by color and employment status of the woman: United States, 1960

Age of woman and employment status	White			Nonwhite		
	Children ever born per 1,000		Percent childless among ever-married women	Children ever born per 1,000		Percent childless among ever-married women
	Total women	Ever-married women		Total women	Ever-married women	
25-29						
Labor force	1,160	1,524	29.4	1,684	2,179	22.1
Employed	1,132	1,498	30.0	1,648	2,144	22.6
Worked 35+ hours	960	1,337	35.1	1,439	1,935	25.0
Worked under 35 hours	1,664	1,907	16.9	2,130	2,579	17.6
Unemployed	1,670	1,938	19.5	2,032	2,493	17.9
Not in labor force	2,360	2,424	5.7	2,902	3,216	8.8
Last worked 1959-60	1,862	1,920	13.9	2,772	3,078	10.7
Last worked 1955-58	2,102	2,118	4.6	2,666	2,869	7.7
Last worked 1954 or earlier	2,783	2,802	2.0	3,314	3,537	6.1
Never worked	2,569	2,806	5.2	2,893	3,314	9.6
35-39						
Labor force	1,880	2,145	16.5	2,277	2,519	24.1
Employed	1,863	2,129	16.6	2,261	2,502	24.2
Worked 35+ hours	1,678	1,985	19.8	2,015	2,261	26.0
Worked under 35 hours	2,332	2,454	9.5	2,759	2,970	20.8
Unemployed	2,258	2,448	13.8	2,475	2,727	22.3
Not in labor force	2,839	2,893	6.8	3,640	3,833	13.9
Last worked 1959-60	2,543	2,592	10.7	3,819	4,010	14.8
Last worked 1955-58	2,401	2,429	11.1	3,161	3,306	14.7
Last worked 1954 or earlier	2,878	2,899	5.0	3,513	3,648	12.7
Never worked	3,216	3,391	6.0	3,853	4,141	14.2
45-49						
Labor force	1,817	2,042	20.4	2,239	2,408	30.4
Employed	1,802	2,027	20.5	2,226	2,395	30.6
Worked 35+ hours	1,692	1,944	22.5	2,026	2,206	32.1
Worked under 35 hours	2,112	2,245	15.5	2,556	2,698	28.2
Unemployed	2,197	2,364	18.1	2,440	2,594	27.9
Not in labor force	2,532	2,602	14.5	3,201	3,336	22.7
Last worked 1959-60	2,409	2,471	16.4	3,560	3,664	21.2
Last worked 1955-58	2,163	2,207	19.7	2,799	2,898	24.9
Last worked 1954 or earlier	2,316	2,356	15.1	2,727	2,840	25.0
Never worked	3,026	3,168	11.3	3,654	3,854	20.2

Source: U.S. Bureau of the Census, 1960 Census of Population, Women by Number of Children Ever Born, PC(2)-3A, Table 30.

Three groups, two of which were in the labor force and one of which was not, tended to exhibit fairly similar levels of fertility. These were the part-time workers, the unemployed, and those not in labor force who had last worked in 1959-60. The unemployed tended to fall between the other two classes with respect to fertility: they tended to have higher fertility than the part-time workers and

lower fertility than those who were not in the labor force at the ti
of the 1960 census but had last worked in 1959 or 1960. These th
groups also tended to exhibit similar patterns of childlessness.

Among the ever-married women who were not in the labor for
those who had last worked in 1955-58 tended to exhibit lowest fe
ity rates and those who had never worked tended to exhibit high
fertility rates.

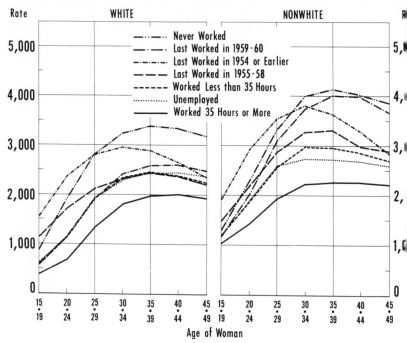

Fig. 11.1. Number of children ever born per 1,000 ever-married white and n
white women 15-49 years old, by employment status and age of woman: Uni
States, 1960.

When fertility rates for a simple two-fold division of ever-marri
women in the labor force were compared, the rates were consisten
higher for the unemployed than for the employed. This held true
all ages, for both white and nonwhite women, and in each type
residence. However, the fertility rates for unemployed women we
much lower than those of women not in the labor force. It see
likely that the higher fertility rates for the unemployed than for t
employed women of the labor force may be due partly to their bei
of lower socioeconomic status and partly to the greater difficulty
finding work if one has one or more young children.

Broad Occupation Groups of Employed Women. The excess of the fertility of nonwhite ever-married women over that of their white counterparts is especially large for employed women at young ages. This appears to be due largely to the greater concentration of the employed nonwhite ever-married women in the manual working classes, where fertility rates are high. When the fertility rates for employed women of given age and broad occupational class are compared, the differences by color are fairly narrow except among professional women, in which case the fertility of nonwhite women is much lower than that of white women, and among farmers and farm laborers, in which case the excess fertility of the nonwhite women is considerable (Table 11.7).

Table 11.7 Occupation of ever-married employed women in relation to number of children ever born per 1,000 white and nonwhite women of specified ages: United States, 1960

Occupation of employed woman	White		Nonwhite	
	35–44	45–54	35–44	45–54
Professional, technical, and kindred workers	1,973	1,702	1,627	1,308
Mgrs., off., and proprietors, exc. farm	1,879	1,733	1,897	2,018
Clerical and kindred workers	1,787	1,595	1,747	1,606
Sales workers	2,206	1,997	2,111	1,970
Craftsmen, foremen, and kindred workers	1,959	1,838	1,884	1,968
Operatives and kindred workers	2,309	2,307	2,161	2,156
Service workers, exc. private household	2,545	2,544	2,567	2,355
Private household workers, total	2,836	2,846	2,864	2,546
Private household workers, living in	1,817	1,931	1,352	1,697
Private household workers, living out	2,906	2,956	2,913	2,579
Laborers, except farm and mine	2,496	2,585	2,584	2,181
Farmers and farm managers	3,017	2,841	5,296	5,153
Farm laborers and foremen	3,165	3,086	5,001	4,436

Source: U. S. Bureau of the Census, 1960 Census of Population, *Women by Number of Children Ever Born*, PC(2)-3A, Tables 35 and 36.

It will be noted that among ever-married professional women 35-44 and 45-54 years of age, the fertility rates of the nonwhite were considerably lower than those of the white women. For women 35-44, the nonwhite rates were somewhat lower within the clerical, sales worker, craft, and operative classes. They were somewhat higher for nonwhite than for white women within the proprietary, service worker, and unskilled laborer (except farm) classes. At ages 45-54 the fertility of nonwhite employed ever-married women exceeded that of white employed ever-married women in the proprietary, clerical, and craft classes. The rates for nonwhite farmers and farm laborers

were much higher than those for white agricultural workers in e
of the two age groups considered (Table 11.7).

Specific Occupation of Employed Women. The fertility rates
employed women of specific occupational classes are of inter
Among ever-married white employed professional women 35
years of age, the cumulative fertility rates were relatively low for
social scientists; accountants and auditors; designers and draftsm
college presidents and professors; and lawyers and judges. They w
relatively high for authors, editors, and reporters; teachers of elem
tary school; registered nurses; and musicians and music teachers. "
variety of professional occupations in which women were emplo
in sufficient numbers to be represented in the fertility tabulati
was narrower for the nonwhite than for the white women. Howe
among nonwhite professional women, fertility rates were relativ
low for teachers and relatively high for professional nurses
medical and dental technicians. (See source note, Table 11.7.)

Among both white and nonwhite married women 35-44 years
employed as proprietors and managers and officials, those descri
as "salaried" exhibited higher fertility rates than those described
"self-employed."

Among the employed white married women 35-44 and 45-54 ye
old in the "clerical and kindred worker" class, the lowest ferti
rates were for secretaries and stenographers and the highest for t
ists and cashiers. Since 10 year age spans are utilized, it may be t
the secretaries and stenographers were younger than the typists
cashiers. Also, it is possible that since the occupation of cashiers r
require less skill than those of secretaries and typists, the forr
occupational group may have a larger representation of mature wor
who re-enter employment after having their children. On the ot
hand, it must be admitted that the differences among those repor
in the census as secretaries, stenographers, and typists are not at
clear. Thus the number of white married employed women 35
years old reported as secretaries (258,869) was over six times as la
as the number reported as stenographers (42,020) and over th
times as large as the number of typists (73,581). Among the nonwl
married women employed in the clerical class, the lowest ferti
rate was the one for stenographers in the 35-44 age group and
secretaries in the 45-54 group. In both age groups, as with the wl
women, the nonwhite cashiers exhibited the highest fertility rate.

white and nonwhite employed women of both age groups, the fertility rate of the sales workers was higher than that of the clerical and kindred workers (exclusive of sales workers).

Within the broad group of craftsmen, fertility rates are shown only for foremen and other craftsmen. The fertility rates were relatively low for the women employed as foremen.

Within the group of white female operatives, that is, semi-skilled workers, of both age groups the lowest fertility rates were those for checkers, examiners, and inspectors, and assemblers, while the highest were for textile spinners and weavers, and operatives in laundry and dry cleaning. The above holds for nonwhite women, too, except for the substitution of "operatives, NEC" for textile spinners and weavers. The fact that textile spinning and weaving is concentrated largely in the South and that textile trades in the South have in the past been virtually closed to Negroes may account at once for the relatively high fertility rate of white female textile workers and the absence of its representation in the data for nonwhite women. It should be emphasized that the fertility rate for white textile workers was high only with reference to that for other semi-skilled workers. Among the white female textile employees, the average number of children ever born was only 2.5 per married woman for those aged 35-44 and 2.8 per married woman for those aged 45-54. The employment of women in textiles is a frequently used illustration of a type of employment conducive to spread of knowledge of family limitation in that the women employees have an opportunity to talk despite the hum of the spinning frames or the clatter of the looms.

The service workers are divided into two main categories—those working in private households and those working elsewhere. As a group, those working in private households consistently had higher fertility than the others. The private household workers in turn are subdivided into two groups on the basis of whether they "live in." The relatively small group of private household workers who "live in" was consistently characterized by quite low fertility. This probably was due largely to selection. Only those without children or without young children are likely to "live in" with their employers.

Among service workers not working for private households, relatively low fertility rates are found for hairdressers and cosmetologists, and housekeepers and stewardesses. Relatively high fertility rates are found for charwomen, attendants in hospitals, and cooks, among white and nonwhite women of both age groups.

Housing Characteristics

The characteristics of housing available for studies in relation to average number of children ever born as reported in the 1960 census include tenure of home, value of owned home and gross monthly rent of rented homes, condition of housing unit and plumbing facilities, and number of rooms. The data are presented in Table 11.8 for ever-married women 35-44 years old, by color and residence. These characteristics are believed to be related closely to socioeconomic status. Another characteristic, number of dwelling units, is also considered below.

Tenure of Home. Tabulations were provided from the 1960 census on number of children ever born to married women according to value of owner-occupied one-unit nonfarm structures and gross monthly rental in rented nonfarm units.

Table 11.8 Housing characteristics in relation to number of children ever born per 1,000 ever-married women 35-44 years old, by color and specified type of residence: United States, urbanized areas, rural nonfarm areas, and the South: 1960

Housing characteristics	White				Nonwhite			
	United States	Urbanized areas	Rural nonfarm	South	United States	Urbanized areas	Rural nonfarm	South
Value of property								
Total in owner-occupied one-unit nonfarm structures	2,556	2,468	2,770	2,488	3,033	2,666	4,161	3,261
$25,000 or more	2,520	2,506	2,506	2,454	2,551	2,457	a	2,343
20,000 - 24,999	2,400	2,384	2,418	2,295	2,266	2,226	a	2,057
15,000 - 19,999	2,399	2,380	2,465	2,260	2,303	2,184	3,598	2,295
10,000 - 14,999	2,467	2,439	2,577	2,275	2,498	2,440	2,916	2,485
5,000 - 9,999	2,679	2,625	2,796	2,473	2,952	2,839	3,711	2,934
Less than $5,000	3,381	3,191	3,459	3,407	4,041	3,486	4,551	3,997
Gross rent								
Total in rented nonfarm units	2,585	2,264	3,357	2,963	3,124	2,647	4,814	3,742
$150 or more	2,271	2,159	2,776	2,452	2,964	2,959	a	a
100 - 149	2,355	2,210	2,884	2,423	2,800	2,784	a	3,405
80 - 99	2,412	2,220	3,068	2,516	2,659	2,555	3,786	3,210
60 - 79	2,472	2,258	3,089	2,615	2,586	2,506	3,129	2,857
40 - 59	2,709	2,337	3,388	3,092	2,988	2,735	4,040	3,341
20 - 39	3,479	2,701	3,878	3,896	3,679	2,979	4,640	3,825
Less than $20	4,103	2,768	4,239	4,367	4,835	a	5,205	4,891
No cash rent	3,165	2,547	3,584	3,589	4,569	2,393	5,283	5,086
Condition of housing unit and plumbing								
Sound	2,467	2,340	2,639	2,445	2,644	2,391	3,553	2,953
With all plumbing facilities	2,433	2,339	2,559	2,364	2,445	2,383	2,725	2,538
Lacking only hot water	3,093	2,757	3,218	3,244	3,189	2,897	4,111	3,100
Lacking other plumbing facilities	3,226	2,361	3,368	3,363	3,863	2,337	4,273	4,145
Deteriorating	3,570	3,152	3,896	3,756	3,916	3,061	4,848	4,407
With all plumbing facilities	3,334	3,127	3,547	3,307	3,150	3,041	3,734	3,313
Lacking only hot water	3,794	3,630	3,964	3,928	3,571	3,122	5,025	3,685
Lacking other plumbing facilities	4,110	3,259	4,298	4,257	4,720	3,110	4,988	4,944
Dilapidated	4,512	3,837	4,884	4,779	4,787	3,710	5,460	5,151
Number of rooms in housing unit								
8 rooms or more	3,331	3,195	3,476	3,120	3,762	3,469	4,879	4,173
7 rooms	2,983	2,818	3,185	2,852	3,732	3,246	5,210	4,481
6 rooms	2,738	2,580	3,002	2,726	3,617	3,015	5,072	4,347
5 rooms	2,467	2,286	2,781	2,570	3,279	2,730	4,366	3,834
4 rooms	2,214	1,930	2,640	2,617	3,263	2,402	4,477	3,887
3 rooms	1,853	1,403	2,697	2,501	2,645	1,911	4,025	3,185
2 rooms	1,922	1,410	2,470	2,507	2,231	1,486	3,928	2,700
1 room	1,863	1,265	2,619	2,442	2,746	1,210	4,856	2,054

Source: U. S. Bureau of the Census, 1960 Census of Population, Women by Number of Children Ever Born, PC(2)-3A, Tables 41,42.

[a]Rate not shown where base is less than 1,000.

The relation of tenure per se to number of children ever born varies by residence and color. For the United States as a whole, the average number of children ever born tended to be lower for home owners than for home renters in nonfarm structures (Table 11.8). This was true for white and nonwhite women in the 35-44 and 45-54 age groups (latter not shown). In this gross comparison the lower fertility rates for the owners than for the renters probably reflects the higher economic status of the owners.

In view of the likelihood that home owners tend more than renters to live outside large central cities, it is clearly advisable to do the analysis by type of residence. By definition, the home owners are largely restricted to those in one-unit dwellings, but a large proportion of those renting homes in large cities are in apartments and multiple-family dwellings.

In urbanized areas the fertility of home owners was *higher* than for home renters among white wives of both age groups and among nonwhite wives 35-44. In such areas the average rental value of the home was also higher for owners than for renters, on the assumption that monthly rent represents approximately 1 percent of the value of owned homes. It is possible that the higher fertility of owners partly reflects the higher fertility of residents of suburbs than of residents of central cities; and the higher fertility of residents of single-family homes than of apartment-house dwellers. In other urban areas and in rural nonfarm areas the fertility rates were lower for owners than for renters; and this was true for white and nonwhite wives of both age groups. The data are not given for rural farm areas since the analysis is restricted to nonfarm structures, owned or rented.

The higher average number of children among owners than among renters in urbanized areas and the reverse type of relation in other urban and rural nonfarm areas tended to persist when rental value of the home was controlled.

Further, within the United States as a whole the fertility rates for the owners tended to exceed those for renters in homes of approximately similar rental value. This again suggests that the control of economic status may serve to uncover the influence of a selective factor. Couples with children or a large family probably tend to be more interested in having a home of their own than those without children or a large family.

Value and Rental of Home. In general, the 1960 census data portray an inverse relation of fertility to value of owned homes and to gross monthly rental of rented homes.[7] However, the relation tended to be weak or nonexistent above given value and rental levels. It tended to be rather strong in the lower value and rental levels. Among white women 35-44 years old in urbanized areas, fertility rates varied but little by value of home above the $10,000 level. However, they increased sharply from 2,439 per 1,000 white women in the $10,000-$14,999 group to 3,191 for those in homes valued at less than $5,000. The variations in fertility by value or rental tended to be sharper in rural nonfarm than in urbanized and other urban areas. They tended to be more pronounced for nonwhite than for white women (Table 11.8).

Condition of Housing and Plumbing. The 1960 census data provide evidence of a wide range of variation in fertility rates by the jointly considered factors of condition of housing and presence of plumbing facilities. The classification provides three categories for condition of housing: sound, deteriorating, and dilapidated. The first two categories are subdivided into three classes according to presence of plumbing facilities: with all plumbing facilities, lacking only hot water, lacking other plumbing facilities (Table 11.8).

Among white ever-married women 35-44 years of age in the United States, the number of children ever born extended from 2,433 per 1,000 wives living in sound houses with all plumbing facilities to 4,512 for those in dilapidated houses. As with value and rental value, the range of variation tended to be wider in rural nonfarm areas than in urbanized or other urban areas and wider for nonwhite than for white women.

Number of Rooms in Housing Unit. For purely selective reasons, the average number of children ever born tends to increase rather sharply with number of rooms in the dwelling unit. There doubtless are many cases of the coincidence of high fertility and overcrowding among the poor but apparently not enough to overcome the tendency for families to procure larger living quarters as the family grows. This may mean leaving a small apartment and finding a home in the suburbs; it may mean moving to another area of the city where rents are cheaper (Table 11.8).

Number of Dwelling Units. The relation of fertility to type of house is mentioned here because of its relevance to the foregoing discussion of tenure in relation to fertility. In general, highest fertility rates were found for residents of detached one-family houses. Lowest rates were found for occupants of houses with five or more dwelling units. In urbanized areas there was a fairly regular relation of this type, with successively lower rates for those in houses with one, two, three, four, and five or more units. The occupants of trailers were rather uniformly characterized by relatively low fertility rates. The selective factor here is lack of room in the trailer for a family with children (Table 11.9).

Characteristics of Housing and Fertility by Color

Whether or not all of a series of housing characteristics were present appeared to be an important factor in the direction of fertility differentials by color in 1960. The characteristics considered were direct access, kitchen or cooking equipment, sound (as opposed to deteriorating) condition, flush toilet and bath for exclusive use, hot piped water, and less than 1.01 persons per room. The number of children ever born per 1,000 women 35-44 years old, married and husband present, are available from the 1960 census according to color of wife, occupation of husband, and whether or not all of the above characteristics were present. The tabulations were specific with reference to urban-rural residence and number of housing units in the structure. For those reporting all characteristics present, the tabulations were also broken down by income of the husband.

In general, among couples living in homes with all characteristics present, the fertility rates tended to be higher among the white than nonwhite couples. This tended to hold true at various income and occupational levels, in structures with one, two to four, and five or more housing units, and among couples in urbanized, other urban, and rural-nonfarm areas. Among couples in homes that were lacking one or more of the specified characteristics, the fertility rates tended to be higher among the white than the nonwhite in professional, managerial, and other white-collar occupations and lower among the white than among the nonwhite in the manual or blue-collar occupations.[8]

Religion in Relation to Fertility

Although a question on religion has long been asked in censuses of

Table 11.9 Number of housing units in structures in relation to
number of children ever born per 1,000 ever-married
women, by color and specified age of woman, United
States, urbanized areas, and the South, 1960

Age of woman and number of housing units in structure	White			Nonwhite		
	United States	Urban-ized areas	South	United States	Urban-ized areas	South
15-19						
1 unit	781	780	759	1,271	1,258	1,293
Detached	794	803	774	1,255	1,206	1,284
Attached	691	688	643	1,349	1,358	1,353
2 units	669	664	603	1,192	1,209	1,215
3 or 4 units	624	638	568	1,313	1,318	1,299
5 or more units	587	592	562	1,276	1,268	1,307
Trailer	612	572	586	a	a	a
25-29						
1 unit	2,292	2,182	2,231	2,966	2,644	3,156
Detached	2,313	2,205	2,243	3,045	2,652	3,228
Attached	2,039	1,996	2,057	2,649	2,625	2,760
2 units	1,870	1,825	1,835	2,521	2,437	2,806
3 or 4 units	1,757	1,707	1,644	2,445	2,430	2,656
5 or more units	1,557	1,506	1,628	2,406	2,386	2,645
Trailer	1,896	1,747	1,890	1,919	a	a
35-39						
1 unit	2,720	2,538	2,714	3,454	2,835	3,805
Detached	2,736	2,548	2,728	3,580	2,822	3,938
Attached	2,475	2,421	2,465	2,882	2,865	2,994
2 units	2,285	2,224	2,341	2,540	2,468	2,818
3 or 4 units	2,175	2,116	2,037	2,436	2,394	2,658
5 or more units	1,891	1,846	1,993	2,484	2,465	2,796
Trailer	1,943	1,784	1,909	a	a	a

Source: U. S. Bureau of the Census, 1960 Census of Population,
Women by Number of Children Ever Born, PC(2)-3A, Table 43. Data relate
to ever-married women in households, not to any residing in group
quarters.

aRate not shown where base is less than 1,250.

some other countries of the world, it has never been included in a
regular decennial census of the United States. The question was asked in the March 1957 Current Population Survey. Some of the broad
results were published in the 1958 issue of _Statistical Abstract of the
United States._ Apparently there was negligible objection to the question by people enumerated, and some consideration was given to the
inclusion of the question in the regular 1960 census. However, rather

strong objections from certain organizations brought an end to any prospects of including the question of religion in the 1960 census. Fortunately, data regarding religion in relation to fertility have been collected in several private investigations during the past decade. These will be considered briefly in the present analysis.

The population covered in the Current Population Survey is a small but carefully designed probability sample of the entire country. According to the CPS of March 1957, approximately two-thirds (66.2 percent) of the population 14 years of age and over were Protestants, about one-fourth (25.7 percent) were Catholic, and about 3.2 percent were Jewish. The remainder were in the category "other religion, no religion, and religion not reported."

Age-specific fertility rates for Protestants, Catholics, and Jews in the United States as a whole and in urban areas are presented in Table 11.10 on the basis of data from the Current Population Survey. Both sets of data indicate higher fertility for Protestants than for the Catholics at ages under 30 and higher fertility for the latter than for the former after age 30. Jewish couples are conspicuous for their low fertility. Within the United States Protestant group, the previously published fertility rates standardized for age per 1,000 women 15-44 years of age were 1,922 for Presbyterians, 1,967 for Lutherans, 2,115 for Methodists, and 2,381 for Baptists (see source note Table 11.10). These variations reflect differentials by color, residence, and socioeconomic status.

Three factors help to explain the apparently higher fertility of Protestants than of Catholics at ages under 30 and the lack of greater excess of Catholic fertility at older ages. In the first place, the analysis is not controlled for color, and the chief nonwhite group, the Negroes, are predominantly Protestant. In the second place, Catholics are more predominantly urban than Protestants. This factor applies mainly to the data for the United States as a whole. Even in the data for urban areas the fact remains that Catholics are more concentrated in the large cities. Finally, age at marriage tends to be later, on the average, for Catholic than for Protestant brides, a factor that obviously has greater influence on the fertility of women under 30 than on that of older women.

Freedman, Whelpton, and Campbell, in their Growth of American Families Study, found results strikingly in agreement with those reported above insofar as similarity of fertility rates for Protestants and Catholics are concerned.[9] They stated: "The fact that the Catholic

Table 11.10 Children ever born per 1,000 women 15-49 years old, by religion reported, age, and marital status: United States and urban areas, March 1957

Subject	15-19	20-24	25-29	30-34	35-39	40-44	45-49
UNITED STATES							
Number of women (thousands)							
Total	5,747	5,324	5,788	6,281	6,074	5,770	5,307
Protestant	3,870	3,544	3,850	4,112	3,970	3,797	3,577
Baptist	1,342	1,251	1,298	1,354	1,247	1,143	1,022
Lutheran	340	346	377	409	395	389	414
Methodist	778	662	739	820	831	863	806
Presbyterian	283	263	316	362	349	344	299
Other Protestant	1,127	1,022	1,120	1,167	1,148	1,058	1,036
Roman Catholic	1,545	1,466	1,628	1,764	1,737	1,552	1,318
Jewish	145	106	146	205	166	226	226
Other, none, and not reported	187	208	164	200	201	195	186
Children ever born per 1,000 women (including single)							
Total	108	971	1,900	2,249	2,457	2,342	2,237
Protestant	129	1,070	2,002	2,299	2,459	2,394	2,241
Baptist	148	1,241	2,215	2,482	2,585	2,619	2,600
Lutheran	79	861	1,748	2,191	2,203	2,049	2,002
Methodist	118	941	1,962	2,212	2,391	2,244	2,127
Presbyterian	74	703	1,788	2,130	2,034	2,151	2,033
Other Protestant	144	1,110	1,928	2,239	2,590	2,479	2,132
Roman Catholic	61	774	1,754	2,204	2,539	2,313	2,319
Jewish	14*	434*	1,178*	1,785	1,946	1,752	1,624
Other, none, and not reported	123	952	1,591	2,085	2,114	2,251	2,323
Children ever born per 1,000 women ever married							
Total	672	1,368	2,139	2,425	2,612	2,514	2,401
Protestant	713	1,419	2,205	2,428	2,571	2,526	2,376
Baptist	682	1,625	2,404	2,639	2,699	2,696	2,720
Lutheran	771*	1,187	1,905	2,274	2,339	2,190	2,109
Methodist	760*	1,264	2,164	2,314	2,512	2,394	2,313
Presbyterian	700*	1,069	1,928	2,209	2,139	2,327	2,187
Other Protestant	720	1,418	2,181	2,391	2,683	2,628	2,243
Roman Catholic	540	1,261	2,061	2,512	2,770	2,569	2,558
Jewish	333*	780*	1,433*	1,839	2,139	1,877	1,799
Other, none, and not reported	590*	1,338*	1,864*	2,254	2,471	2,613	2,512
URBAN							
Number of women (thousands)							
Total	3,527	3,580	3,650	3,979	3,837	3,730	3,601
Protestant	2,042	2,095	2,196	2,326	2,182	2,154	2,158
Baptist	661	714	730	752	681	636	584
Lutheran	211	230	225	237	221	230	279
Methodist	410	389	384	451	431	453	469
Presbyterian	193	188	225	226	195	216	211
Other Protestant	567	574	632	660	654	619	615
Roman Catholic	1,222	1,252	1,196	1,324	1,368	1,234	1,086
Jewish	142	106	135	193	155	217	225
Other, none, and not reported	121	127	123	136	132	125	132
Children ever born per 1,000 women (including single)							
Total	97	837	1,692	2,040	2,238	2,090	1,961
Protestant	129	940	1,803	2,085	2,159	2,080	1,904
Baptist	165	1,176	2,030	2,113	2,153	2,167	2,164
Lutheran	76	687	1,533	2,059	1,991	1,987	1,692
Methodist	132	851	1,805	2,151	2,255	1,949	1,883
Presbyterian	98	585	1,662	1,951	1,872	1,912	1,896
Other Protestant	115	923	1,685	2,064	2,246	2,181	1,772
Roman Catholic	50	706	1,572	2,022	2,437	2,165	2,142
Jewish	14*	434*	1,185*	1,777	1,929	1,724	1,627
Other, none, and not reported	132*	772*	1,439*	1,809*	1,841*	2,136*	1,977*
Children ever born per 1,000 women ever married							
Total	600	1,240	1,972	2,240	2,416	2,281	2,139
Protestant	662	1,290	2,026	2,229	2,288	2,223	2,046
Baptist	637	1,538	2,245	2,293	2,273	2,241	2,277
Lutheran	555*	1,006	1,716	2,188	2,178	2,176	1,788
Methodist	783*	1,199	2,094	2,266	2,382	2,097	2,118
Presbyterian	633*	1,147	1,833	2,051	2,005	2,140	2,041
Other Protestant	596	1,227	1,909	2,207	2,362	2,340	1,892
Roman Catholic	445	1,185	1,938	2,348	2,682	2,440	2,386
Jewish	333*	780*	1,441*	1,834*	2,121*	1,851	1,830
Other, none, and not reported	533*	1,153*	1,825*	2,050*	2,189*	2,567*	2,212*

Source: Current Population Survey, March, 1957. For standardized fertility rates for women 15-44 years old, see U. S. Bureau of the Census, Statistical Abstract of the United States, 1958, p. 41; Donald J. Bogue, The Population of the United States (Glencoe, Ill.: Free Press, 1958), p. 696.

*Rates marked with asterisks based on fewer than 150,000 women. See text of Current Population Reports, Series P-20, No. 79 (February 2, 1958) for information on composition of category "Other, none, and not reported" and for data on distribution by color within each religion.

wives had borne no more children than the Protestant wives by the time of the interview is due primarily to the higher age at marriage of the Catholics. Because the Catholics had married when they were an average of 1.5 years older than the Protestants, they had spent fewer years in marriage by the time of the interview and consequently had fewer years in which to bear children. If we compare the average number of children borne by Protestants and Catholic women in each cohort who married at the same age, we find that the Catholics have generally been more fertile than the Protestants."[11]

The field work of the Growth of American Families Study to which the above statement related was carried out in 1955, two years before the 1957 Current Population Survey. It was done among "2,713 white married women between the ages of 18 and 39 (inclusive) . . . selected in such a way as to constitute a scientific probability sample of the approximately 17 million wives in our national population having the indicated characteristics in March, 1955." However, as with the CPS of 1957, the similarity of the fertility rates for the Protestants and Catholics probably arose in part from the fact that the latter are more densely concentrated in large cities.

Several studies relating to specific cities or to metropolitan areas have yielded evidence of higher and more striking increase of fertility rates among Catholics than Protestants. The household survey data from the Indianapolis Study of Social and Psychological Factors Affecting Fertility indicated virtually similar fertility rates of Protestants and Catholics for wives under 25 years old but sharply higher rates for the latter at older ages.[10]

Westoff, Potter, and Sagi, on the basis of the first two phases of the Princeton Fertility Study, found that "religious preference, that is, preference for the Protestant, Catholic, or Jewish faith, is the strongest of all major social characteristics in its influence on fertility."[11] The Princeton Fertility Study relates to a sample of white women in seven of the eight largest metropolitan areas who had their second child in September 1956. They were interviewed first in 1957 and a second time in 1960. According to the authors, "Catholic couples want the most and Jewish couples the fewest children, with Protestants in an intermediate position." The authors believe that the Catholics have more children than the Protestants because they want more. However, they also present evidence that Catholics' family planning is less effective than the Protestants'. "The influence exerted by religion operates primarily through its effect on the number of children desired and only secondarily through family-planning success . . . [The] comparatively ineffective fertility planning [of the Catholics] should be viewed mainly in terms of child-spacing. The assumption . . . is that once their larger family ambitions are realized, their success in controlling family size improves."[12]

Several students have reported evidence of a persistent widening of differences in fertility by religion despite the narrowing of fertility differentials by geographic area, urban-rural residence, and socioeconomic status. With available data from the Official Catholic Directory[13] regarding number of Catholics and annual number of baptisms, Kirk estimated the crude birth rates of Catholics for the years 1910-53. Comparing these with the birth rates for the total United States for the same years, he found that "(1) the Catholic population of the United States continues to have a substantially higher birth rate than the non-Catholic population; (2) the narrowing of religious differentials predicted in the 1930's has not in fact occurred; (3) the Catholic population has contributed disproportionately to the sustained high birth rate in the United States since the second world war."[14]

In their recent comparison of data from the 1955 and 1960 Growth of American Families Studies and from surveys conducted by the Survey Research Center of the University of Michigan in 1962, Freedman, Goldberg, and Slesinger stated: "In contrast to the contraction of fertility differentials for most of the variables discussed here, religious differences in fertility are large and apparently growing larger.[15]

After dividing the rural townships in 15 counties of Northeastern Wisconsin into two groups, (a) those in which the population was known to be over 50 percent Catholic, and (b) those in which the population was under 50 percent Catholic, Neusse computed and compared standardized fertility ratios for the two sets of areas from census data for 1940, 1950, and 1960. He reported a "maintenance of religious differentials [of child-woman ratios] in the region and . . . a probable renewal of their importance during the 20 years from 1940 to 1960."[16]

In general, therefore, whereas differentials in fertility have narrowed by geographic area, urban-rural residence, and socioeconomic status, they have increased by color, and probably also by religion, within the United States.

Summary

The relation of income of the husband during 1959 to number of children ever born to white women, married and husband present, differed sharply by age of woman. The relation was direct at ages under 25, absent at ages 25-29, and inverse at ages 30 and over. A plausible interpretation of this is that young people of high income are more likely than people of low income to concentrate their childbearing into a relatively short period after marriage. Being more adept at family planning, they are in position to do this.

Fertility rates among white women 35-44 and 45-54 years old, married once and husband present, were analyzed in relation to three simultaneously considered socioeconomic characteristics of the husband (income, education, and occupation). These were made separately for wives marrying at ages 14-21 and at ages 22 and over. The relation of fertility to one socioeconomic variable when the other two were held constant tended to be inverse for wives marrying at ages 14-21 and direct for those marrying at ages 22 and over. The direct relation was more frequently found among urban than among rural women and more commonly found among couples of high than of low socioeconomic status according to the two "control" variables of socioeconomic status.

Age at marriage also appeared to be a critical factor in the tendency for the fertility of nonwhite women to fall below that of white women of high socioeconomic status. Among women marrying at ages 22 and over, there was a rather frequent tendency for the fertility of nonwhite women to fall below that of white women of specific status with reference to income, occupation, and education of the husband. This tendency was virtually absent for wives marrying at younger ages, even those of high status with respect to income, occupation, and education of the husband.

Fertility rates were conspicuously lower for women in the labor force than for those not in the labor force. Among those in the labor force, fertility rates were lower for the employed than for the unemployed. Among the employed women, the fertility rates were lower for the full-time than for the part-time workers. Among women not in the labor force, the fertility rates tended to be lowest for those who had last worked 2-5 years earlier and highest for those who had never worked. The above statements tend to hold true for nonwhite as well as for white women.

There tended to be a relation of fertility to tenure of home, rental value of home, and various housing characteristics when selective factors such as urban-rural residence were controlled.

As for religion, fertility rates tended to be highest for Catholics, intermediate for Protestants, and lowest for Jews, according to unofficial data specific for color and type of residence. According to the Current Population Survey data for 1957, among the urban Protestants the fertility rates standardized for age were relatively low for Presbyterians and Lutherans and relatively high for Methodists and Baptists. These variations reflect differentials by color, residence, and socioeconomic status.

12 / The Relation Between Fertility and Economic Conditions

Whether or not there is a relation between fertility and economic conditions is a question that has thus far been answered somewhat ambiguously. On the one hand, the impressive century-long historical record of the United States and other industrially developed countries suggests that economic progress and declining fertility go hand in hand. Consistent with the historical record are studies showing that couples with high incomes have fewer children than those with low incomes. On the other hand, short-range observations of year-to-year fluctuations suggest that fertility rises and falls in concert with changes in economic conditions. These apparently contradictory findings have not yet been reconciled in any general theory about the relation between fertility and economic well-being.

As a first step in understanding the kinds of phenomena involved in the relation, it is necessary to distinguish between cohort and period measures of fertility, a topic that will be treated in greater detail in the next chapter. Cohort measures relate to the cumulative childbearing of a group of women as they move through the childbearing years of life. The most useful cohort measures are the cumulative fertility rates by age, which describe how many children a cohort of 1,000 women had borne up to the age specified.[1] Period measures of fertility, in contrast, relate only to the births occurring during a limited period of time—usually 1 calendar year. The births occurring in 1 year represent the combined fertility of the 35 (approximately) cohorts having children in that year. Their experience can be summarized by a number of measures; the most common are age-specific birth rates, the gross reproduction rate, the total fertility rate, the general fertility rate, and the crude birth rate.

For present purposes, the important distinction between the cohort and period measures is that variations in these measures represent different aspects of fertility. Year-to-year changes in period measures tend to represent shifts in the timing of births. However, cohort-to-cohort changes in cumulative rates, especially those for the later childbearing ages (approximately 30 and over), represent primarily changes in completed fertility (i.e., the average number of children that the women of the cohort will ever have).

Inasmuch as these two aspects of fertility are largely independent of each other, they can, and often do, show different trends. For example, the rapid increase in age-specific birth rates at the younger ages following World War II did not reflect an equally rapid increase in the completed fertility of cohorts, but a decline in the age of child-bearing. In studying the relation between fertility and economic conditions, therefore, it is important to recognize the particular aspects of fertility that are reflected by the measures under study.

The Relation between Completed Fertility and Economic Conditions
Is there any evidence that the completed fertility of cohorts (average number of children ever born by the end of the childbearing period per 1,000 women) moves in response to the economic conditions experienced by the cohorts during the main portion of the childbearing period? So far, this question has received little attention. Although all aspects of the problem cannot be explored within the limitations of the present report, some of the basic data bearing on the problem will be presented.

Figure 12.1 shows two trend lines: one represents the completed fertility of the cohorts of 1876-40; the other shows average gross national product (in constant dollars, comparable in purchasing power) during the years when those cohorts were 20-24 years of age (in this

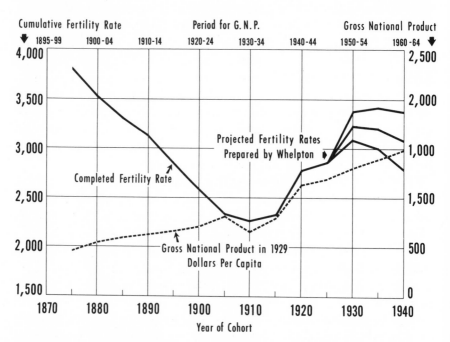

Fig. 12.1. Completed fertility rate for cohorts of 1875-1940 and gross national product per capita (1929 dollars), 1895-1964.

country, the ages of highest fertility). For example, the chart relates average gross national product during 1930-34 to the 1910 cohort because the members of this cohort reached ages 20-24 in these years.

The general picture presented here suggests that the two variables are independent of each other. Completed fertility declined rapidly for the cohorts of 1886 to 1905, although economic conditions during the prime childbearing years of these cohorts were gradually improving. On the other hand, completed fertility increased for the cohorts of 1910 to 1935 or 1940, and so did the per capita gross national product during the years when these cohorts were 20-24 years of age.

Important as these considerations are, the evidence for a lack of relation between fertility and economic conditions must be regarded as superficial. It must be recognized that gross national product is a limited measure of economic conditions. Although it is correlated with such measures as personal income, percent employed, and industrial production, even these measures relate only to limited and easily quantified aspects of economic conditions. They tell us little or nothing, for example, about the changing distribution of wealth, changing arrangements for financial security during periods of unemployment or after retirement, or changing access to credit. All of these aspects of the broad variable "economic conditions" could have important influences on couples' decisions to have or not to have additional children.

The thorough exploration of the relation between the completed fertility of cohorts and the economic conditions that may have influenced their childbearing has not yet been done. At present, one can only say that the nature of the relation, if it exists, is not obvious.

The Relation between the Timing of Fertility and Economic Conditions

A number of studies have demonstrated the relation between annual fluctuations in fertility and in economic conditions.[2] In terms of the context suggested at the beginning of this chapter, these studies demonstrate the connection between the *timing* of fertility and economic conditions. Couples tend to delay births during depressions and have them during periods of prosperity. It is not possible to estimate what proportion of the couples in the childbearing years of life regulate conception according to changes in economic conditions, but even if only a minority of couples do so, their decisions are sufficient to cause substantial variation in annual measures of fertility.

This section of the present chapter describes a study conducte at the Scripps Foundation for Research in Population Problems 1959 and 1960 that has not been published previously. The purpo: of this study was to investigate the hypothesized direct relation b tween annual measures of fertility and economic conditions by tl most rigorous means feasible. This involved the use of newly availab measures of fertility (age-parity-specific birth probabilities), sever measures of economic conditions (income, unemployment, and indu trial production), and an attempt to reduce to a minimum the infl ence of serial correlation (which will be explained later). The fertilit rates used in this study relate to the period 1917-57. Before descril ing the results of the study, the methods employed will be summarize

Birth Probabilities. As noted above, birth probabilities rather tha birth rates were used. The birth probability is defined as the prol ability that a women who has had N births as of the beginning of year of age will have an (N + 1)th birth during the year of age.

The birth probability is superior to the age-order-specific birth rat (births of order N to women age x per 1,000 women age x) becau: it eliminates the influence on the latter rate of changes in the numbe of women eligible to have an N-order birth. For example, the *rate* fc second order births to women 30-34 years old declined from 26.5 t 21.5 per 1,000 between 1948 and 1957. However, in the same perio· the *probability* that a one-parity woman 30-34 years old would hav a second birth increased from 111 to 123 per 1,000. The rate decline only because the number of one-parity women 30-34 years old d· clined relative to the number of second-order births at ages 30-3·

It would also be desirable to eliminate the influence of variatior in the duration of parity, but this is not feasible because of lack c data.

Probabilities were computed for each order of birth, one throug seven, and eighth and higher orders combined.

Two sets of probabilities were computed for first births, one base on all zero-parity women and one based only on zero-parity marrie women. The probabilities for zero-parity married women are undoub edly too high, especially at the younger ages, because they are base on the assumption that all first births occurred to married womer which is obviously not the case. In fact, some of the probabilities ar above 1,000 at ages 15-19. Nevertheless, these probabilities were use· in the analysis because the fluctuations in the inaccurate probabilitie were assumed to reflect largely (though not wholly) fluctuations i the actual probabilities. There was greater interest in the fluctuations of the probabilities than in their absolute levels.

Probabilities were computed for 5-year age groups, 15-19 through 40-44, for each year 1917-57. However, probabilities were not computed for age-order groups where births are rare—that is, ages 15-19 for fourth and higher order births, ages 20-24 for seventh and higher order births, and ages 40-44 for first and second births.

The Measurement of Economic Conditions. It was considered desirable to use indicators that reflect the most visible and general changes in the economy—that is, changes that directly affect the lives of millions of people or at least encourage or frighten them about their financial prospects.

One highly visible measure of economic conditions is the proportion of persons who are unemployed. One may reasonably expect not only that couples' family plans may change if the breadwinner loses his job but also that widespread unemployment will alarm those who still have their jobs. Conversely, periods of nearly full employment brighten couples' prospects. Accordingly, one measure of economic conditions used in this study is the proportion of the civilian labor force that is unemployed.

Another important aspect of personal financial security is income. Changes in income may not be as dramatic as changes in employment, but they should be sufficiently obvious to have some effect on decisions about childbearing. To express income, personal disposable income in constant dollars (1947-49 price levels) per capita was chosen. The Department of Commerce provides the basic data for 1929 and later years, but for no years before 1929. Several sets of data are available for 1916-28. For this period it was decided to modify the Department of Commerce figures for Gross National Product with the use of adjustments provided by Goldsmith.[3]

To complete the picture of economic conditions, an index of industrial production was used. This has the advantage of being a very general indicator of the health of the economy, but the disadvantage of being less visible to most people than either employment or income.

The Allowance for Secular Trend. In order to use correlation analysis on time series it is necessary to eliminate the influence of secular trend. If secular trend is not eliminated, it is impossible to tell whether high correlation coefficients result from a real association between the two variables under study or from the fact that both variables fluctuate little around their central trend lines. For example, let us suppose that each of two variables moves up or down along a straight line during a given time period. The correlation coefficient will be 1.0 if the lines go in the same direction, and –1.0 if they go in opposite directions. But the fact that both variables moved in a straight line may have been purely coincidental and not due to any real causal links between them.

One need not use straight lines to illustrate the point, however. Any two series that move smoothly (i.e., in which adjacent values tend to be *about* the same, even though there may be wide secular swings) will tend to yield high correlation coefficients. This tendency produces "nonsense correlations," such as the coefficient of .9512 between the proportion of marriages that were performed in the Church of England and the standardized mortality rate for England and Wales in the period 1866-1911. High values in one series were related to high values in the other, because such values occurred at about the same time; low values were similarly associated.[4] Yet the high correlation coefficient cannot be construed as demonstrating a close causal association between the two sets of rates. They simply happened to decline at the same time.

Trends in neither fertility nor economic conditions in the United States have been as unidirectional or as smooth as those in the two series cited above, but the same kind of problem exists: economic conditions were good and fertility was high in the 1920's, both series were low during the depression, and both series were high after World War II. Are these similar movements causally linked, or is this association in time fortuitous? Correlation coefficients between raw values will not give the answer. A more refined technique is needed.

One way of studying relations between time series is to confine attention to deviations from secular trends. Whether or not this procedure provides a rigorous test of the association between two variables depends on how the secular trend is defined. For example, if the secular trend of the income series is defined as a simple curve increasing monotonically from 1916 to 1956, falling below the observations for the 1920's, above those for the 1930's, and below those for the postwar period, and if the measure of income for present purposes in a given year is defined as the extent to which the observation departs from the trend, low values may still be concentrated in the 1930's and high values concentrated in the 1920's and the postwar period. If, in addition, the secular trend of a fertility series is defined in a similar way with similar results, there would have been no great departure from the use of the original observations. It would still be uncertain whether a high correlation coefficient meant that there was a close causal connection between income and fertility.

For the purposes of this study, it was considered desirable to define secular trend in such a way that it followed closely the observed values, sometimes falling above them, sometimes below, but never staying above or below for many years consecutively. Then neither the high nor the low deviations from secular trend would be concentrated in any particular period. Instead, both high and low deviations would occur in all periods regardless of the general level of the observations within periods. In the depression of the 1930's, for example, some of the income deviations will be high, and in the more prosperous 1950's some of the income deviations will be low.

Secular trends of this type are often provided by moving averages. These have the advantage of assuring the user that positive and negative deviations will occur within relatively short periods of time, depending on how many years are included in the definition of the moving average. Three definitions of deviation from moving average were tried.

1. *Absolute deviation from average for previous 3 years.* On the assumption that people usually judge their present economic status and their prospects for the future in terms of the recent past, it was thought that a good measure of current economic conditions would be the extent to which they departed from average conditions for the previous 3 years. The same definition was used for the fertility series on the assumption that current fertility was regarded as high or low largely in relation to the recent past. Although some preliminary research was done using this definition, it was eventually rejected because high values were found to cluster with high values, and low values with low values, which was the disadvantage to be overcome.

The measure used to determine the extent of such clustering was the serial correlation coefficient—that is, the correlation coefficient obtained by relating a value for one year in a series with the value for the previous year in the same series. A high serial correlation coefficient indicates that similar values tend to occur in adjacent years, while a low correlation coefficient indicates that this tendency does not exist. A majority of the serial correlation coefficients (for birth probabilities and economic indicators) were above 0.60.[5]

2. *Percent deviation from average for previous 3 years.* It was thought that relative deviations might eliminate more of the secular trend than did absolute deviations. However, the serial correlation

coefficients for relative deviations were as high as those for absolute deviations.

3. *Absolute deviation from 5-year moving average.* Although it was difficult to give up the theoretical advantage of the deviation from previous 3 years (i.e., that it reflects the fact that people judge current conditions in terms of the recent past), it was necessary to find some method of measurement that would yield low serial correlation coefficients. To do this, the absolute deviation from the 5-year moving average was computed. For example, the deviation for 1922 is the original value for 1922 minus the average of the original values for the 5 years 1920 through 1924.

In order to use as many years as possible in the analysis, 5-year moving averages were computed for birth probabilities in 1915-19 and 1916-20, even though original values were missing for 1915 and 1916, by assuming that the averages for 1915-19 and 1916-20 were on a straight-line extension of averages for 1917-21, 1918-22, and 1919-23. Similarly, the moving averages were extended forward to 1954-58 and 1955-59 by extrapolation from 1951-55, 1952-56, and 1953-57. These extensions yielded a deviation for every year, 1917-57, for the birth probabilities. Similar extensions were not needed for the economic series because enough observed data were available to compute deviations for 1916-56, the years for which these series were needed.

The use of absolute deviations from 5-year moving averages eliminated secular trend very well, as shown by low serial correlation coefficients. None of the coefficients was above .50, and only rarely did one go above .40. In general, they clustered around zero.

Time Lag. In this study it was assumed that if economic conditions affect fertility, the average gap between the economic stimulus and the fertility response is 1 year. This assumption was made because the economic and fertility data relate to calendar years, so that the time lag must be a whole number of years, and because a gap of 1 year is more appropriate than 2 or more years. The latter reason is supported by the following considerations: (1) Fluctuations of fertility rates are caused largely by couples who control their fertility; the large group who do not try to control their fertility or who do so ineffectively show much less variation in fertility than the former group. (2) Those planners who wish to have more children begin to try to become pregnant when economic conditions and prospects are favorable. (3) The median length of time required to become pregnant after stopping contraception is about 4 months.[6] (4) Four months trying to conceive plus 9 months of pregnancy give 13 months for the time between deciding to have a child and having one. Another way of stating this is to say that planned births represent attempts to conceive that were begun about 13 months previously. (5) Thirteen months is much closer to 1 year than to 2 years; hence, 1 year is the best choice. Even though it may be possible to justify an average gap between first attempt to conceive and eventual birth of more than 13 months, it is not possible to justify more than 18 months. Therefore, regardless of what reasonable assumptions are made, 1 year is still the best choice when alternatives are limited to whole numbers of years.

Time Periods Studied. The years 1917-57, to which the birth probabilities relate, were divided into three major periods. This was done in order to find out whether the strength of the relation between fertility and economic conditions varied under different general circumstances. The criteria for defining the periods were the times of occurrence of major changes that could affect the family plans of most of the childbearing population. The three periods are as follows: (1) 1917-30. This is the pre-depression period. Although the depression began in late 1929 or early 1930, the planned births of 1930 resulted largely from decisions made in 1929, the last year of prosperity. (2) 1931-41. These are the years of depression and recovery. It was thought desirable to end the period with 1941 or 1942, in order to exclude the war period. On this basis alone, it would have been reasonable to end with 1942, inasmuch as the planned births of this year resulted from attempts to conceive begun in 1941, when the country was at peace for 11 months. However, it was decided to end the period with 1941 because 1942 births may have been influenced not so much by economic conditions as by the threat of war and the draft. (3) 1947-57. This is the postwar period. The period begins with 1947 because the planned births in that year resulted from decisions made in 1946, the first full year of peace. The decision to include 1947 was probably a poor one, however, because births in this year were still unduly influenced by the many new marriages that followed the rapid demobilization of the armed forces in 1945 and 1946. It would probably have been more reasonable to have started the postwar period with 1948.

The span of years 1917-57 could have been divided into shorter periods, but this would have made the number of years in each period too small to obtain significant results. As it is, there are only 14 years in 1917-30, 11 years in 1931-41, and 11 years in 1947-57. However, the study retained several years during which family plans were probably influenced less by economic conditions than by other events. For example, 1918-20 was included in the pre-depression period even though childbearing decisions in those years may have been influenced by mobilization and demobilization associated with World War I and by the severe influenza epidemic of 1918-20. Similarly, 1951-53 was retained in the postwar period in spite of the possible effects of the Korean War on numbers of births during those years.

Procedure Followed in Correlation Analysis. Correlation coefficients were computed for each of the three time periods (1917-30, 1931-41, and 1947-57) using deviations from 5-year moving averages for each of 44 sets of birth probabilities and each of three sets of economic indicators. Thus, 3 x 44 = 132 coefficients were computed for each period. In addition, coefficients were computed for the following combinations of periods: 1917-41, 1931-57 (excluding 1942-46), and 1917-57 (excluding 1942-46). Coefficients were computed for these summary groups in case the coefficients for the shorter period would be sufficiently alike to warrant summary presentation. Altogether, 6 x 132 = 792 correlation coefficients were computed. They are shown in Tables 12.1, 12.2, and 12.3.

Findings. The median values of the correlation coefficients for the three broad periods under study are shown below for the three economic indicators. Each median is computed from a distribution of coefficients for 44 birth probabilities.

	Median value of r for relation between birth probabilities and:		
Period	Unemployment	Income	Production
1917-30	−.41	.20	.40
1931-41	−.24	.19	.38
1947-57	.04	.32	−.22

Table 12.1 Coefficients of correlation between age-parity-specific
birth probabilities and percent unemployed of the civilian labor force, 1917-57

(Both variables are measured by deviation from 5-year moving averages)

Age and parity of woman	1917 to 1957	1917 to 1930	1931 to 1941	1947 to 1957	Summaries 1917 to 1941	Summaries 1931 to 1957
15-19: 0 (Ever married)	.48	.18	.71	.68	.47	.70
0 (Total)	-.25	-.27	-.71	.12	-.37	-.27
1	-.18	-.52	-.02	.37	-.30	.05
2	-.13	-.38	.27	-.24	-.13	.18
20-24: 0 (Ever married)	.00	-.07	.19	.18	-.03	.11
0 (Total)	-.16	-.17	-.68	.19	-.29	-.16
1	-.24	-.36	-.41	.19	-.40	-.13
2	-.37	-.56	-.14	.05	-.41	-.13
3	-.40	-.58	-.12	-.42	-.40	-.18
4	-.41	-.72	.06	-.55	-.40	-.09
5	-.31	-.48	-.07	-.51	-.29	-.17
25-29: 0 (Ever married)	-.11	-.12	-.61	.17	-.22	-.14
0 (Total)	-.11	-.10	-.79	.20	-.28	-.15
1	-.21	-.37	-.60	.21	-.53	-.18
2	-.27	-.35	-.24	.08	-.33	-.16
3	-.25	-.40	-.05	-.01	-.28	-.04
4	-.35	-.47	-.13	-.42	-.34	-.19
5	-.38	-.49	-.24	-.27	-.39	-.22
6	-.35	-.36	-.44	-.27	-.36	-.38
7+	-.30	-.44	-.10	-.48	-.28	-.17
30-34: 0 (Ever married)	-.13	-.07	-.74	.02	-.33	-.16
0 (Total)	-.13	-.16	-.80	.16	-.44	-.14
1	-.20	-.26	-.42	.13	-.41	-.17
2	-.36	-.53	-.27	-.04	-.47	-.17
3	-.34	-.51	-.11	-.11	-.39	-.10
4	-.42	-.65	-.18	-.07	-.49	-.14
5	-.29	-.45	-.10	-.01	-.32	-.06
6	-.33	-.43	-.13	-.25	-.34	-.16
7+	-.29	-.40	-.14	-.41	-.28	-.18
35-39: 0 (Ever married)	-.17	-.36	-.56	.17	-.44	-.10
0 (Total)	-.16	-.29	-.70	.25	-.47	-.13
1	-.29	-.43	-.53	.26	-.52	-.17
2	-.34	-.44	-.48	.10	-.49	-.21
3	-.33	-.41	-.43	.07	-.44	-.22
4	-.37	-.47	-.40	-.01	-.44	-.23
5	-.44	-.63	-.34	.31	-.51	-.19
6	-.39	-.67	-.24	.17	-.51	-.09
7+	-.49	-.54	-.49	-.30	-.52	-.43
40-44: 2	-.22	-.41	.30	.02	-.28	.06
3	-.18	-.39	.25	-.11	-.24	.02
4	.01	-.24	.35	.44	-.08	.28
5	-.15	-.49	.21	.11	-.21	.16
6	-.16	-.22	-.02	-.33	-.14	-.09
7+	-.36	-.50	-.24	-.10	-.41	-.19

Source: Scripps Foundation for Research in Population Problems.

Table 12.2 Coefficients of correlation between age-parity-specific birth probabilities and personal disposable income, 1917-57

(Both variables are measured by deviations from 5-year moving averages)

| Age and parity of woman | 1917 to 1957 | 1917 to 1930 | 1931 to 1941 | 1947 to 1957 | Summaries | |
					1917 to 1941	1931 to 1957
15-19: 0 (Ever married)	-.34	-.38	-.63	.37	-.51	-.30
0 (Total)	.16	-.02	.57	.30	.13	.38
1	.28	.34	.04	.49	.22	.26
2	.11	.37	-.20	-.38	.16	-.24
20-24: 0 (Ever married)	.00	-.19	-.31	.61	-.18	.22
0 (Total)	.17	-.11	.58	.44	.06	.41
1	.35	.21	.42	.56	.30	.47
2	.34	.38	.08	.68	.29	.32
3	.29	.39	.16	.25	.30	.19
4	.15	.46	-.11	-.31	.25	-.17
5	.16	.38	.02	-.15	.23	-.04
25-29: 0 (Ever married)	.16	-.15	.53	.55	-.00	.46
0 (Total)	.17	-.18	.66	.46	.04	.42
1	.43	.28	.56	.65	.46	.55
2	.27	.10	.21	.72	.16	.46
3	.20	.11	-.01	.72	.08	.29
4	.16	.17	.08	.30	.14	.16
5	.15	.19	.23	-.06	.18	.10
6	.11	.13	.34	-.34	.18	.10
7+	.01	.14	.07	-.35	.11	-.11
30-34: 0 (Ever married)	.15	-.12	.64	.22	.17	.25
0 (Total)	.24	-.07	.66	.43	.23	.39
1	.37	.08	.35	.64	.30	.49
2	.41	.41	.26	.49	.39	.38
3	.28	.31	.06	.39	.25	.22
4	.37	.46	.22	.27	.39	.24
5	.20	.22	.12	.23	.20	.14
6	.21	.20	.12	.33	.19	.20
7+	.16	.20	.17	.11	.17	.14
35-39: 0 (Ever married)	.30	.07	.43	.58	.22	.44
0 (Total)	.31	.04	.63	.54	.28	.47
1	.30	.18	.47	.28	.35	.34
2	.29	.21	.44	.23	.33	.31
3	.25	.23	.30	.18	.29	.24
4	.29	.27	.30	.28	.29	.28
5	.44	.47	.27	.74	.40	.45
6	.30	.53	.18	-.06	.41	.06
7+	.37	.33	.47	.38	.37	.44
40-44: 2	.10	.29	-.41	-.18	.19	-.17
3	.18	.26	-.24	.24	.17	.08
4	-.04	.14	-.46	-.17	.00	-.25
5	.12	.28	-.30	.27	.07	-.03
6	.12	.08	.04	.41	.05	.20
7+	.35	.29	.09	.83	.24	.43

Source: Scripps Foundation for Research in Population Problems.

Table 12.3 Coefficients of correlation between age-parity-specific birth
probabilities and index of industrial production, 1917-57

(Both variables are measured by deviations from 5-year moving averages)

Age and parity of woman		1917 to 1957	1917 to 1930	1931 to 1941	1947 to 1957	Summaries	
						1917 to 1941	1931 to 1957
15-19:	0 (Ever married)	-.50	-.19	-.47	-.76	-.39	-.59
	0 (Total)	.07	.29	.73	-.32	.38	-.01
	1	-.02	.43	.14	-.45	.28	-.18
	2	-.03	.15	-.22	-.01	-.04	-.13
20-24:	0 (Ever married)	-.06	.15	.07	-.37	.14	-.21
	0 (Total)	-.05	.22	.75	-.45	.34	-.16
	1	.04	.43	.71	-.47	.53	-.12
	2	.32	.56	.42	.07	.45	.26
	3	.40	.53	.33	.62	.40	.41
	4	.43	.73	.07	.60	.39	.32
	5	.23	.36	-.01	.48	.15	.23
25-29:	0 (Ever married)	-.08	.19	.68	-.44	.28	-.18
	0 (Total)	-.14	.18	.76	-.51	.34	-.23
	1	-.06	.34	.77	-.50	.65	-.15
	2	.18	.44	.47	-.30	.43	.03
	3	.24	.42	.30	.02	.35	.15
	4	.36	.47	.36	.42	.37	.38
	5	.39	.51	.38	.54	.39	.45
	6	.30	.35	.44	.31	.33	.36
	7+	.39	.63	.16	.45	.36	.30
30-34:	0 (Ever married)	-.10	.00	.82	-.36	.38	-.14
	0 (Total)	-.16	.19	.78	-.48	.49	-.23
	1	.01	.32	.58	-.40	.55	-.09
	2	.12	.35	.47	-.25	.40	-.01
	3	.21	.45	.33	-.10	.37	.07
	4	.32	.60	.48	-.08	.53	.17
	5	.29	.55	.29	.04	.41	.16
	6	.36	.44	.28	.52	.35	.39
	7+	.32	.34	.39	.50	.31	.41
35-39:	0 (Ever married)	-.07	.50	.20	-.34	.39	-.20
	0 (Total)	-.16	.25	.47	-.49	.39	-.25
	1	-.02	.50	.50	-.57	.55	-.23
	2	.10	.50	.46	-.41	.51	-.12
	3	.12	.40	.54	-.36	.46	-.03
	4	.15	.34	.48	-.25	.37	.03
	5	.20	.40	.44	-.22	.37	.12
	6	.18	.46	.37	-.21	.41	.03
	7+	.42	.41	.62	.42	.46	.51
40-44:	2	.09	.39	-.22	-.11	.23	-.10
	3	-.04	.16	-.24	-.16	.09	-.15
	4	-.27	.14	-.25	-.65	.03	-.51
	5	-.03	.41	-.36	-.13	.04	-.22
	6	.07	.03	.20	.10	.06	.13
	7+	.25	.33	.36	.14	.32	.24

Source: Scripps Foundation for Research in Population Problems.

These low values alone suggest that the relation between fertility and economic conditions is direct, but not very strong. The highest median value of $r = .4$, for example, is consistent with a prediction index of .08, which indicates that the prediction of fertility is improved by only 8 percent if one takes economic conditions into account. However, the strength of the relation varies considerably with the particular economic index used, the period of time considered, the number of children already born, and age.

The direct relation between economic conditions and fertility was found to be strongest for first birth probabilities for all zero-parity women in 1931-41. The correlations with unemployment ranged from −.68 to −.80; with income, from .57 to .66; and with industrial production, from .47 to .78. The strength of these relations can be explained partly by high correlations between the marriage rate and economic conditions and between the first birth rate and the marriage rate.

When variations due to changes in the marriage rate are eliminated by confining attention to the first birth probability for zero-parity married women, the values of the correlation coefficients during 1931-41 are reduced. In fact, at ages 15-19, the correlations are reversed, suggesting that very young married women are more likely to have a first birth when economic conditions are poor than when they are good. This reversal is evidently spurious, and probably results from the fact that in the computation of the first birth probability for zero-parity married women, *all* first births were assumed to have occurred to married women. The proportion married at ages 15-19 responded much more vigorously to changing economic conditions than did the first birth rate. In effect, then, both the numerator and the denominator of the first birth probability for zero-parity married women behaved in accordance with the hypothesis, but the quotient itself was inconsistent with the hypothesis. If data were available on the number of first births to married women only, it is possible that the first birth probability for very young zero-parity married women would vary directly with economic conditions.

The arrays of correlation coefficients shown in Tables 12.1, 12.2, and 12.3 show few definite patterns. No one indicator of economic conditions is clearly better than another as a predictor of fertility. In 1917-30 unemployment and industrial production show the strongest relations with fertility. In 1931-41 industrial production was the best predictor, and in 1947-57 income was most closely related to fertility.

Generally, the relations were strongest in 1917-30 and weakest in 1947-57.

As noted earlier, the correlation coefficients were highest for first births to zero-parity women during 1931-41. Aside from this finding, however, birth probabilities for the older women (up to 35-39) and the higher orders of birth tended to vary more in accordance with economic conditions than did the probabilities for younger women and lower birth orders. (Women 40-44 are an exception to this generalization; their birth probabilities showed poor agreement with economic conditions, except for the probability for eighth and higher births).

The tendency for the higher order birth probabilities to vary with economic conditions was greatest in 1917-30 and 1947-57, least in 1931-41.

It may seem anomalous for the higher order birth probabilities to show closer association with economic conditions than the lower order ones. If it is assumed, as seems reasonable, that birth probabilities vary largely because of wider variations among births to planners than to nonplanners, and if planners are more likely to respond to economic changes than are nonplanners, then the closest relation between birth probabilities and economic conditions should be found among the groups with more planners. Lower order births (after the first) are more often planned than higher order births.[7] Therefore, lower order birth probabilities should vary more directly with economic conditions than higher order birth probabilities. The fact that they do not requires explanation.

A possible reason for this unexpected finding is that of the many influences affecting couples' family planning decisions, the economic influence is dominant among couples who already have several children. Noneconomic factors may be just as important or more important among couples with fewer children. Therefore, among low-parity couples, the impact of economic conditions is mixed with other influences, and the relation of fertility to economic conditions is relatively weak. Among high-parity couples, however, the economic influence may be virtually the only one operating. Therefore, it is relatively unhampered by other factors.

It must be recognized that this is an *ad hoc* hypothesis constructed to explain an unexpected finding. Perhaps it is useful only in suggesting questions for further research.

In general, the findings reported above are consistent with the hypothesis that the timing of fertility varies directly with economic conditions. However, except for specific instances, the association is not close, and there are apparently other influences that have stronger effects.

Easterlin's Hypothesis

A major attempt to relate long-term cycles in fertility and economic conditions has been made by Richard A. Easterlin.[8] The evidence he reviews suggests that long-term movements in fertility rates are consistent with long-term movements in economic activity. The main impact of economic conditions on fertility comes about through the mechanism of the labor market, particularly as it affects the entrance of younger workers to the labor force. When the demand for labor is high and the supply is low, the economic conditions of younger couples are relatively good, and their fertility is relatively high. The postwar baby boom, according to Easterlin, is not unique in the sense that it resulted from new forces, but was due to the coincidence of three trends: an unusually strong economic expansion accompanied by a demand for more labor, restricted immigration, and relatively small numbers of young people at the ages of usual entrance to the labor force. The latter two factors limited greatly the supply of labor-force entrants, and enabled those who were available to find relatively well-paying jobs.

An implication of this hypothesis, noted by Easterlin, is that when the children born during the baby boom became old enough to enter the labor force, the supply-demand picture would be relatively less favorable for young entrants to the labor force and fertility would decline.[9] In a later paper, published in 1966, the recent evidence for this hypothesis is reviewed and found to be consistent with it.[10] Fertility has declined during the early 1960's, and the economic conditions of young people have not improved as rapidly as those for older members of the labor force.

The fertility cycles investigated by Easterlin are long-term movements of 15 to 20 years' duration. As will be shown in Chapter 13, such changes are mixtures of trends in completed fertility and shifts in the timing of births. These two elements composing the long-term movements in period fertility rates have operated so as to reinforce, rather than dampen, each other, so that the movements in period fertility rates are considerably greater than the movements that would have occurred if only one dimension of fertility had changed. Figure 13.1, for example, compares actual trends in the total fertility rate (a period measure) for 1920-64 with hypothetical trends that would have been observed if the timing of fertility had remained constant. The hypothetical series shows much less variation than the actual series.

So the question arises, To which aspect of fertility does the Easterlin hypothesis relate? Does the changing economic environment affect primarily the timing of fertility (that is, the ages at which women have children) or the eventual number of children that couples have? Easterlin faced this problem in a paper in which he speculated that the decline in period fertility rates observed in the early 1960's was due primarily to a decline in completed fertility, although he noted that at ages over 30 changes in timing also had tended to reduce period measures of fertility.[11]

It is entirely possible and plausible that the relations documented by Easterlin operate both with respect to the timing of fertility and completed fertility. This is consistent with current speculation, noted again in Chapter 13, that postponement of childbearing to later ages often results in a lower average family size.

Easterlin's hypothesis is the most successful attempt to date to relate economic conditions and fertility on the basis of observed data. However, certain aspects of the hypothesis, particularly those relating to the distinction between timing and completed fertility, clearly require more research. Unfortunately, the time series of data that should be used in such studies are not yet very long. So the full investigation of the relation hypothesized by Easterlin still lies in the future.

Summary

Although the century-long records of fertility and economic conditions in the industrially developed countries suggest that fertility declines as economic conditions improve, recent evidence suggests that other things being equal, there is a direct relation between fertility and economic conditions.

The main evidence for a direct relation is found in studies of the relation between short-term fluctuations in fertility and economic conditions. These studies are interpreted as demonstrating primarily a relation between the timing of births and economic conditions. In other words, couples tend to delay births when economic conditions are poor and have them when economic conditions are favorable.

The relation between the completed fertility of cohorts and the economic conditions experienced by cohorts during the main years of the childbearing period has not yet been thoroughly investigated.

A study of the relation between annual fluctuations in age-parity-specific birth probabilities and three economic indicators is described. This study confirms the direct association between fertility and economic conditions.

A major hypothesis to explain the direct association between long-term movements in fertility and economic conditions has been proposed by Richard A. Easterlin. So far, the main features of this hypothesis have been strongly supported by the available evidence, although more research is needed to investigate it fully.

13 / Cohort Fertility

In describing trends and differentials in fertility, it is often useful to distinguish between two types of fertility measures: period measures and cohort measures. Period measures relate to limited periods of time—usually 1 year. Examples of such rates are the general fertility rate, gross and net reproduction rates, and age-specific birth rates. Cohort measures, on the other hand, are designed to follow the fertility of groups of women as they proceed through the childbearing years of life. In other words, period rates focus on the experience of specific calendar years, but cohort rates focus on the experience of groups of women over a number of years.

We may think of the cohort approach as an attempt to study the continuing *process* of changing fertility rates as they are observed throughout the reproductive period rather than to compare points within the process as if they were isolated from each other. Cohort analysis proceeds on the assumption that rates at various stages of the reproductive period are not isolated in reality, but strongly influence one another. What happens early in the process affects what happens later. Cohort analysis tries to make these relations explicit.

The most common ways of identifying groups of women studied in cohort analysis are by the year of their birth and the year of their first marriage. The former method analyzes the fertility of groups called birth cohorts; the latter studies marriage cohorts. Since each approach has unique advantages, both will be discussed. The first part of this chapter deals with birth cohorts and the second part with marriage cohorts.

Birth Cohorts
Technical features of cohort fertility tables have been treated elsewhere.[1] Rather than try to cover this ground again in detail, this chapter will describe some of the practical uses of cohort fertility tables for interpreting current trends in fertility and for making short-range forecasts. For readers who are not familiar with the cohort approach, a brief description of commonly used cohort measures and concepts is presented in Appendix A.

In the first half of this chapter cohort fertility rates that have been computed from vital statistics data are used. However, it should be noted that it is also possible to obtain roughly comparable rates from census and survey data. For example, average numbers of children ever born to women in specified age groups, from reports in a census or survey, are equivalent to cumulative birth rates by age based on vital statistics data. Also, parity distributions by age can be computed from both data sources.

Comparisons of cumulative fertility rates based on vital statistics data with those based on census data for 1940 and 1950 were made by Pascal K. Whelpton.[2] He showed that both sets of rates were in close agreement. Cumulative fertility rates from the two sources frequently differed by less than 2 percent and seldom differed by more than 5 percent. Similar comparisons for 1960, presented in Table B.3, also show relatively close agreement. Most of the major differences were expected on the basis of knowledge about probable biases.

The Conceptual Framework of Cohort Analysis. The number of children borne by a cohort in a particular year may be regarded as the product of two variables: the number of children the women of the cohort will have by the end of the childbearing period, and the proportion of children they have in the specified year. If it were known, for example, that the women of the 1930 cohort would have 3,100 births per 1,000 women by the end of the childbearing period and that they would have 2 percent of these births during age 35, attained in 1965, then one would know that the central birth rate for the 1930 cohort during 1965 would be 62 births per 1,000. In brief, cohort analysis views annual fertility rates as the resultant of two factors: completed fertility and the distribution of births over the ages of the reproductive period.

In the process of analyzing trends in fertility, attempts are made to state the extent to which changes in each of these factors are responsible for changes in annual measures of fertility. A method of separating the effects of these two components is described below.

Completed Fertility and Total Fertility. For the purposes of this discussion, annual fertility is measured by the *total fertility rate.* This is the sum of age-specific birth rates for all ages in the reproductive span, observed in a given calendar year.

An important conceptual advantage of the total fertility rate is that it states the number of births 1,000 women would have if they experienced a given set of age-specific birth rates throughout the reproductive age span. The rate of 3,331 for 1963, for example, means that if a hypothetical group of 1,000 women were to have the same birth rates at each single year of age that were observed in the entire childbearing population in 1963, they would have a total of 3,331 children by the time they reached the end of the reproductive period, taken here as age 50, assuming that all of them survive to that age.

This rate is useful because it can be compared with the past and projected reproductive performance of actual groups of women as they proceed through the reproductive period of life. Such comparisons give some idea of the extent to which fertility in a given year may be distorted by factors that can have only a temporary effect. For example, the total fertility rate for 1957 was 3,724. This was the highest rate observed in this country since the beginning of the series in 1917. However, there was evidence from an interview survey of married women that no actual group of women then in the childbearing population expected to have as many as 3,700 children per 1,000 women by the end of their reproductive period.[3] This survey suggested that women then in the prime reproductive ages of 20-24 would have no more than 3,300 births per 1,000 women. This comparison means that the 1957 rate of over 3,700 was "distorted" in the sense that such a high rate could not be maintained for a long time if women in the main reproductive ages were going to have no more than 3,300 births. The total fertility rate would soon have to descend to a level more compatible with the experience of actual groups of women living through the childbearing period.

The measure with which the total fertility rate is compared in the above example is known as the *completed fertility rate*. It is the total number of children ever born to the women of a cohort by the time they reach the end of the reproductive period, which is assumed to be 50 years of age. In the above example, the rate of 3,300 is a projection of the average completed fertility rate for women in the cohorts of 1931-35.

Table 13.1 shows both the total fertility rate (averages for 5-year periods) and the completed fertility rate (averages for 5-year cohort groups). The total fertility rates are shown in the top row of the table, and the completed fertility rates are shown in the last column. The rest of the rates in Table 13.1 are averages of central rates (see Appendix A for a description of the age groups to which these rates relate). These rates are the additive components of both the total fertility rates and the completed fertility rates. When the central rates are added vertically (within 5-year calendar periods), they yield the total fertility rate. When they are added horizontally (within 5-year cohort groups) they yield the completed fertility rate.

Table 13.1 Central birth rates during 5-year calendar periods specified, by groups of cohorts

Cohort group	Calendar years (Jan. 1 to Dec. 31)									Completed fertility rate
	1920-24	1925-29	1930-34	1935-39	1940-44	1945-49	1950-54	1955-59	1960-64	
Total fertility rate	3,200	2,788	2,307	2,156	2,429	2,884	3,284	3,640	3,454	...
1951-55	...	...	...	...	...	...	...	...	...	...
1946-50	...	...	...	...	...	...	...	...	86	...
1941-45	...	...	...	...	...	...	...	101	787	...
1936-40	...	...	...	...	...	...	98	870	1,153	...
1931-35	...	...	...	...	...	86	771	1,178	782	...
1926-30	...	...	...	...	61	631	1,019	797	423	...
1921-25	...	...	...	58	511	872	748	457	185	...
1916-20	...	...	53	445	735	658	426	198	37	...
1911-15	...	60	439	619	569	406	184	38	1	2,316
1906-10	63	510	637	489	347	189	37	1	...	2,273
1901-05	565	752	525	318	165	40	1	...	...	2,421
1896-1900	850	634	368	176	38	2	...	...	...	2,675
1891-95	734	457	217	47	3	...	...	...	...	2,963
1886-90	545	285	62	4	...	...	...	...	...	3,208
1881-85	335	81	6	...	...	...	...	...	...	3,391
1876-80	99	9	...	...	...	...	...	...	...	3,636
1871-75	9a	...	...	...	...	...	...	...	...	...

Source: National Center for Health Statistics, Vital Statistics of the United States, selected volumes.

aEstimated.

The Timing of Fertility. When it is possible to compute or estimate the completed fertility rate for a cohort (or group of cohorts), the distribution of central rates by age of mother or by calendar year of birth can also be computed. For example, from the rates in Table 13.1 one can compute the proportion of births to the 1911-15 cohorts that occurred in the period 1935-39, when the cohorts progressed from exact ages 20-24 to 25-29. This proportion is 26.7 percent (619 divided by 2,316 and multiplied by 100). Percent distributions of central rates, computed in this manner, are used to express the "timing" component in cohort analysis.

Before such percent distributions can be computed, it is necessary to have an estimate of the total number of children that a cohort or cohort group will have altogether, that is, an estimate of completed fertility. Such estimates are difficult to make for cohorts that have not yet completed the childbearing period. In order to prepare such estimates for this discussion of the timing of births, projections prepared by Whelpton in 1963 have been modified by procedures described in the footnote of Table 13.2.

In brief, Whelpton's three series of projected cumulative birth rates, by cohort, for January 1, 1965, were compared with the observed rates for that date. Ratios of actual to observed rates were computed

Table 13.2 Estimated completed fertility rates based on projections by Whelpton, cohorts of 1916–20 to 1946–50

Cohort	Whelpton's projections[a]			Adjusted projections[b]			Average of adjusted projections
	Low	Medium	High	Low	Medium	High	
1946–50	2,484	2,930	3,395	2,638	2,652	2,702	2,664
1941–45	2,682	3,024	3,378	2,698	2,843	2,976	2,839
1936–40	2,898	3,135	3,378	3,028	3,157	3,277	3,154
1931–35	3,118	3,295	3,474	3,227	3,338	3,443	3,336
1926–30	3,056	3,168	3,281	3,087	3,158	3,229	3,158
1921–25	2,866	2,895	2,924	2,852	2,866	2,880	2,866
1916–20	2,546	2,565	2,584	2,552	2,552	2,552	2,552

Source: National Center for Health Statistics, Vital Statistics of the United States, selected volumes.

[a]Pascal K. Whelpton, Arthur A. Campbell, and John E. Patterson,
Fertility and Family Planning in the United States, Table 210.

[b]Estimated by multiplying Whelpton's projections of completed
fertility by ratios of actual to projected cumulative fertility rates
for 1965. The ratios are shown in the last three columns of Table
13.3.

as shown in the last three columns of Table 13.3. These ratios were
then multiplied by Whelpton's projections of completed fertility rates,
by cohort, as set forth in the first three columns of Table 13.2, in
order to obtain a revised estimate of the completed rate. The revised
estimates of completed rates were computed for each of the three
series, and the three resulting rates were averaged to obtain a central
estimate that is used as the estimate of the completed fertility of cohort group.

An interesting by-product of this procedure is an evaluation of
Whelpton's fertility projections up to 1965. His medium series was
quite close for the older cohorts (1936-40 and earlier), but his low
series was closest for the younger cohorts (1941-45 and 1946-50).
The ratios of actual to projected rates in Table 13.3 show the details.

Table 13.4 shows how the distribution of births by age within cohorts has changed over time. Women in the cohorts of 1891-1930 had
48 to 57 percent of their births before reaching exact ages 25-29.
More recent cohorts, however, are having substantially higher pro-

portions of their births before ages 25-29. The proportions projected for the cohorts of 1936-45 are around 67 percent.

How have the timing changes shown in Table 13.4 affected annual birth rates in the past 45 years? One way of answering this question is to compute hypothetical total fertility rates that would have been observed in 5-year calendar periods if there had been no changes in timing, and then to attribute the difference between the observed and hypothetical rates to changes in timing.

Table 13.3 Comparison of actual cumulative rates, by age, with projections by Whelpton for 1965

Cohort	Age	Whelpton's projected rates for current ages on 7-1-65[a]			Projected rates adjusted to exact ages on 1-1-65			Actual[b] 1-1-65	Ratios of actual to projected rates		
		Low	Medium	High	Low	Medium	High		Low	Medium	High
1946-50	15-19	118	137	156	81	95	108	86	1.062	.905	.796
1941-45	20-24	1,000	1,070	1,142	883	945	1,008	888	1.006	.940	.881
1936-40	25-29	2,128	2,209	2,291	2,030	2,107	2,186	2,121	1.045	1.007	.970
1931-35	30-34	2,782	2,844	2,908	2,721	2,781	2,844	2,817	1.035	1.013	.991
1926-30	35-39	2,933	2,972	3,012	2,901	2,939	2,979	2,931	1.010	.997	.984
1921-25	40-44	2,846	2,861	2,875	2,846	2,861	2,875	2,831	.995	.990	.985
1916-20	45-49	2,546	2,565	2,584	2,546	2,565	2,584	2,552	1.002	.995	.988

[a]Pascal K. Whelpton, Arthur A. Campbell, and John E. Patterson, Fertility and Family Planning in the United States (Princeton: Princeton University Press, 1966), Table 210.

[b]National Center for Health Statistics, Vital Statistics of the United States, 1964, Vol. I, Natality, Tables 1-17.

Table 13.4 Percent distribution of completed fertility rates by 5-year age groups, cohorts of 1876-80 to 1941-45

Cohort	Completed fertility rate	Percent of completed fertility occurring at ages								Summary	
		10-14 to 15-19	15-19 to 20-24	20-24 to 25-29	25-29 to 30-34	30-34 to 35-39	35-39 to 40-44	40-44 to 45-49	45-49 to 50-54	10-14 to 25-29	25-29 to 50-54
1876-80	3,636	----	----	----	----	----	----	2.7	0.2	----	----
1881-85	3,391	----	----	----	----	----	9.9	2.4	0.2	----	----
1886-90	3,208	----	----	----	----	17.0	8.9	1.9	0.1	----	----
1891-95	2,963	----	----	----	24.8	15.4	7.3	1.6	0.1	50.8	49.2
1896-1900	2,675	----	----	31.8	23.7	13.8	6.6	1.4	0.1	54.4	45.6
1901-05	2,421	2.3	23.3	31.1	21.7	13.1	6.8	1.7	0.0	56.7	43.3
1906-10	2,273	2.8	22.4	28.0	21.5	15.3	8.3	1.6	0.0	53.2	46.7
1911-15	2,316	2.6	19.0	26.7	24.6	17.5	7.9	1.6	0.0	48.3	51.6
1916-20	2,552	2.1	17.4	28.8	25.8	16.7	7.8	1.4	0.0	48.3	51.7
1921-25[a]	2,866	2.0	17.8	30.4	26.1	15.9	6.5	1.3	0.0	50.2	49.8
1926-30[a]	3,158	1.9	20.0	32.3	25.2	13.4	6.0	1.2	0.0	54.2	45.8
1931-35[a]	3,336	2.6	23.1	35.3	23.4	10.2	4.5	0.9	0.0	61.0	39.0
1936-40[a]	3,154	3.1	27.6	36.6	19.5	8.6	3.8	0.8	0.0	67.3	32.7
1941-45[a]	2,839	3.6	27.7	36.3	19.3	8.5	3.8	0.8	0.0	67.6	32.4
1901-45 average	2,768	2.6	22.0	31.7	23.0	13.2	6.2	1.3	0.0	56.3	43.7

Source: National Center for Health Statistics, Vital Statistics of the United States, selected volumes.

[a]The method of estimating completed fertility rates for these cohorts is described in Table 13.1. The percentages below the diagonal line, which represent fertility after January 1, 1965, are estimates based on the assumption that the age distribution of the remaining fertility of a given cohort group is the same as that for the preceding cohort group at comparable ages.

In order to do this, some timing pattern is needed to use as a model in computing hypothetical rates. The model timing pattern used here is the average of the percentages in Table 13.4 for the cohorts of 1901-45 (shown on the bottom row of the table).

The Interplay of Timing and Completed Fertility, 1920-65. If all of the cohorts in the reproductive years of life in the 45-year period 1920-64 were to have distributed their births by age according to the model chosen, the total fertility rates of each of the 5-year periods would have been the hypothetical values shown in Table 13.5 and Fig. 13.1.

Since the hypothetical trend line is not affected by changes in timing, it shows changes due to completed fertility only. Without shifts in timing, total fertility would have fallen from about 2,800 in 1920-24 to 2,400 in the 1930's, and would then have risen to 3,000-3,100 in the 1950's and early 1960's.

Table 13.5 Actual and hypothetical total fertility rates, by 5-year periods, 1920-69

| Period | Total fertility rates | | Percent actual above or below hypothetical |
	Actual	Hypothetical[a]	
1965-69	----	2,954	---
1960-64	3,454	3,089	12
1955-59	3,640	3,118	17
1950-54	3,284	2,986	10
1945-49	2,883	2,755	5
1940-44	2,429	2,539	- 4
1935-39	2,156	2,417	-11
1930-34	2,307	2,432	- 5
1925-29	2,788	2,577	8
1920-24	3,200	2,802	14

Source: National Center for Health Statistics, Vital Statistics of the United States, selected volumes.

[a]The hypothetical rates are those that would have been observed if fertility within cohorts had been distributed by age in accordance with the average timing pattern for the cohorts of 1901-45. This pattern is shown in the bottom row of Table 13.4.

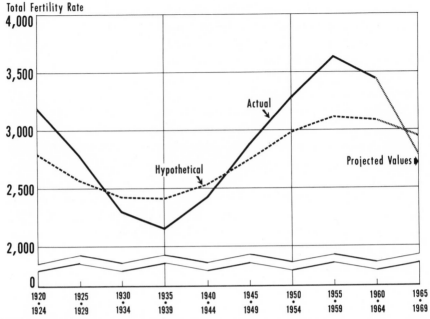

Fig. 13.1. Actual and hypothetical total fertility rates, by 5-year periods, 1920-69. Hypothetical rates are based on the assumption of a constant distribution of births by age of mother within cohorts. See text for details.

Actual total fertility rates followed the general direction of these movements, but the amplitude of the cycle was much wider. Actual rates were above hypothetical rates in the 1920's, below them in 1930-44, and above them in 1945-64. These deviations are due to shifts in the timing of actual births.

The much steeper decline of actual than of hypothetical total fertility rates in the 20-year period 1920-39 was due to a shift away from the younger ages of childbearing. The reversal of this trend during the next 20-year period resulted from a combination of two distinct movements: (1) a shift toward the older ages of childbearing for the cohorts of 1911-20, and (2) a shift toward younger ages of childbearing for later cohorts.

Although the first of these movements did not have as much impact on the total fertility rate as the second, it should be noted carefully, because it illustrates the main point of cohort fertility analysis: the fertility of the earlier years of the childbearing period strongly influences the fertility of the later years. The women of the 1911-15 cohorts, for example, had borne only 48.3 percent of their children by 1940, when they had reached 25-29 years of age, compared with

53.2 percent by the same ages for the preceding cohort group (1906-10). This simply meant that a larger proportion of the births of the 1911-15 cohorts were delayed until 1940 and later years. Similar shifts occurred for the 1916-20 cohorts. They postponed (in effect) some births before 1945 only to have them later and inflate the total fertility rates of the postwar period.

The women of the 1921-25 cohorts began the shift toward younger ages of childbearing. They reached ages 20-24 in 1945, and had relatively high birth rates in the immediate postwar period. Later cohorts had higher and higher proportions of their children at the younger childbearing ages. The trend apparently reached its culmination with the 1936-45 cohorts. Recently observed rates for younger cohorts suggest that a reverse movement has begun, although this is not yet certain.

It is important to note that the changes in the timing of births over the 45-year period under study have tended to exaggerate the movements due to changes in completed fertility. In other words, when completed fertility was declining (as in the 1920's), the age distribution of fertility rates shifted toward later childbearing, which made the decline steeper than it otherwise would have been. Later, when completed fertility was rising, the age distribution of fertility shifted toward earlier childbearing and made the rise in total fertility more rapid than it would otherwise have been.

Theoretically, at least, changes in timing could have operated to dampen the movements due to changes in completed fertility rather than to exaggerate them. If falling completed fertility rates had been accompanied by a trend toward earlier childbearing, and if rising completed fertility rates had been accompanied by a trend toward later childbearing, the changes in period total fertility rates would have been much gentler than the movements that actually occurred.

The experience of the 1920-64 period, then, suggests that whatever factors cause completed fertility to decline, whether they are economic or of some other nature, also cause the age distribution of childbearing to shift toward later ages. Conversely, the factors that bring about a rise in completed fertility also cause a trend toward earlier childbearing.

It is also possible, of course, that there is a direct causal connection between completed fertility and age at childbirth, Freedman speculates, for example, that later childbearing may bring about a decline in completed family size.[4] If such a relation does indeed exist, we can expect variations in period measures of fertility to continue to exceed those in cohort measures. Perhaps total fertility rates will fluctuate almost as much in the next 50 years as they did in the past 50.

Implications for Fertility in 1965-69. The shift toward younger childbearing on the part of the cohorts of 1921-45 has meant an inevitable decline in the proportion of children borne at the older childbearing ages; the total fertility rates of the period 1965-69 are bound to reflect this reaction.

In effect, this means that the average total fertility rate for 1965-69 will probably fall below the hypothetical rate of 2,954 computed on the basis of cohort projections for this period. It is reasonably certain that actual percentages of children borne at ages 25-29 and later will be below those used in the model (compare, for example, the last two rows of Table 13.4). Also, it seems quite possible that the proportions of children borne at the younger childbearing ages will fall below the levels estimated for the 1936-40 and 1941-45 cohorts. On balance, it now seems reasonable to expect a total fertility rate of about 2,800 for the 1965-69 period.

Such an expected figure should be regarded primarily as a model against which to view actual changes in fertility. If actual fertility is well above or well below the expected level, projections of completed fertility or assumed timing patterns would have to be revised further. However, it is only by making such a priori estimates on the basis of what is known to date that one can refine the procedures used in cohort analysis.

Marriage Cohorts

For present purposes a marriage cohort is defined as a group of women who *first* married in a given calendar period, regardless of subsequent widowhood, divorce, or remarriage. Because of the mores of our society, the fertility history of women generally dates from their first marriage. The tabulations may, however, be separate for that part of a cohort that is still in an unbroken first marriage and for that part that is not. The date of first marriage is the one reported for a woman and may in some instances involve a consensual marriage rather than a legal marriage. The relatively few children born to women before marriage are included with those born after marriage to the extent that illegitimate children are reported. Since most women eventually marry, most illegitimate children, if reported, would eventually be assigned to a marriage cohort.

Availability of Data. Data on the number of children ever born to women classified by years since first marriage have been tabulated from the censuses of 1910, 1940, 1950, and 1960, and from the March 1962 Current Population Survey. The period in which the woman first married can, of course, be determined by subtraction of the years since marriage from the survey date. But such materials yield only the fertility status of a marriage cohort as of the survey date. In order to follow the experience of a given cohort through successive marriage durations, data on fertility are needed for more than one date. Birth dates of children yield fertility data on a retrospective basis, but such fertility histories have rarely been compiled. At this writing, tabulations made from the August 1959 Current Population Survey comprise the most extensive data presently available for the United States on the fertility progressions of marriage cohorts. Similar tabulations from the June 1965 Current Population Survey are not yet available. It may be said, therefore, that only a beginning has been made in research into the fertility of marriage cohorts for the United States. Several European countries have done more, notably the British in their "family census" of 1946. Also, some countries have long recorded date of marriage on their birth registration forms, whereas that item is not available on the standard birth registration forms used in the United States.

Distribution of Cohorts by Age at Marriage. Marriage cohorts comprise women of all ages at first marriage, including a relatively small number who marry at too old an age to have children. The distribution of the members of a cohort by age at marriage is therefore part and parcel of the makeup of the cohort. Typically, however, most women marry at an age that is sufficiently young for them to have many children if they so desire. Table 13.6, based on 1960 census data, provides an understated indication of how the ability to bear children varies by age. It is evident from the table that even women who married in their forties were often capable of having at least one child after marriage. About three-tenths of the women 40-44 years old who had been married only 1.0 to 1.9 years had a first child. Undoubtedly, some of the other women who married at such an advanced age were capable of having children even though they had none.

Figure 13.2 illustrates how some marriage cohorts of white women have varied in the initial distribution of their members by age at marriage. The data shown include restorative allowances, made with the

Table 13.6 Percentage of women who have had a first child, for women married 1.0 to 1.9 years, by color and age of woman: United States, 1960

Age in 1960 (years)	White		Nonwhite	
	Total women	Percent with first child	Total women	Percent with first child
15	4,933	65.5	775	87.1
16	17,351	69.2	2,911	83.2
17	43,233	70.8	6,223	83.0
18	74,635	70.4	10,858	83.8
19	123,646	66.5	14,444	80.4
20	141,214	64.6	14,216	77.9
21	123,541	63.0	13,337	73.4
22	102,906	61.0	11,816	73.3
23	82,500	58.1	8,907	72.4
24	59,904	56.1	8,637	68.2
25–29	119,764	56.1	22,513	64.8
30–34	39,686	50.9	8,586	61.0
35–39	19,475	43.7	4,731	51.3
40–44	9,418	31.5	2,674	43.0

Source: Derived from U.S. Bureau of the Census, 1960 Census of Population, Women by Number of Children Ever Born, PC(2)-3A, Tables 21,22.

aid of life tables, for those women who died between the marriage date and the August 1959 survey date. The marriage ages shown have a terminal group of 30 and over, not because such women cannot bear children but because relatively few women marry for a first time at such ages. The cohorts differ very little from one another in the proportion of their members married at age 30 and over. The largest differences between cohorts occur in the proportions married by age 20 and by age 22. Because most women marry by age 25, relatively smaller differences between cohorts occur by that age than by younger ages.

The white marriage cohorts of 1955-59 and 1950-54 are notable for their relatively high proportions of women who married by age 20 or 22 as compared with earlier marriage cohorts. Those high proportions reflect a trend towards a younger average marriage age that began after World War II and culminated with the cohort of 1955-59.[5] There is evidence from other surveys (not shown) that the average age at first marriage increased between 1960 and 1964. The cohorts

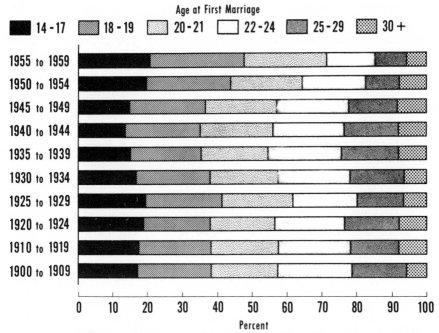

Fig. 13.2. Distribution by age at first marriage for specified white marriage cohorts: United States. Retrospective data from August 1959 Current Population Survey; data include life table allowances for effect of mortality since marriage date.

of 1955-59, 1950-54, and 1925-29 were the ones that deviated most from the general levels of distribution by age at first marriage for cohorts over the half-century covered by the chart. The other cohorts in the 50-year period have a very high degree of similarity of distributions by age at first marriage.

The cohort of 1925-29 married 7 to 11 years after World War I. Its distribution by age at marriage closely resembles that of the 1950-54 cohort, which married 5 to 9 years after World War II. This similarity suggests that economic and other conditions favorable to young marriages tend to be abnormally strong a few years after a major war. Probably it is easier for a young man to get a job and marry a young girl during the time that the economy is making up for wartime postponed production of consumer goods. The full effect of a postwar economy on a young average marriage age most likely is not felt immediately after a war but a few years later. In the immediate postwar years, war veterans making up for postponed marriages, with brides correspondingly older, tend to increase the average age of brides.

The economic depression of the 1930's is characterized in the literature as having led to some postponement of marriages to a later age than would otherwise have been the case. The cohort that married in 1935-39 had a smaller proportion of its members married at young ages than any other cohort, perhaps reflecting some making up of marriages postponed from 1930-34, but its distribution by age at marriage does not differ much from that of the cohorts of 1940-44 and of 1920-24.

Data for nonwhite cohorts are shown in Fig. 13.3. Because sampling variability is considerable for the relatively small numbers of nonwhites interviewed in the 1959 sample, the nonwhite cohorts are grouped by 10-year periods rather than 5-year periods. The nonwhite cohorts have far greater proportions of members married at age 14 to 17 than the white cohorts, as may be seen by comparing Figs. 13.2 and 13.3. Whereas the recent white cohorts exhibited a trend towards younger average marriage ages as compared with the earlier cohorts, nonwhites had a trend towards an older average age. To some extent, that may mean that the nonwhites are becoming more like whites in

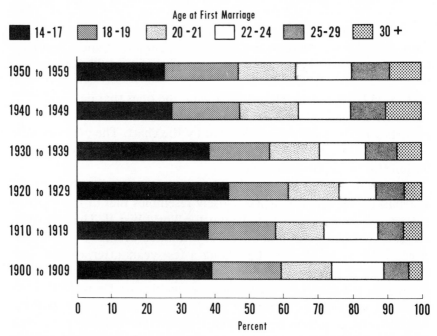

Fig. 13.3. Distribution by age at first marriage for specified nonwhite marriage cohorts: United States. Retrospective data from August 1959 Current Population Survey; data include life table allowances for effect of mortality since marriage date.

respect to marriage age distributions, by reducing their formerly very high proportions married at age 14 to 17. Confirmation of at least a small decline in proportion of nonwhite girls marrying before age 18 may be found in decennial census data (not shown) for 1960 and 1940, on the proportion of nonwhite girls under 18 who have married. But much of the decline shown by Fig. 13.3 may reflect a bias in the data rather than a reality. The data for the 1950-59 nonwhite marriage cohort are roughly in line with expectations from 1950 and 1960 census data on the marital status of young women, but those for earlier cohorts, especially the pre-1940 cohorts, appear to overstate the proportion of nonwhite women married at ages 14-17. In the 1940 census, for example, 29 percent of nonwhite girls 18 years old were reported as having been married, whereas the data from the August 1959 survey indicated that 38 percent of the 1930-39 nonwhite cohort married at ages 14-17, while 44 percent of the 1920-29 cohort did so. We speculate that some members of the earlier nonwhite cohorts surveyed in 1959 tended to misreport a date of first "experience" as a date of first marriage. The speculation is based in part on trends in illegitimate first births, discussed later. No biases of similar magnitude appear in data for white women.

Effect of Mortality. As a marriage cohort progresses through life, its older members are continuously subject to higher mortality than its younger members. Accordingly, survey data for surviving members of a cohort become somewhat selective in favor of those members who married at a young age. The bias from mortality can be allowed for with the aid of life tables, as was done for the data shown in Figs. 13.2 and 13.3. However, that allowance involves data tabulated by age at marriage. Most of the fertility data currently available for marriage cohorts are not cross-classified with age at marriage. The bias from the selective effect of mortality is generally small for many years after the marriage date, but its existence should be kept in mind when studying fertility data. By the way of illustration, Table 13.7 shows how the age at marriage distribution differs for members initially in a marriage cohort (figured with the aid of life tables) and for surviving members, for two cohorts that are long past the marriage date. It may be noted from the table that the white cohort of 1925-29 differs in rather small degree in terms of data for initial members and data for members surviving 30 to 34 years after the marriage date. More recent cohorts than the one of 1925-29, not shown, are in much closer agreement. But for the cohort of 1900-09, which was

50 to 59 years past the marriage date by 1959, quite sizable differences exist, as would be expected in view of the fact that many of the survivors were in their 70's or 80's by 1959.

Table 13.7 Distribution by age at first marriage for women initially in marriage cohort and women surviving to August 1959, for white women first married in 1925-29 and 1900-09: United States

Color and age at first marriage	Cohort of 1925-29		Cohort of 1900-09	
	Initially in cohort	Survivors in 1959	Initially in cohort	Survivors in 1959
Women (thousands)	4,341	3,870	6,642	2,925
Percent, 14 and over	100.0	100.0	100.0	100.0
14-17	19.6	20.2	17.2	22.6
18-19	21.9	22.4	21.0	25.3
20-21	20.1	20.3	19.2	20.8
22-24	18.6	18.5	21.1	19.4
25-29	13.1	12.6	15.6	10.4
30 and over	6.7	5.9	5.9	1.5
Median age at marriage	20.8	20.7	21.2	20.2

Source: U. S. Bureau of the Census, Current Population Reports, Series P-20, No. 108, Table 14.

Stability of First Marriages. A few examples from the August 1959 Current Population Survey will suffice to provide some information about the stability of marriage, and particularly about the stability of marriage during the childbearing period.

The cohort of 1945-49 was 10 to 14 years past the first-marriage date by 1959. The importance of that time interval can perhaps best be indicated by the fact that roughly seven-tenths of a woman's lifetime childbearing occurs by 10 years after marriage. Among survivors in 1959, 85 percent of white women first married in 1945-49 were living with their first husbands. It is estimated that 2 percent more were in an intact first marriage with the husband being employed or otherwise living elsewhere for reasons other than marital discord. Nine percent of the marriage cohort had remarried, and the remaining 4 percent were currently separated, divorced, or widowed.

Among white women first married in 1935-39, who on the average were about 40-44 years old in 1959 and thus were of virtually completed fertility, 75 percent were still living with their first husbands and 15 percent had been married more than once.

The stability of first marriages varies with the age at marriage. In the 1935-39 cohort (who as of 1959 were 20 to 24 years past the date of first marriage), 64 percent of white women who first married at ages 14-17 were still living with their first husbands, compared with 76 percent of those who married at ages 18 and 19, 79 percent of those who married at ages 22-24 and also of those who married at ages 25-29, and 69 percent of those who married at age 30 and over. Although marriages at ages 14-17 were relatively unstable compared with those at ages 18-29, it appears that roughly two-thirds of the early marriages remained intact. Women who first married at age 30 and over were subject to a greater risk of widowhood than women who married at a younger age.

To a considerable extent the breakup of first marriages during the childbearing period is offset by subsequent remarriage, so that fertility does not necessarily come to an end. Among white women in the 1935-39 cohort who were not living with their first husbands in 1959, 77 percent of those who first married at ages under 20 had remarried by 1959, compared with 62 percent among those first married at ages 20 and 21, 51 percent among those first married at ages 22-24, and 44 percent at ages 25-29.

Among nonwhite women, only 73 percent of women first married in 1950-59 were living with their first husbands as of August 1959. Among nonwhite women first married in 1930-39, the corresponding proportion was only 46 percent. In the latter cohort, 55 percent of those not living with their first husbands had remarried. Because first marriages are less stable on the average for nonwhite than for white women, the nonwhite women have more remarriages per marriage cohort, overall. But if the comparison is limited to data for women not living with their first husbands instead of including data for an entire marriage cohort, then the proportions remarried tend to be smaller for nonwhite women than for white women, age for age. The slim chances of remarriage for nonwhite women may be related to men of low average income being reluctant to marry a woman who already has a considerable number of children by a prior marriage. The costs of divorce may also be a factor, preventing some women whose first husbands have left them from obtaining a divorce in order to remarry.

Fertility of Marriage Cohorts: An Overall Point of View. As of 1959, the cohorts through 1939 were the ones for which completed or virtually completed fertility experience was available. (For younger cohorts, some clues as to the outlook for completed fertility were available.) Presented below are rates of children ever born per 1,000 women for marriage cohorts of completed or virtually completed fertility:

Cohorts	White	Cohorts	Nonwhite
1935-39	2,512	1930-39	3,244
1930-34	2,393	1920-29	2,767
1925-29	2,474	1910-19	3,262
1920-24	2,697	1900-09	4,447
1910-19	3,148		
1900-09	3,862		

Before discussing the figures given above, it may be well to provide a historical perspective. The cohort of 1900-09 is far from being indicative of much higher levels of fertility that once existed. It is estimated that in Colonial times white women of completed fertility had averaged about eight children ever born per woman, and that fertility declined steadily after about 1810.[6] The census of 1910 showed a rate of 5,278 children ever born per 1,000 white women ever married 70-74 years old; those women largely married just before the War Between the States. For nonwhite women the comparable rate from the 1910 census was 6,957, but some younger groups of women had higher rates. Slavery conditions did not always permit Negroes to reproduce at will. Given the benchmark figures just mentioned, it is obvious that trends in the fertility of marriage cohorts as shown above represent a partial continuation of declines that set in long before 1900-09, but which ended with one or another of the cohorts shown. It should be kept in mind that the rates for the 1900-09 cohort may be a little too high for a fair comparison with rates for younger cohorts because the surviving women in the 1900-09 cohort were more selective of women who married at a young age than in the case of data for younger cohorts.

Among white women, the rate of 2,393 children ever born per 1,000 women for the cohort of 1930-34 represents a nadir in the trend of completed fertility for successive cohorts of women. The cohort of 1930-34 married at a younger average age than the one of 1935-39, as previously noted, but the cohort of 1935-39 had more children (rate of 2,512). This is additional evidence that variations in fertility are somewhat independent of variations in age at marriage.

Among nonwhite women, the lowest level in completed fertility appears to have occurred with the marriage cohort of 1920-29 instead of with the cohort married in the economic depression of the 1930's. We do not know the full story of why the nadir occurred earlier for nonwhite than for white women. One clue exists in 1960 census data on the percentage of nonwhite women who have borne no children. That percentage was at a maximum (28) among nonwhite women ever married 50-54 years old, many of whom probably belonged to the 1925-29 marriage cohort. In contrast, only 13 percent of nonwhite women 85 years old and over in 1960, ever married, were childless, and only 14 percent of those 26 years old. According to data for marriage cohorts from the 1959 survey, 26 percent of women in the 1920-29 nonwhite marriage cohort, which had completed its childbearing, were childless. In contrast, the 1950-59 nonwhite cohort was already down to 12 percent childless by 84 months after marriage. Much of the nonwhite childlessness in the past is thought to have been of an involuntary nature because private studies indicated that few Negroes practiced contraception before birth of their first child. Also, certain diseases that cause sterility are thought to have reached a peak about 10 years after World War I; their occurrence was reduced by various public health measures during the 1930's and even more after the advent of antibiotics during the 1940's.

As marriage cohorts of 1940-44 through 1950-54 (and perhaps also the cohort of 1955-59) complete their childbearing, they are expected to continue the upward trend in completed fertility for successive cohorts that began with the nadirs just mentioned. This may be seen by examining the number of children born thus far for cohorts of incomplete fertility and by dividing that number by an assumed proportion of lifetime fertility completed by a given interval since first marriage. For example, the white cohort of 1950-54 already had a rate of 2,069 children ever born per 1,000 women by 84 months after marriage. If it is assumed that the women had completed about 65 percent of their eventual lifetime fertility by 84 months after marriage, then division of the observed rate of 2,069 by the assumed 65 percent yields a projected completed fertility rate of about 3,200. The figure of 65 percent is, of course, only a rough approximation. It comes by noting (see next section) that the cohorts of 1910-19 through 1935-39 completed 57 to 60 percent of their lifetime fertility by 84 months after marriage and by allowing somewhat for the effect of earlier childbearing in the 1950-54 cohort than in older cohorts. Evidence on the earlier childbearing for the 1950-54 cohort exists in data that show this cohort has already had more first-, second-, and third-child births by 84 months after marriage than the older cohorts had had by that interval.

The 1955-59 cohort had more children by 18 months after marriage than any older cohort had had by that interval, but that is too short an interval to indicate the prospects for completed fertility.

Among nonwhite women, rates of children ever born are much higher for the 1950-59 cohort than for earlier cohorts at comparable intervals since first marriage. For example, the nonwhite cohort of 1950-59 had already borne 1,772 children per 1,000 women by 48 months after marriage, as compared with a low of 1,019 for the cohort of 1920-29 by that interval since marriage, and a previous high of 1,320 for the 1940-49 cohort, considering the 50-year marriage cohort span for which data are available. The assumption that the cohort of 1950-59 had completed less than 45 percent of its lifetime childbearing by 4 years after marriage implies that the ultimate complete fertility rate will exceed 4,000.

Proportion of Lifetime Fertility Completed by Successive Intervals since First Marriage. White marriage cohorts of 1910-19 through 1935-39 had remarkably similar relative proportions of lifetime fertility completed by successive intervals since first marriage (Table 13.8). About 10 percent of their lifetime fertility occurred by 12 months after marriage, with additional increments of about 10 percent in each of the next 2 years after marriage, for a total of about 30 percent by 36 months after marriage. In those first 3 years there was no slowing down of birth production as a proportion of lifetime fertility. By 60 months (5 years) after marriage, the proportion of lifetime fertility already produced was 45 to 48 percent. The median, or halfway mark, occurred by 63 to 70 months after marriage. By 10 years, or 120 months, after marriage the women had already completed about seven-tenths of their lifetime fertility. Only about 15 percent of lifetime fertility was added in the interval between 10 and 15 years and a final 12 percent after 15 years. That description does not fit the white marriage cohort of 1900-09, which bore relatively more of its children at long intervals after marriage (and which had much higher fertility than the succeeding cohorts). Nonwhite cohorts also have a pattern of relatively many children at long intervals after marriage, which appears stronger than that of the white cohort of 1900-09, but they also have a larger proportion of their lifetime children by 12 months after marriage as compared with data for white cohorts.

The near-stability of proportions of lifetime fertility completed by successive intervals since first marriage as shown in Table 13.8 should not be taken as evidence that similar patterns will also apply to oncoming cohorts that have not yet completed fertility. It is quite likely that the proportions of lifetime fertility completed by 5 years and by 10 years after marriage will prove to be much higher for the white marriage cohorts of 1945-49, 1950-54, and 1955-59 than those shown for older cohorts. The oncoming cohorts have already produced first,

Table 13.8 Percentage of lifetime fertility completed by specified intervals since first marriage, for cohorts of completed fertility, by color: August 1959

Interval since first marriage, months	White					
	1935–1939	1930–1934	1925–1929	1920–1924	1910–1919	1900–1909
12	10.2	10.1	11.1	11.1	10.7	8.2
24	21.0	21.3	22.6	22.0	21.1	16.9
36	29.7	30.6	31.9	31.5	29.8	24.7
48	37.8	39.0	40.2	40.1	37.6	31.7
60	45.4	45.8	47.7	47.5	44.9	38.0
84	58.5	57.2	59.4	59.8	57.1	49.6
120	73.0	71.6	72.2	73.5	71.1	63.8
180	88.7	88.5	87.4	88.3	87.2	82.0
241+	100.0	100.0	100.0	100.0	100.0	100.0

Interval since first marriage, months	Nonwhite			
	1930–1939	1920–1929	1910–1919	1900–1909
12	14.4	14.3	12.7	7.4
24	23.0	22.4	20.3	14.5
36	29.9	30.7	29.2	21.7
48	37.3	36.8	35.2	28.8
60	43.2	42.8	40.2	33.7
84	52.6	52.0	50.6	43.5
120	64.6	63.5	63.9	57.0
180	81.5	80.2	79.2	76.0
241+	100.0	100.0	100.0	100.0

Source: U. S. Bureau of the Census, Current Population Reports, Series P-20, No. 108, Tables 16,17.

second, and third births in large proportion by 5 to 10 years after marriage, so fewer members are left who have not yet had such children. It is assumed here that there will be no return to the large-family system of yore. If half of lifetime fertility is completed by 5 to 6 years after marriage, as in data for white cohorts of 1910-19 through 1935-39, then it may be expected that in 5 or 6 years half of the nation's annual births will come from women not married at the present time.

First Births. Among white marriage cohorts of completed fertility, the rate of first births per 1,000 surviving women in 1959 varied from 898 in the cohort of 1900-09 (the oldest cohort for which data are available) to 831 in the cohort of 1930-34. For nonwhite women, the corresponding variation was from 871 in the cohort of 1900-09 to 744 in the cohort of 1920-29. The white cohort of 1950-54 had already attained a rate of 876 by 84 months after marriage and may augment that by about 40 points, for a total of roughly 920, by the time it completes its childbearing. Perhaps the 1955-59 white cohort will have more children than the 1950-54 cohort; the 1955-59 cohort already had a rate of 613 first births per 1,000 women by 18 months after marriage, as compared with a corresponding rate for that marriage interval of 501 for the 1950-54 cohort and of 466 for the 1900-09 cohort. The nonwhite cohort of 1950-59 had a rate of 884 by 84 months after marriage.

The median interval between marriage and first birth was 16.7 months in the white cohort of 1910-19. This is the lowest median for any white cohort of completed fertility for which data are available. The median increased to 21.6 for the cohort of 1930-34. Although they have not yet completed their childbearing, it is already known that the women of the 1950-54 cohort will have a median interval of about 15 months and that the women of the 1955-59 cohort will have a median interval of about 13 months. The cohort of 1955-59 had already attained a cumulated first-child birth rate of 494 by 14 months after marriage; doubling of that rate would yield a too high ultimate rate of 988, so it is evident that the halfway, or median, interval was achieved before the end of 14 months after marriage.

Among nonwhite women, the lowest median interval between marriage and first birth for cohorts of completed fertility was 12.6 in the cohort of 1930-39. The median interval was 14.0 in the cohort of 1920-29 (which had the lowest first-birth rate of any nonwhite cohort on record). It now appears that when the 1950-59 cohort completes its childbearing it will have a median of about 10 months.

All the above medians for the interval between marriage and first births are based on data that include illegitimate first births as well as first births occurring after marriage. In tabulations made from the August 1959 survey, children born before the marriage of the mother were included with data for children born less than 1 month after marriage. Data on cumulated first births (including illegitimate births) per 1,000 women for selected months in the first year after marriage are presented in Table 13.9.

By subtraction of the cumulated rate for less than 1 month from the cumulated rates for subsequent intervals, some information on legitimate first births can be obtained. For white cohorts, the rates

Table 13.9 Cumulated first births per 1,000 women by selected intervals since marriage, by color, for cohorts: August 1959

Color and cohort	Interval since marriage					
	Less than 1 month	6 months	7 months	8 months	9 months	12 months
WHITE						
1955-59	32	85	127	160	223	420
1950-54	24	71	96	119	175	331
1945-49	26	57	77	103	156	310
1940-44	19	44	61	80	114	234
1935-39	22	51	68	86	118	233
1930-34	26	54	69	90	123	225
1925-29	17	44	56	81	122	256
1920-24	16	48	59	83	127	285
1910-19	25	55	69	89	139	308
1900-09	24	45	57	74	133	298
NONWHITE						
1950-59	220	356	379	413	436	531
1940-49	148	237	266	294	336	429
1930-39	111	207	235	255	293	391
1920-29	117	180	190	218	262	341
1910-19	92	168	189	207	250	355
1900-09	63	90	102	118	188	294

Source: U. S. Bureau of the Census, Current Population Reports, Series P-20, No. 108, Tables 16, 17.

for less than 1 month are too low to affect appreciably the median intervals between marriage and first births that were cited above. But for nonwhite women, the medians are considerably altered when illegitimate first births are excluded. For example, the nonwhite cohort of 1930-39 would have had a median interval of about 18 months between marriage and first birth if births through less than 1 month after marriage were eliminated, as compared with the cited median of 12.6 months for data involving all first births.

Figure 13.4 shows the pattern of rates of first births occurring in specified months after marriage per 1,000 white women childless at the beginning of the month, for three marriage cohorts. It should be kept in mind that this type of rate involves only legitimate births for

First Births Per 1,000 Childless Women

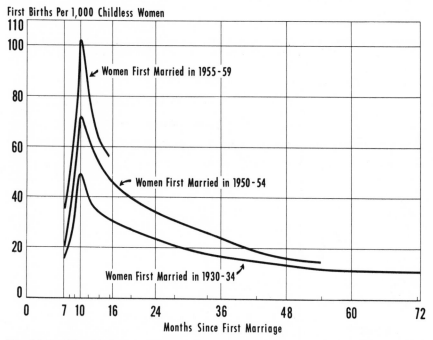

Fig. 13.4. First births in successive months since first marriage per 1,000 women childless at beginning of the month, for specified marriage cohorts of white women: United States.

the numerator and that the denominator excludes women who have already had a first child. The cohorts of 1955-59 and 1950-54 had higher first-birth rates in the first few years after marriage than have been observed for any older cohort for which data are available (back to the one of 1900-09), whereas the cohort of 1930-34 had the lowest rates. Other cohorts, not shown, have rates of intermediate magnitude.

The patterns for the three cohorts shown in Fig. 13.4 suggest that cohorts which have high rates at very early intervals after marriage tend to maintain relatively high rates at much later intervals, instead of reducing them by the way of partial compensation for early childbearing. This holds only for rates based on women who are childless. For marriage cohorts as a whole, including mothers as well as childless women, it is obvious that early childbearing reduces the proportion of women at longer intervals who are not yet mothers.

The cohorts exhibit remarkably similar trends of rates by successive intervals since first marriage in the sense that within each cohort the rates increase to a maximum at 10 months after marriage and then decline, with the decline being especially steep between 10 months and 16-18 months of marriage with some tapering off thereafter. It should be noted, however, that the 1955-59 and 1950-54 cohorts had rates at intervals well past 10 months that exceeded the 10-month peak rate for the 1930-34 cohort.

Typically, about nine out of ten first births (including illegitimate births) occur by 5 years (60 months) after first marriage, among white and nonwhite women alike. Women who have their first child at a long interval since first marriage are more apt to stop with that child than women who have their first child at a short interval. Partly for that reason, the median interval between marriage and first birth tends to be longer for women who stop at one child than for women who go on to have more than one child. For example, in the white marriage cohort of 1935-39 the median interval between marriage and birth of the first child was 37.4 months when the first child was the only child the women ever had. But it was 19.3 months for those women who went on to have additional children after the first child.

Births of Second Order. By 84 months (7 years) after marriage the white cohort of 1950-54 had 700 second children per 1,000 women, compared with corresponding rates of 424 for the cohort of 1930-34 and of 613 for the cohort of 1900-09. The latter two cohorts completed their childbearing with second-child birth rates of 643 and 760, respectively. It would appear, therefore, that the chances are excellent that the cohort of 1950-54 will surpass the cohort of 1900-09 in respect to eventual lifetime production of births of second order. The younger cohort has already surpassed the lifetime rates for cohorts between 1920-24 and 1935-39. As of 48 months after marriage, the 1950-54 cohort had a rate of 434; doubling of that rate would yield a much too high "target" value of 868 for purposes of computing a median interval between marriage and birth of the second child. It would seem, therefore, that the true median will be less than 48 months. Among white cohorts of completed fertility, the median interval between marriage and birth of the second child varied from 48 months in the cohorts of 1900-09 and 1910-19 to 62 months in the cohorts of 1930-34 and 1935-39. It is clear that in recent cohorts second births, like first births, have been coming earlier after marriage than was the case among older cohorts.

It may be of interest to note that the second-birth rate of 700 per 1,000 women for the 1950-54 cohort by 84 months after marriage was 80 percent as large as the cumulated first-birth rate of 876 for the same interval. This means that many of the women who had a first child went on to have a second child. Comparable ratios for 84 months after marriage are 55 percent for the cohort of 1930-34 and 74 percent for the cohort of 1900-09. Because most first births have already occurred by 84 months after marriage, although that is not the case for second births, the ratios cited understate the proportion of women who progress from first to second births during their life-time. In the cohorts of 1900-09 through 1920-24 about 20 percent of second-child births occurred after 84 months since marriage, and in the cohort of 1930-34 about 35 percent. The cohort of 1930-34 evidently postponed some second births to a long interval after marriage.

Among nonwhite cohorts, it appears that the cohort of 1950-59 will have a median interval of roughly 30-33 months between marriage and birth of the second child, as compared with observed medians of 41 to 45 months in cohorts of 1900-09 through 1935-39. However, those higher medians for cohorts before 1940 may be partly biased upwards from some misreporting of the marriage date. Partly because of a high proportion childless in pre-1940 cohorts, the nonwhite cohorts of completed fertility had lower rates than white cohorts of second children per 1,000 women. The rate varied from 722 in the nonwhite cohort of 1900-09 to 534 in the nonwhite cohort of 1920-29. All indications available suggest that the women of the nonwhite cohort of 1950-59 will surpass the rate of 722 for the 1900-09 cohort by the time they complete their childbearing. Lower rates of first- and second-child births among nonwhite than among white women do not conflict with the fact that nonwhite women are more fertile than white women, overall. The nonwhite women have relatively more births of high order.

Births of Third and Higher Order. By 84 months (7 years) after marriage, the white cohort of 1950-54 had borne 345 third children per 1,000 women. That rate was more than twice a nadir of 151 for the same marriage duration in the cohort of 1930-34. It probably represents a higher level of fertility (in terms of third births) than for any prior cohort for which data are available. The white cohort of 1900-09 had an observed rate of nearly the same size (340) by 84 months after marriage, but that rate is biased upwards from the effect of selective mortality. Thus, the production of third births, like that of first and second births, has been more rapid after marriage in the 1950-54 white cohort than in others preceding it by as much as half a century.

The 1930-34 white cohort completed its childbearing with only 382 third children per 1,000 women, with a median interval of about 100 months between marriage of the women and the birth date of their third child, whereas the 1900-09 cohort completed its child-bearing with an observed rate of 597 third children per 1,000 women and a median of 79 months. The earlier rate is biased upwards from the effect of selective mortality and the median of 79 months is biased downwards. It is possible that the cohort of 1950-54 merely had many of its third children sooner after marriage than that of 1900-09, in which case it will not necessarily overtake the cohort of 1900-09 in respect to lifetime production of third births, although it certainly will exceed that of cohorts intermediate between 1950-54 and 1900-09.

Data now available do not provide satisfactory information on the production of births of fourth and higher order for marriage cohorts of 1950 and later because those cohorts had not been married long enough as of 1959 to have had many births of such high orders. On the basis of data for marriage cohorts of 1900-09 through 1935-39, it appears that roughly 10 percent of births of fourth or higher order occur by 84 months after marriage, and half by 150 to 160 months. Perhaps the best that can be done at this time is to note the previous estimate that the white cohort of 1950-54 will complete its child-bearing with a total of about 3,200 children (of all birth orders) per 1,000 women, or about the same as for the 1910-19 white cohort (rate of 3,148) but less than that for the 1900-09 cohort (rate of

3,862). From this, coupled with the fact that the 1950-54 cohort will surpass the 1910-19 cohort with respect to production of first, second, and third births, one may infer that the 1950-54 cohort will have fewer births of fourth and higher order than the cohort of 1910-19. The 1910-19 white cohort completed its childbearing with 1,069 births of fourth and higher order per 1,000 women, far fewer than a corresponding rate of 1,607 for the 1900-09 cohort. It seems fairly certain, therefore, that the white cohort of 1950-54 will have fewer than 1,069 births of fourth and higher order by the time it completes its childbearing. A return to the large-family system of previous eras is unlikely. On the other hand, the white cohort of 1950-54 may be safely visualized as eventually surpassing the nadir of 537 births of fourth and higher order that occurred in the white cohort of 1930-34. Among nonwhite cohorts, the cohort of 1940-49 was ahead of the one of 1910-19 in respect to births of fourth and higher order per 1,000 women by 120 months (10 years) after marriage, and it may or may not surpass the lifetime rate of 1,439 for the 1910-19 cohort but probably will fall far short of the comparable rate of 2,267 for the nonwhite 1900-09 cohort. Not enough observations are available to provide numerical values for the nonwhite cohorts of 1950 and later in terms of births of fourth and higher order.

Summary

Fertility rates for birth cohorts are essential in analyzing trends in annual (or period) fertility rates. The trend in annual measures of fertility is determined by trends in two components of fertility: completed fertility (the number of children born by the end of the childbearing period) and the age distribution of fertility rates throughout the reproductive period of life. Changes in either of these components affect the level of annual fertility rates.

The high fertility rates observed in the United States during the period 1946-63 resulted from changes in both of these components. The first was a rise in completed fertility. The average number of children ever born rose from approximately 2,300 births per 1,000 women for the cohort of 1906-15 to an estimated 3,300 for the cohort of 1931-35. Although this was certainly an important factor in the maintenance of high annual fertility rates during the postwar period, two additional changes in the timing of fertility also contributed to high fertility.

The first of these changes was an upward shift in the age distribution of fertility rates for the cohorts of 1916-25 (approximately). The women in these cohorts had had relatively low age-specific birth rates during the depression and war years, when they were in the younger childbearing ages. They compensated for this low fertility by having relatively high rates at the older childbearing ages in the years immediately following World War II.

The second change in the timing of fertility rates was a downward shift in the age distribution of fertility rates for younger women (those in the cohorts of 1925-40, approximately). They married at younger ages than the women in preceding cohorts and had their children sooner after marriage. Both of these changes in the age distribution of fertility rates inflated annual measures of fertility well above the levels that would have been observed if the only change had been the increase in completed fertility.

Over the 45-year period 1920-65, changes in completed fertility and the timing of fertility have reinforced each other so as to produce much wider variations in period fertility rates than those that would have resulted solely from changes in completed fertility.

In the 1960's the United States entered a new phase of the long-term fertility cycle, in which changes in the age distribution of fertility rates are producing relatively depressed annual measures of fertility. The women who were having high rates at the younger ages in the 1950's are now having relatively low rates at the older childbearing ages. In addition, the age distribution of rates for the younger cohorts appears to be shifting toward the older ages. This also has a depressing effect on annual measures of fertility. It is possible, too, that recent cohorts will have lower completed fertility than the cohorts of the 1930's, but one cannot yet be certain of the influence of this factor because these cohorts are still in the early portion of the reproductive period.

A marriage cohort is defined as a group of women who *first* married in a given calendar period. Typically, the fertility of women begins after marriage, and the first few years are the most productive. In the United States roughly half of the lifetime childbearing of women occurs by about 5 years after marriage, and roughly seven-tenths by 10 years after marriage. This has important implications for projections of births because within a short time the bulk of the nation's annual births will come from women who are not now married and who may differ somewhat from those now married in respect to the number of children they want and the timing of the births.

Data from the August 1959 Current Population Survey show clearly that the marriage cohorts of 1955-59 and 1950-54 have had their first children at a shorter average interval since marriage than older cohorts, and that relatively high proportions of the more recent cohorts had married by age 20 or 22 as compared with older cohorts. Keeping in mind the high proportion of lifetime number of children born in the first 10 or so years after marriage, it is of some interest to note that in the marriage cohort of 1945-49, 85 percent of white women were living with their first husbands at the time of the 1959 survey and an additional 9 percent had remarried and were living with a subsequent husband. The stability of marriages varies with age at marriage, being less at both very young ages and very late ages than at the more usual ages of marriage. Despite the hazards of teenage marriages, two-thirds of the white women who married in 1935-39 were in intact first marriages 20 to 24 years later.

The data for marriage cohorts show that a woman's last child is typically born at a much later interval since marriage than other children of the same birth order whose mothers went on to have yet more children.

The marriage cohort of 1930-34 is the one with the lowest average number of children ever born. It had a slightly younger average age at marriage than the cohort of 1935-39 but spent more of its childbearing period under economic depression conditions. The marriage cohort of 1955-59 had more children in shorter intervals than any prior cohorts dating back to 1900-09.

In the preceding pages the authors have attempted to describe the recent trends in fertility among different elements of the population of the United States. The chief data utilized were the registration data from the National Center for Health Statistics and the United States census data regarding number of children ever born in relation to various demographic and socioeconomic characteristics. However, other materials have been used, particularly those relating to fecundity and family planning from the Growth of American Families Studies, with which one of the authors was formerly associated.

In the demographic world setting the United States is conventionally classified as a country of low fertility, along with countries of Europe, Oceania, Canada, Japan, and Uruguay. It was not always so. As described in the 1950 census monograph, *The Fertility of American Women,* fertility rates in Colonial America were among the highest in the world. Conventional estimates place the average number of offspring at eight per woman of completed fertility during the early part of the Colonial period. Malthus used population data for Colonial America to illustrate the principle of geometric increase. However, the high fertility of young pioneers in a frontier society where industrious offspring could clear land and start their own families was obviously not a social problem of the type that is associated with high fertility in the densely settled underdeveloped areas of today.

Whatever the reasons for the high fertility in Colonial America, there was a virtually continuous decline in fertility ratios of white women in the United States during the long period 1810-1940. Then, contrary to all the carefully prepared forecasts and projections, World War II was followed by a sustained increase in fertility rates in countries of "low fertility." This proved to be of longer duration in the United States than in most other modernized countries. However, there have been declines in the annual birth rate in this country since 1957.

Although human fertility is heavily influenced by existing institutions, culture, customs, and socioeconomic factors, reproduction is basically a biological process. Over the centuries fertility rates in preindustrial societies have tended to be high not merely because fertility was uncontrolled but also because high fertility had survival value for the species. High rates of infant mortality and fetal deaths necessitated many confinements in order to have a few children. Conversely, the marked improvement that has come about in the saving of infant lives and the reduction of fetal deaths has been frequently cited as a factor partly responsible for the decline in pregnancy rates in modern nations. In a broader context, declines in infant mortality have permitted family planning, and family planning has helped to reduce infant mortality.

Advances in medicine, public health, and health education have, of course, increased the possibility for successfully completed pregnancies. For instance, the reduction in the incidence of venereal disease after World War II has probably been a factor in the increased fertility and decreased childlessness among nonwhite families in the past two decades. There have been marked declines in infant and maternal mortality and in fetal deaths in modernized countries. High death rates in these categories are associated with poverty, high order of pregnancy, and plurality of births. All are higher among nonwhite than among white persons and among illegitimate than among legitimate conceptions. (There is also a higher rate of infant mortality and of fetal deaths among males than among females.)

The few studies of the relation of mental illness to fertility suggest that marital fertility rates of women with schizophrenia are much like those of the general population. However, because of relatively low marriage rates in this group, its general fertility rates are lower. The female inmates of correctional institutions tend to be of lower fertility than the general population.

The Growth of American Families Studies of 1955 and 1960 and the National Fertility Study of 1965 and other investigations have provided information regarding fecundity and family planning. Almost one-third (31 percent) of white couples with wives 18-39 years old in the 1960 G.A.F. Study were classified as Subfecund—i.e., below normal in the ability to reproduce. In about one-third of the Subfecund white couples (or one-tenth of all white couples in the 1960 G.A.F. Study) the wife or husband had undergone operations which made it impossible to conceive. Over half of these operations were contraceptive in intent.

Although fecundity impairments probably were more common among urban Negroes than among white persons in this country during the interwar period, there now appears to be little difference between white and nonwhite persons with respect to fecundity.

With regard to family planning, a majority of married white couples (87 percent) have used or expect to use some form of limitation on their fertility. According to the 1960 Growth of American Families

Study, the proportion was 76 percent for nonwhite couples. Between 1955 and 1960 there was a trend toward earlier use of contraception.

Although the average number of children ever born per 1,000 women of given age in the childbearing period generally was higher in 1960 than in 1950 for all classes, the rates of increase varied. As a result of these variations the fertility differentials by region, urban-rural residence, and socioeconomic status became narrower during the 1950-60 decade but those by color, and probably also those by religion, were enhanced.

By region, the Northeast still ranks lowest and the South highest with respect to fertility of the women residents. However, the top position of the South in 1960 was due to the high fertility of non-white women in that region. Among white women under 40 years old in 1960, those in the North Central States exhibited higher fertility on the average than those in the South. The relative variations in fertility by region tended to be sharper for nonwhite than for white women. This arises from the situation of higher fertility among the nonwhite women than among their white counterparts in all regions except the Northeast.

Because of sharper increases in the fertility of nonwhite than of white women during the 1950-60 decade, the fertility differential by color increased at all ages of the 15-49 span and especially at ages 25-39. Thus, the average number of children ever born per 1,000 ever-married women 30-34 years old was 12 percent higher for nonwhite than for white women in 1950 and 23 percent higher in 1960.

Among the nonwhite population of the United States as a whole, the American Indians exhibited highest fertility rates at all ages within the 25-49 span. The Negroes held top position at ages under 25. The lowest fertility rates tended to be those of women of Japanese and Chinese ancestry. Among white women, those of Mexican and Puerto Rican birth or origin exhibited conspicuously high fertility. With respect to foreign white stock other than Mexicans, fertility rates were relatively high for Canadians and relatively low for those reporting Norway, Sweden, Germany, and Austria as countries of birth or ancestry.

Because the 1950-60 increases in average number of children ever born tended to be higher in urban than in rural areas, the fertility differentials by urban-rural residence generally were much smaller in 1960 than in 1950. Thus, among ever-married white women 30-34 years old, the percent excess of the fertility rate for women in rural nonfarm areas over that of comparable urban women was 28 percent in 1950 and 14 percent in 1960. The excess of the rate for white rural-farm ever-married women over urban women was 50 percent in 1950 and 26 percent in 1960.

The narrowing of the urban-rural differential in fertility also occurred among nonwhite women during the decade, but in both 1950 and 1960 the urban-rural differential was wider for nonwhite than for white women. The fertility differential by color tended to be smallest in urban areas and largest in rural farm areas.

The relation of fertility to migration is a complex one and depends much upon types of migrants and migration considered. The 1960 census data on number of children ever born to married women in relation to migration status (as determined by replies to a question regarding residence 5 years previously) rather consistently portrayed lower fertility among those involved in at least intercounty migration (including interstate and interregional) than among those not so involved. Similarly, ever-married women experiencing at some time during their lives a change of residence across broad regional lines were rather consistently of low fertility relative to women who continued to live in the region of birth.

The same data revealed no consistent tendency for the fertility rate for migrants to fall between the indigenous fertility rates of the region of origin and the region of destination. It was most likely to be lower than rates for either region. Although fertility rates of migrants are low with reference to those of nonmigrants left behind, migrants may carry with them patterns of high or low fertility with reference to communities into which they move.

The proportions of women who marry, their ages at marriage, and the timing of their births have considerable influence on period fertility rates. Thus, the rash of early marriages immediately following World War II and the postwar pattern of completing the family early in married life contributed heavily to the increase of fertility and its maintenance at a high level in this country. In addition, there was a substantial increase in completed size of family. That this occurred in the face of widespread acceptance of family planning suggests that after the war young couples wanted larger families than their parents in the preceding generation had wanted. They wanted larger families and they wanted them completed at an earlier age.

Since 1957 there may have been a reversal of the trends described above. Again, the chief component probably is one of period fertility, but the factor of eventual decline in completed cohort fertility may also be involved. The trend toward earlier average age at marriage appears to be ending with the birth cohorts of the late 1930's or early 1940's. Data from the Current Population Survey indicate that as of 1965 women under age 25 have been having fewer children than women of similar ages in surveys for past dates. Also, the numbers of children that young white women in the 1960 G.A.F. Study said they wanted and expected to have were a little smaller on the average than those wanted and expected by young women in the 1955 G.A.F. Study.

Age at marriage of the wife is a factor of prime importance in the trends and variations in human fertility. Examination of the 1960 census data on number of children ever born by wife's age at marriage and color suggests that a 2-year shift upwards or downwards is likely to change the average number of children ever born by roughly 8 percent for white women and 24 percent for nonwhite women. The difference by color probably is due in part to more family planning among white women.

It should also be recognized that for both white and nonwhite women, age at marriage tends to be directly associated with socioeconomic status. Thus, a 2-year lowering in age at marriage would be associated with a lowering of socioeconomic status. Nevertheless, there is no doubt that wife's age at marriage is a determinant of fertility of prime importance in its own right; it persists in groups that are alike with respect to either family planning or socioeconomic status. At certain ages selective factors are present. It is known, for instance, that a high proportion of premarital conceptions are involved among girls marrying before they are 18 years old.

An example of the importance of age at marriage is the finding that the nature of the relations of fertility to socioeconomic status and also to color are reversed when one shifts from early age at marriage to late age at marriage. Even on the basis of 1910 census data for the United States, Notestein found a direct relation of fertility of wife to occupational status of husband among native white couples with wives marrying at ages 25 and over. The 1960 data tabulated by wife's age at marriage and husband's education, occupation, and income tended to yield an inverse relation of fertility to socioeconomic status for wives marrying under age 22 and a direct relation for those marrying at ages 22 and over. The data generally affirmed the closer relevance of age at marriage than of socioeconomic status to fertility.

In data controlled for age and education of wife but not for age at marriage, the average number of children ever born tended to be higher for nonwhite than for white ever-married women at all educational levels except the highest (college 4+). However, when the data were restricted to women married at ages 22 and over, the fertility rate for white women was frequently higher than for nonwhite women at the same levels of education.

To some extent, the interval between marriage and first birth emphasizes the trend toward early family formation. The lowest median interval between marriage and first birth on record for marriage cohorts of completed fertility was 16.7 months for the white marriage cohort of 1910-19. From that date there was an increase to 21.6 for the marriage cohort of 1930-34, associated with the conspicuous decline of the birth rate during 1910-34. Although the white women in the marriage cohort of 1950-54 have not completed their childbearing, it is already known from data in the August 1959 Current Population Survey that the median interval between marriage and first birth will be only about 15 months for this group. It will be about 13 months for the 1955-59 marriage cohort of white women.

Intervals between marriage and first birth by color also provide a rough gauge of the relative number of premarital conceptions for white and nonwhite women and of the trends for each group. Thus, the cumulative rate of first births occurring less than 1 month after marriage was 32 per 1,000 white women and 220 per 1,000 nonwhite women in the marriage cohorts of 1955-59. The corresponding figures for the 1900-09 marriage cohorts were 24 per 1,000 white women and 63 per 1,000 nonwhite women. These rates include births before marriage insofar as they were reported.

The various measures of illegitimacy from registration data also point to considerably higher rates of illegitimacy among nonwhite than among white women, and to increases in illegitimacy rates for both color groups. However, there are many weaknesses in the data, including the presence of hidden factors which may have important effects on trends and variations in illegitimacy.

During the decade 1950-60 there was among married white women 25-49 years old a marked narrowing of the differentials in fertility by educational attainment of the woman and by occupation group of the husband. Thus, among urban white ever-married women 30-34 years of age, the average deviation of the fertility rates of the various educational classes from the average for the age group was 11.3 percent in 1950 and 8.5 percent in 1960. Comparable deviations for urban white women of this age (married and husband present) were 7.4 percent in 1950 and 5.3 percent in 1960.

In contrast to the rather marked and consistent narrowing of fertility differentials by socioeconomic status among white women 25-49 years of age was the enhancement of the differentials among nonwhite women during the 1950-60 decade.

The fertility rates of nonwhite women reporting 1 or more years of college tended to be below those of white women of this educational level. At other educational levels the fertility of nonwhite women tended to exceed that of white women and the percent excess tended to be inversely related to educational level. Similarly, among wives of professional men, the average number of children was frequently lower for nonwhite than for white women. For other occupational classes the fertility rate tended to be higher for nonwhite than for white women, and this excess was largest among wives of laborers.

Available evidence from unofficial sources suggests a widening of fertility differentials by religion in the United States in recent years. This appears to arise from sharper increases in the fertility of Catholics than of non-Catholics. The rationalization of accidental pregnancies may be a factor, but these studies suggest that Catholic couples have more children than non-Catholics primarily because they want them. The studies definitely indicate that Catholics practice family planning less frequently and less effectively than non-Catholics.

The studies consistently indicate lowest fertility for Jews, intermediate position for Protestants, and highest fertility for Catholics. By specific denomination of Protestants, the Episcopalians and Presbyterians tend to have lowest fertility and the Methodists and Baptists the highest. The foregoing ranking of Protestant sects reflects variations in fertility by color, urban-rural residence, and socioeconomic status. However, conspicuously high fertility rates are found for Mormons and Hutterites, who are exclusively white and well above average economically. There is definite need for more adequate data on the relation of religion to fertility in the United States. Census data for Canada suggest some narrowing of the Catholic–non-Catholic differentials in fertility in that country.

The relation of both period fertility and cohort fertility to economic trends is a subject on which more research is badly needed. Historically, studies have indicated that despite the inverse relation of socioeconomic status to proportions married at early ages, marriage rates tend to increase sharply with improving economic conditions. Probably mainly for this reason there tends to be also some rise in birth rates with improving economic conditions. Under conditions of planned fertility it seems likely that annual natality levels will tend to follow cyclical trends more closely.

The world population crisis that has developed since World War II has prompted unprecedented interest in population. This has been manifested not only in the formation of social action groups involving "Madison Avenue" approaches but also in the heavy endowment of research and in the expressed readiness of the United States Government, the United Nations, and other government and international organizations to participate in or support research and action in this field. On the family planning front during the last decade there have emerged two new devices, the oral pill and the intrauterine device, both of which have the advantages of simplicity and no interference with the sex act. These have opened up a considerable number of opportunities for social action and research.

United States government agencies are increasing their research in fertility in this country and in the collection and analysis of pertinent data. The National Institutes of Health, for example, contracts for such research with various universities, medical research organizations, and foundations. The Office of Economic Opportunity is supporting family-planning clinics and research in many poverty areas. The Bureau of the Census and the states are constantly seeking to improve their projections of population for long-range planning needs of government and the public. Many of these projects require benchmark data and new information from the Bureau of the Census and the National Center for Health Statistics. The National Center for Health Statistics has established a mail follow-up of a sample of birth registration records to obtain data not available on the standard registration records. The National Center for Health Statistics is also exploring possibilities of carrying out periodic surveys for the collection of data not now available in birth registration. The Bureau of the Census for some years has been planning a revised "standard package" of annual tabulations from the Current Population Survey which, among other things, will permit annual data on women by own children under 1 year old and under 5, by characteristics of the population. It also is preparing tabulations from the June 1965 CPS which go well beyond the invaluable types of information on childspacing and marriage cohorts obtained in the August 1959 CPS, and it has detailed plans for collecting data from future surveys and the 1970 census, resources permitting. The outlook for an ever-improving fund of data on fertility is therefore very good.

Appendix A. Concepts and Measures Used in Cohort Fertility Analysis Based on Vital Statistics

Birth Cohort

A birth cohort is a group of women born in the 12-month period centering on January 1 of the year by which the group is identified. For example, the cohort of 1900 was born between July 1, 1899 and June 30, 1900. The reason for defining birth cohorts on the basis of 12-month periods centering on January 1 rather than on the basis of conventional calendar years is that it makes more convenient the analysis of fertility trends by age and calendar year.

Using this definition of a cohort, most of the mothers who gave their age as 20 (meaning that they had reached age 20 on their last birthday) in 1920, for example, belonged to the 1900 birth cohort. The following table illustrates this point:

Date women gave birth at age 20	Possible dates of birth of women bearing children on date specified	Percentage of women belonging to cohorts[a] of		
		1899	1900	1901
Jan. 1, 1920	Jan. 2, 1899-Jan. 1, 1900	50	50	-
June 30, 1920	July 1, 1899-June 30, 1900	-	100	-
Dec. 31, 1920	Jan. 1, 1900-Dec. 31, 1900	-	50	50
Average percentage for year		12.5	75.0	12.5

[a]Assuming that birth dates are evenly distributed throughout the year.

Thus, approximately 75 percent of the 20-year-old women who gave birth in 1920 belonged to the 1900 birth cohort. In computing age-specific birth rates for the 1900 cohort, the denominator of the rate is actually a weighted average of the 1899, 1900, and 1901 cohorts. (The weights are .125, .750, and .125, respectively.)

The relation between age, cohort, and the year in which age is attained is straightforward. Where c is the cohort, a is age, and y is the year in which age a is attained, $y = c + a$. Until the introduction of cohort analysis, it was customary to present time series of age-specific birth rates in tables that may be represented by the formulation ($a \times y$). That is, age of mother was shown on one axis and year of birth on the other. Rates for cohorts could be followed only on the diagonals of such tables. The cohort approach, however, uses tables that may be represented by ($a \times c$) or ($y \times c$). Such tables make it possible to see in one row or one column all of the rates for a specified cohort. Table 13.1, for example, can be represented by the formulation ($y \times c$).

Central Birth Rate

The rate from which all other cohort measures are eventually derived is the central birth rate, specific for age. This is the number of births per 1,000 women for a specified cohort, year of age, and calendar year. For example, the central birth rate of the 1947 cohort during age 17 in 1964 is 62.4 births per 1,000 women. Central birth rates are also computed for each order of birth from the first through the seventh and for eighth and higher-order births combined.

Cumulative Birth Rate

Cumulative birth rates are sums of central birth rates from age 14 (assumed to be the age at which the childbearing period begins) up to an age specified for a given birth cohort. For example, the cumulative birth rate for the 1947 birth cohort by exact age 18 on January 1, 1965, is 109.7. This is the sum of the following central birth rates:

Age	Year of birth	Central birth rate
14	1961	4.0
15	1962	11.7
16	1963	31.6
17	1964	62.4
		109.7 = cumulative rate for exact age 18 on Jan. 1, 1965

Cumulative rates are generally specified for an exact age and for January 1 of a particular year. This is done in order to indicate that the cumulative rate includes all births that have occurred up to the beginning of a particular year of age and a particular calendar year. Central birth rates, in contrast, are always specified for a current age (i.e., age at last birthday) and an entire calendar year. Cumulative birth rates are also computed for births of each order.

Parity Progression Ratio

Parity progression ratios are derived from cumulative birth rates. They show the proportion of women with at least N births who have also had N + 1 births. For example, 17.9 percent of the women in the 1947 birth cohort who had at least one child also had at least one more child by January 1, 1965, when the ages of the women in the cohort average exactly 18 years. The parity progression ratio is computed by dividing the cumulative rate for N + 1 births by the cumulative rate for N births. The figure cited above was computed by dividing the cumulative rate for second births (16.3) by that for first births (91.1) and multiplying by 100.

In the computation of parity progression ratios, the cumulative birth rate is interpreted as a proportion of women who have ever had a birth of the order specified. In the example cited above, the fact that there were 91.1 first births per 1,000 women also means that 9.11 percent of all the women in the 1947 cohort had borne at least one child, since a woman can, by definition, have no more than one first birth. Similarly, the cumulative rate for second births (16.3 per 1,000) also means that 1.63 percent of the women in the 1947 cohort had borne two or more children.

Parity Distribution

This way of looking at cumulative birth rates leads to another cohort measure, the parity distribution. This is a distribution of all the women in a cohort by the number of children they have ever borne. These proportions are found by subtracting cumulative rates for adjacent orders of birth. In the example used above, if 9.11 percent of the women in the 1947 cohort have had one or more births, and if 1.63 percent have had two or more, then 9.11 − 1.63 = 7.48 percent have had only one birth. Further, if 9.11 percent have had one or more births, then 100.00 − 9.11 = 90.89 percent have had no births.

Birth Probabilities

Finally, an age-parity-specific birth probability shows the probability that a woman who has attained N parity by exact age x will have an (N + 1)th birth during age x. These probabilities are computed by dividing central birth rates for order N + 1 by the proportion of women with N births at the beginning of the year. For example, 36.8 per 1,000 (or 3.68 percent) of the women of the 1947 birth cohort had borne only one child by age 17, attained on January 1, 1964. During age 17 in 1964, the women of this cohort had 11.3 second births per 1,000 women. It is assumed that all of these second births occurred to women who had borne one child before 1964.

Therefore, the probability that a 17-year-old one-parity woman would have a birth during 1964 was 307 per 1,000 (11.3 divided by 36.8 and multiplied by 1,000).

Cohort Groups

For convenience, some cohort fertility measures are frequently presented for 5-year groups of cohorts, ages, and calendar years. This was done in Chapter 13. Such condensations save a great deal of space and emphasize the broad movements in fertility measures. The space-saving advantage can be appreciated by a comparison of a summary table showing central birth rates for 5-year cohort and age groups, with the detailed table from which it was derived. Each of the rates in the summary table is an average of 25 rates in the detailed table (five ages by five cohorts). Therefore, the reduction from the detailed to the summary table can be represented by the ratio of 25 to 1. In other words, the summary table occupies only 4 percent of the space that the detailed table would occupy.

While such summary presentations are useful for many purposes, they require the use of age groups that are not familiar to many users. For example, the women of the 1931-35 cohorts attained ages 15-19 in 1950 and ages 19-23 in 1954. Therefore, the central rate for the 1931-35 cohorts during the period 1950-54 is an average of central rates for different 5-year age groups in each year of the period. Instead of specifying age groups in conventional 5-year groups (15-19, 20-24, etc.), therefore, it is necessary to designate them in other ways. In Table 13.4, for example, the age groups are designated by the exact ages attained by the beginning and end of the 5-year period. This convention introduces some awkwardness in the representation of age groups, but the resulting disadvantages are easily outweighed by the economy of summary presentation.

Appendix B. Quality of Data on Children Ever Born in the 1960 Census and in Current Population Surveys

In the censuses and population surveys taken through 1965 the question on children ever born usually has been asked only of women who are reported as ever married. The relatively small loss of information from not asking never-married women about children ever born will be discussed later. In the tabulations never-married women are treated as having borne no children.

Nonresponse Rates

The question on children ever born was one of the few for which the nonresponse rate was considerably lower in the 1960 census than in the 1950 or 1940 censuses. Among women ever married, 6.0 percent of those 14 years old and over in 1960 had no report on children ever born as compared with 9.0 percent for women 15-59 years old in the 1950 census and 12.7 percent for women 14-74 years old in the 1940 census. The reduction in the nonresponse rate from census to census mainly reflects the effect of changes in enumeration procedures. In the 1960 census much of the sample information was obtained on a 25-percent basis in a "Stage II" enumeration that had no apparent indication on the enumeration form that any sample question was more or less important than any other question. In the 1950 census the basic enumeration form asked some questions on a 100-percent basis, some on a 20-percent basis, and some (including a question on children ever born) on a 3 1/3-percent basis, with the result that some harried enumerators and some field offices evidently regarded the different sample sizes as indicating the relative importance of the questions and hence of the relative need to make call-backs to pick up missing information. In the 1940 census not only was a question on children ever born asked at a third (5-percent) level of coverage on the same enumeration form as other questions asked at higher levels of coverage, but there was also no check box for entries of "none" for the item on children ever born, with the result that some enumerators simply left the item blank for a woman who was childless instead of entering a zero. In the Current Population Surveys, where special efforts are made to obtain answers to all questions, the nonresponse rate for data on children ever born has varied in different surveys from less than 1 percent to about 2 percent.

In the censuses of 1960 and 1950 allocations were made of the number of children ever born when women ever married had no report on that item. The allocations generally were made in a manner that took account of number of own children of the woman present in the home and allowed for some women having children absent from home or deceased, with control on age, marital status, and other characteristics of the woman. The 1960 census allocations were made by the electronic computer which temporarily stored data for the most recent woman of given characteristics who did have a report on children ever born and then assigned the same value to a next woman with no report on children but who had the same given characteristics. The 1950 allocations were made in a manual operation and were based on distributions for reporting women of specified characteristics obtained from a special national sample of about 60,000 women enumerated in that census.

Data on children ever born published in the 1940 census reports on fertility had no allocations for nonresponses, but the rates of children ever born were computed in a manner that gave nearly correct results for all women (including never-married women). However, those shown for ever-married women in the 1940 census reports are a little higher than they would have been had allocations for nonresponses been made. Subsequent Current Population Survey reports and some reports from later censuses present revised rates from the 1940 census for comparison which include allowances for nonresponses, based largely on ratios of young children in the household for women with and without a report on children ever born. As an example of the effect of the revision, the 1940 census unrevised data show 2,501 children ever born per 1,000 women 40-44 years old in the United States and 2,801 per 1,000 women ever married in this age group; the revised rates are 2,490 and 2,754, respectively.

The Current Population Survey also makes allocations of children ever born when there is no entry for that item. The allocations are made by the electronic computer when the fertility supplement is not complex; they are made manually when the supplement also has items on birth dates of children ever born or a fertility history.

Some information on the quality of allocations for nonresponses is available. A content evaluation study of the census (CES) made in 1960 by reinterview methods obtained information on children ever born for a sample of women who had no report on that item in the 1960 census. Table B.1 presents data from the CES in column 1

Table B. 1 Distribution of women ever married 14 years old and over
by number of children ever born as reported or as allocated:
United States, 1960

| Number of children reported or allocated | Women with no report on children ever born in the 1960 census | | Women with a report on children ever born in 1960 census |
	Report obtained in CES reinterview (1)	Data as allocated in 1960 census (2)	(3)
Total	100.0	100.0	100.0
No children	23.9	23.6	16.4
1 child	26.1	21.7	18.7
2 children	20.1	20.3	24.2
3 children	10.4	13.4	16.7
4 children	5.0	8.1	9.7
5 & 6 children	9.9	7.5	8.5
7 or more	4.6	5.4	5.8
Children ever born per 1,000 women ever married	2,136	2,232	2,522

Source: Derived from U. S. Bureau of the Census, 1960 Census of
Population and Housing, Accuracy of Data on Population Characteristics
as Measured by Reinterviews, Series ER 60, No. 4, Table 13; and 1960
Census of Population, Vol. I, Characteristics of the Population, Part 1,
U. S. Summary, Tables 190 and D-1.

and data from the 25-percent sample of the 1960 census in columns
2 and 3 for women with and without an original report on children
ever born. It will be noted that the allocations made in the 1960 census (column 2) are closer to the distribution in column 1 than to that
in column 3, as they should be if the 1960 census allocation procedures had worked well.

Intercensal Comparisons of Data
Comparisons of data on children ever born for women in one census
who are of completed or nearly completed fertility with data from a
following census of women in the same cohort provide a partial check
on quality of data. Information of this type is shown in Table B.2.
The comparisons are not definite evidence of quality of data, because
the women surviving at an older age in the later census may not be
strictly representative of the larger number of women at the earlier

census in view of any differential mortality between women with many children and women with few children, misstatements of age, and other factors such as sampling variability and net emigration or net immigration. Yet the data in Table B.2 indicate that there is a high degree of consistency from census to census in national data on children ever born. Very close agreement can also be found between data from the Current Population Surveys (in which the nonresponse rates are low) and data from censuses when compared in a cohort fashion similar to that in Table B.2.

Table B. 2   Children ever born per 1,000 women 40-64 years old in 1940 by age, and per 1,000 women of correspondingly older age in 1950 and 1960: United States

Census and age of woman	Number of women	Children ever born per 1,000 women
1940: 40-44	4,327,860	2,501
1950: 50-54	4,077,240	2,497
1960: 60-64	3,718,944	2,503
1940: 45-49	4,001,300	2,758
1950: 55-59	3,567,120	2,728
1960: 65-69	3,295,048	2,734
1940: 50-54	3,472,420	2,891
1960: 70-74	2,528,914	2,949
1940: 55-59	2,823,260	3,038
1960: 75-79	1,656,748	3,103
1940: 60-64	2,307,380	3,101
1960: 80-84	877,942	3,159

Source: U.S. Bureau of the Census, 1940 Census of Population, Differential Fertility 1940 and 1910--Fertility for States and Large Cities, Table 3; 1950 Census of Population, Fertility, PE-5C, Table 1; and 1960 Census of Population, Women by Number of Children Ever Born, PC(2)-3A, Tables 4 and 5.

Effect of Not Asking Never-Married Women about Children Ever Born

Mainly for reasons of public relations, the Bureau of the Census has not generally asked never-married women about the number of children ever born to them. The census and survey data are not limited to data on legitimate fertility, however, because most women eventually marry and thus are asked the question on children ever born, and because some women with illegitimate children misreport their marital status as other than never married. On the other hand, the count of illegitimate children undoubtedly is more incomplete than that of legitimate children. According to birth registration data, roughly 5 percent of white babies and 20 percent of nonwhite babies are illegitimate, nationally, but this includes some babies whose mothers were widowed or divorced, not just those with never-married mothers. There are at least two ways in which the effect of not asking never-married women about children ever born can be indirectly evaluated. In one way, cumulations of birth rates for birth cohorts of women from annual vital statistics are compared with census or survey data on children ever born. Table B.3 presents an example of this type of comparison, for women of all races. It will be noted that

Table B. 3 Children ever born per 1,000 women 15-49 years old, by age, from cohort cumulations of vital statistics and from the census: United States, 1960

Age of woman	Vital statistics (to January 1, 1960)		1960 census	Column (2) as percent of column (3)
	As published (by exact age)	Adjusted to match census age detail[a]		
	(1)	(2)	(3)	(4)
15-19	101	146	127	115
20-24	969	1,097	1,032	106
25-29	2,035	2,134	2,006	106
30-34	2,508	2,564	2,445	105
35-39	2,646	2,674	2,523	106
40-44	2,515	2,523	2,409	105
45-49	2,315	2,315	2,245	103

Source: National Center for Health Statistics, Vital Statistics of the United States, 1963, Vol. I, Natality, Tables 1-17, and records; and U. S. Bureau of the Census, 1960 Census of Population, Vol. I, Characteristics of the Population, Part 1, U. S. Summary, Table 190.

[a]Census data relate to persons in a whole year of age, who on the average, are at the midpoint of a year of age instead of at an exact birthday. The figures in column (2) were estimated by averaging the cumulative rates for exact ages in order to make them comparable to the rates based on census data. For example, the rate at ages 15-19 was obtained by averaging the rates at exact ages 15-19 and 16-20.

the 1960 census rates of children ever born are generally 2 to 4 percent lower than those from the vital statistics cumulations, which include illegitimate births. It is thought that the differences largely reflect the effect of not asking never-married women about children ever born and the effect of some married women failing to report illegitimate children in the surveys. It is known from the August 1959 Current Population Survey that some ever-married women do report illegitimate children. In Chapter 13, Table 13.9, the column for "less than one month" since first marriage is roughly representative of births reported as occurring *before* the marriage. In that survey roughly 2 percent of first births to white women ever married were reported as having occurred before first marriage of the mother, and roughly 10 percent of first births to nonwhite women.

The other of the two ways in which the effect of not asking single women about children ever born can be indirectly measured also involves the August 1959 Current Population Survey. That survey obtained birth dates of children ever born for women ever married, which were used to obtain retrospective or reconstructed birth rates for the periods in which the children were born. Those rates in turn could be compared with birth rates from contemporary vital statistics for the same past dates. The data are available by color, age of mother, and birth order. Some summary data are presented in Table B.4. The birth rates from contemporary vital statistics are fully corrected for under-registration of births, but the population bases for those rates are not corrected for a possible undercount, with the result that these birth rates from vital statistics may be overstated by roughly 2 percent for white women and perhaps 6 or 7 percent for nonwhite women. For the former, the rates from the August 1959 survey are comparable in magnitude with those from birth registration data for years since 1959 but fall short by 3 to 5 percent for births in 1930 to 1959. For nonwhite women, the rates from the survey are especially short for recent years and then become less short for later years, as though some nonwhite mothers with illegitimate children eventually married and then were asked the question on children ever born.

Content Evaluation Study for Population Characteristics (CES)
As a part of the program for evaluating data collected in the 1960 Census of Population, the Bureau of the Census reinterviewed samples of the 1960 enumerated population. The reinterviews were conducted in July and October 1960, for probability samples involving about

Table B 4   Average annual births per 1,000 women 15-44 years old
from the August 1959 Current Population Survey (CPS)
and from contemporary vital statistics, by color:
United States, 1930 to 1959

Color and source of data	1955 to 1959	1950 to 1954	1945 to 1949	1940 to 1944	1935 to 1939	1930 to 1934
WHITE						
CPS	115.5	110.2	97.0	81.5	71.1	76.2
Vital statistics	115.2	108.6	100.7	85.1	74.9	79.7
CPS as percent of vital statistics	100.3	101.5	96.3	95.8	94.9	95.6
NONWHITE						
CPS	134.1	126.1	108.3	97.5	97.4	94.8
Vital statistics	160.3	144.5	122.7	107.0	99.7	102.6
CPS as percent of vital statistics	83.7	87.3	88.3	91.1	97.7	92.4

Source: U. S. Bureau of the Census, Current Population Reports,
Series P-20, No. 108, Tables 25 and 26.

15,800 sample persons in approximately 4,750 households. Exhibit
B.1 shows the questions that were asked about fertility for the purpose of checking on the quality of the 1960 census data on children
ever born. Whereas the 1960 census asked only one question on fertility of women ever married, many more questions were asked in the
reinterview in an effort to be sure that the count of children ever
born included all children ever born alive and excluded adoptions,
stepchildren, and other children not born to the woman. The 1960
census question was "How many babies has she ever had, not count-
ing stillbirths? (Do not include adopted children or stepchildren.)"

In most cases, if there was a difference between information reported in the census and the CES interview, the difference was reconciled.
During reconciliation, the interviewer told the respondent about the
difference and asked which answer was correct. The comparisons
could be made, of course, only for those persons who could be located
for the reinterviews several months after the decennial census enumeration. Approximately 9 percent of the CES sample persons were not
interviewed.

INQUIRY VI- NUMBER OF CHILDREN EVER BORNE (LIVE BIRTHS)	1. *Classify by sex and age:* ☐ Female under 14 ⟶ **END INTERVIEW** ☐ Male under 14 ⟶ **END INTERVIEW** ☐ Female 14 and over ☐ Male 14 and over ⟶ *Go to Inquiry VII.*

	2. On April 1, 1960, were you: *(Ask all parts to get exact status)* ☐ Married? ☐ Divorced? ☐ **Never married?** ⟶ *Go to Inquiry VII.* ☐ Widowed? ☐ Separated?

THE FOLLOWING QUESTIONS ARE ONLY FOR WOMEN WHO HAVE EVER BEEN MARRIED

3. Have you ever had a child?
  ☐ Yes   ☐ No ⟶ *(Have you had any children who are no longer living with you?)*
  ☐ Yes   ☐ No ⟶ *Go to Inquiry VII.*

4. Of the children you have borne:	Number
a. How many were living with you on April 1, 1960?...................................	
b. How many were living elsewhere on April 1, 1960?.................................	
c. How many were born alive but died before April 1, 1960?............................	

5. That makes a total of _____ babies born alive as of April 1, 1960. Is that correct?
  ☐ Yes   ☐ No ⟶ *Make corrections in Item 4. Then continue with Item 6.*

6. Have you ever adopted any children or been a foster mother to any children other than your own?
  ☐ Yes ⟶ Are any of them included in the children we have just counted?
  ☐ Yes ⟶ *Make corrections in Item 4. Then continue with Item 7.*
  ☐ No   ☐ No

7. Have you ever been a stepmother to any children?
  ☐ Yes ⟶ Are any of them included in the children we have just counted?
  ☐ Yes ⟶ *Make corrections in Item 4. Then continue with Item 8.*
  ☐ No   ☐ No

8. Have you ever had any children who were adopted by someone else?
  ☐ Yes ⟶ Are all of them included in the children we have just counted?
  ☐ Yes   ☐ No ⟶ *Add to Item 4. Then continue with Item 9.*
  ☐ No

9. I would like to get a few facts about the last child born to you before April 1, 1960:
  a. Was a birth certificate filled out for this child?
    ☐ Yes ⟶ How is the name shown on the birth certificate?
    ☐ No ⟶ What is the name of the child?

Last	First	Middle initial

b. When was he born? ....

Month	Day	Year

c. Where were you living at the time the baby was born?

City or town	County	State

d. Where was the hospital or actual place of birth?

City or town	County	State

FORM 60-PH-EP-17 (REV.) (8-25-60)

Fig. B.1. Questionnaire used for information on children ever born in the Content Evaluation Study for Population Characteristics: 1960.

Among women 14 years old and over, ever married, and reporting on children ever born in both the CES reinterview and in the 1960 census, exact agreement between the two records as to number of children occurred for 91.9 percent of cases. In 5.4 percent the CES record showed more children than the census record, and in 2.8 percent of cases the reverse situation occurred. Many of the differences involved only one child more or less on the one record than on the other. Overall, the total count of children ever born was 1.7 percent smaller according to the census records than according to the CES records. It would appear, therefore, that the extensive questions and probing in the CES did not add relatively many children to the census counts.

Birth Record Check on Children Ever Born: 1960

Nature of the Sample. The CES provided information on where to find the birth record for a woman's latest child. That birth record, when found, was used to check the birth record entry for order of live birth against both the 1960 census entry and the CES reinterview entry for number of children ever born to a woman. The data utilized in this section are based on unweighted hand tallies of materials from the first of the three national samples involved in the full CES interview program. Resources available did not permit the utilization of all three samples for the birth record check of data on children ever born, and furthermore, did not permit a proper weighting of data. It is thought, nonetheless, that the results of the hand tallies are useful indicators of the quality of data on children ever born.

The first CES sample, used as a basis for the present study, was selected in a 148-area sample design of about 4,900 sample persons (all ages, both sexes) in about 1,450 households. The original design was for a multistage probability sample that, when properly weighted, would in itself be representative of the national population. The CES interviews for this sample of the 1960 census enumerated population were conducted in July 1960. The present data, based on hand tallies that give equal weight to all applicable observations, are biased in that some of the sample areas are over-represented and others are under-represented as compared with the results that would be obtained from a proper weighting of data. One comparison is possible of data from the hand tallies for the first CES sample with properly weighted data from the full three-sample CES study. As may be determined from the data in Table B.5, the number of children ever born

Table B. 5 Children ever born to mothers 14 years old and ever
married, by color and age of woman and type of record,
for women in Sample I of the Content Evaluation Study,
1960: United States

(Unweighted data)

Color and age of woman per census record	Mothers with three records giving number of children ever born	Children ever born according to:		
		Census record	CES re-interview record	Birth record for latest child
WHITE				
14-44	456	1,184	1,187	1,189
14-24	74	122	128	125
25-34	186	500	503	506
35-44	196	562	556	558
45 & over	363	1,283	1,330	1,320
45-54	172	531	542	538
55-64	94	352	363	372
65 & over	97	400	425	410
NONWHITE				
14-44	42	165	171	172
45 & over	19	83	85	82

Source: Unpublished data from Evaluation and Research
Program of 1960 Census of Population.

according to hand tallies from census records for mothers ever married age 14 and over is 97.9 percent of the corresponding number of
children ever born from hand tallies of CES records for the identical
women. According to data published elsewhere for the full CES study,
properly weighted, the number of children ever born for mothers
ever married age 14 and over according to census records is 98.3 percent of the number according to the CES reinterview records for the
same women.[1] The hand tally result of 97.9 percent is slightly less
than the one of 98.3 percent from the full weighted CES materials.
The reader should keep in mind that the close agreement of the two
results for mothers 14 and over does not necessarily mean that similarly close agreement would be found in terms of data specific for

[1] The figure of 98.3 percent was derived by computation from data in U.S. Bureau of the
Census, 1960 Census of Population and Housing, *Accuracy of Data on Population Characteristics as Measured by Reinterviews,* Series ER 60, No. 4, Table 13.

fine age detail or for color, but the comparison does show that the unweighted hand tally results are at least roughly indicative of quality of data.

As already stated, the first CES sample contained about 1,450 households. Within these households, the interviews yielded data on 1,157 women ever married who had borne one or more children. The tallies shown here are based on data for 880 women, with a report on children ever born in all three sources of data: the census record, the CES interview record, and the birth record for the woman's latest child. Excluded from the original count of 1,157 cases are 76 cases in which the reinterview did not yield sufficient information to locate the birth record, 9 cases where the birth date of the latest child antedated the state birth registration file, 42 cases where the latest child was born in Massachusetts (in that state the birth record has no item on order of birth), 12 cases where the latest child was born abroad, 45 cases where the census record had no report on children ever born, 74 cases where the birth record could not be found or was an unacceptable match, and 14 cases where the birth record was found but lacked information on order of birth. Also excluded were 5 cases where the census record indicated the women was childless but the CES reinterview record and the birth record indicated the woman had children. This last group of 5 cases was excluded in an effort partly to offset bias that would otherwise result from lack of data for 24 other cases where the census record indicated the woman had borne children but the CES record indicated the woman was childless and therefore gave no information on where to find a birth record. The birth records used in the tallies date back many years; the oldest happens to be for the year 1906.

Net Differences in Reporting on Number of Children Ever Born for Groups of Women. Table B.5 presents data on the number of children ever born as reported for the 880 mothers ever married. For white women 14-44 years old, the number of children ever born according to the census records is 1,184, or less than 1 percent below the corresponding figure of 1,189 obtained from birth records and the 1,187 obtained by the CES reinterview records. For white women 45 years old and over, the number of children ever born according to the census records is 1,283, or 2.8 percent below the number (1,320) obtained from matched birth records, and still further below the number (1,330) from the CES reinterviews. There is a marked tendency in the data for white women for the count of children ever born to be relatively less complete in census data for women at successively older ages, as compared with data from the other two sources. Among nonwhite women, there is evidence of an undercount of children ever born for women aged 14-44 from the census as compared with data from the other two sources, but there are too few observations for nonwhite women in this age group and in the following age group, 45 and over, for a reliable assessment of the net quality of data.

Gross Differences in Reporting on Number of Children Ever Born.
Table B.6 indicates the extent to which data on children ever born

Table B. 6 Agreement on number of children ever born from three sources of data--the census record, the census evaluation study reinterview record, and the birth record for the woman's latest child--for mothers in Sample I of the Content Evaluation Study, 1960: United States

(Unweighted data)

Color and age of woman	Total women	All three records agree	Census and one other record agree	Census differs, other two records agree	All three records differ	Percent with census in agreement with at least one other record
WHITE						
14-44	456	417	20	18	1	95.8
14-24	74	69	2	2	1	95.9
25-34	186	172	7	7	-	96.2
35-44	196	176	11	9	-	95.4
45 & over	363	293	34	29	7	90.1
45-54	172	146	15	10	1	93.6
55-64	94	71	12	10	1	88.3
65 & over	97	76	7	9	5	85.6
NONWHITE						
14-44	42	35	3	3	11	a
45 & over	19	10	7	2	-	a

Source: Unpublished data from Evaluation and Research Program of 1960 Census of Population.

aPercent not shown where base is less than 50.

for individual women from the census record agreed with data from the other two records. Among white mothers 14-44 years old, the reported number of children ever born was identical on all three records for 417 women, or 91 percent of the 456 women in the color-age group, and the census record was in agreement with either (but not both) the CES record or the birth record in an additional 20 cases, or 4 percent. For white women 45 years old and over, agreement occurred on all three records for 81 percent of cases and the census record agreed with one other record in an additional 9 percent. There was much less relative agreement between records for nonwhite than for white women. Only about half of nonwhite women 45 years old and over and about eight-tenths of those 14-44 years old had identical reports of children ever born in all three records.

All three types of records are subject to possible error in the listing of number of children ever born. Some of the oldest birth records, for example, used such wordings as "number of children born to this mother including present birth" or other wording that may have resulted in an inadvertent inclusion of some stillbirths or exclusion of some children who died after birth. Even the CES record, with its rather extensive probing questions on children ever born, was sometimes of dubious accuracy. For example, there was one instance where the CES record indicated seven children ever born, all living, and the same CES record led to finding of a birth record for the woman's last child that indicated only one child ever born, the same as the census record. Possibly the "7" was misread from a poorly written "1."

Table B.5, of course, shows more relative agreement on total counts of children ever born for groups of women than Table B.6 shows for individual women. Some women have overstatements and some have understatements of children in any one type of record, in a manner that causes net counts, as in Table B.5, to be smaller than gross differences, as in Table B.6.

Table B.7 compares the specific number of children ever born as reported for each woman in the census with the number from the birth record, for the sample of 880 mothers. It may be noted from this table that most differences between the two records are on the order of plus or minus one child. The reader who is interested in comparisons of this type for the census record with the full CES materials may wish to consult the CES report mentioned earlier. A similar comparison (not shown) for CES records for 880 women with birth

Table B. 7 Children ever born as reported for mothers in the 1960
census and in the birth record for the latest child,
for women in Sample I of the Content Evaluation Study,
1960: United States

(Unweighted data)

Age of woman and children ever born as reported in 1960 census	Total mothers	Children ever born as reported on matched birth record					
		1	2	3	4	5 & 6	7 or more
MOTHERS 15–44							
Total	498	98	175	115	60	32	18
1 child ever born	102	98	3	–	–	1	–
2 children	178	–	169	9	–	–	–
3 children	112	–	3	104	5	–	–
4 children	57	–	–	2	53	2	–
5 & 6 children	31	–	–	–	2	28	1
7 or more	18	–	–	–	–	1	17
MOTHERS 45 & OVER							
Total	382	71	103	59	52	53	44
1 child ever born	76	65	9	1	–	–	1
2 children	100	4	89	4	2	1	–
3 children	70	1	5	51	9	4	–
4 children	51	1	–	3	39	7	1
5 & 6 children	44	–	–	–	2	39	3
7 or more	41	–	–	–	–	2	39

Source: Unpublished data from Evaluation and Research Program
of 1960 Census of Population.

records indicates that there is a slight tendency for the CES to obtain
more children than are on the birth records, suggesting the possibility
that not all children who died after birth or who were given up for
adoption were included in the birth record report on order of live
birth. Generally speaking, the census record on children ever born
agrees slightly more often with the birth record than it does with the
CES record.

Notes / Bibliography / Index

Notes

Chapter 1. The World Setting

1. Among the exceptions, countries of low fertility in Asia are Japan and Asiatic U.S.S.R; in Latin America, Argentina and Uruguay; and in Africa, the Union of South Africa. Also, it is possible that for medical or other reasons sterility may be high among some of the African countries and tribes. On the other hand, there are pockets of high fertility in the more developed areas, such as Albania in Europe and the rural South in the United States.

2. J. Mayone Stycos and Jorge Arias, eds., *Population Dilemma in Latin America* (Washington, D.C.: Potomac Books, 1966).

3. Bernard Berelson et al., *Family Planning and Population Programs* (Chicago: University of Chicago Press, 1966).

4. National Center for Health Statistics, *The Measurement of Fertility,* Public Health Service Publ. No. 1000, Series 4, No. 1 (November 1965).

5. Bernardo Colombo, "Factors Affecting Fertility in Industrialized Countries," in *Proceedings of the International Population Conference, New York, 1961* (London, 1963), I, 36-39; Clyde V. Kiser, "Social, Economic, and Religious Factors in the Differential Fertility of Low Fertility Countries," in *Proceedings of the World Population Conference, Belgrade, 1965* (New York: United Nations, 1967), II, 219-222.

6. Charles F. Westoff, Robert G. Potter, Jr., and Philip C. Sagi, *The Third Child* (Princeton: Princeton University Press, 1963), pp. 87-90, 237; Gwendolyn Z. Johnson, "Differential Fertility in European Countries," in *Demographic and Economic Change in Developed Countries,* A Report of the National Bureau of Economic Research (Princeton: Princeton University Press, 1960), pp. 36-71; Pascal K. Whelpton, Arthur A. Campbell, and John E. Patterson, *Fertility and Family Planning in the United States* (Princeton: Princeton University Press, 1966), p. 77.

7. United Nations, "World Population Prospects as Assessed in 1963," *Population Studies,* No. 41 (New York, 1966), p. 34.

8. *Ibid.,* p. 33.

9. U.S. Bureau of the Census, "Projections of the Population of the United States by Age and Sex to 1985," *Current Population Reports,* Series P-25, No. 279 (February 4, 1964), p. 4.

10. United Nations, *Population Bulletin,* No. 7 (1963); *Demographic Yearbook, 1965* (New York, 1965), pp. 1-3; *Demographic Yearbook, 1966* (New York, 1967), pp. 200-219.

Chapter 2. Medical and Biological Aspects of Fertility

1. Sam Shapiro, Edward R. Schlesinger, and Robert E. L. Nesbitt, *Infant, Perinatal, Maternal, and Childhood Mortality in the United States* (Cambridge, Mass.: Harvard University Press, 1968).

2. J. Clifton Edgar, "The Education, Licensing, and Supervision of the Mid-wife," *Proceedings of the American Association for Study and Prevention of Infant Mortality* (1915), p. 90. Cited by Paul H. Jacobson, "Hospital Care and the Vanishing Midwife," *Milbank Memorial Fund Quarterly,* vol. 34, No. 3 (July 1956), pp. 253-261.

3. International Standard Classification Codes (seventh revision): Toxemias of pregnancy, 642, 685, 686; Abortions, 650, 651, 652; Hemorrhage, 643, 644, 670-672; Sepsis, 640, 641, 681, 682, 684; Ectopic Pregnancy, 645; Other causes of maternal mortality, 646-648, 660, 673-678, 680, 683, 687-689.

4. Health Information Foundation, "Advances in Maternal Health," *Progress in Health Services,* vol. 7, No. 9 (November 1958), p. 3.

5. National Center for Health Statistics, *Medical Care, Health Status, and Family Income,* Public Health Service Publ. No. 1000, Series 10, No. 9 (May 1964), p. 30.

6. National Center for Health Statistics, *Volume of Physician Visits by Place of Visit and Type of Service: United States, July 1963-June 1964,* Public Health Service Publ. No. 1000, Series 10, No. 18 (June 1965), Table 13.

7. Francis C. Madigan, "Are Sex Mortality Differentials Biologically Caused?" *Milbank Memorial Fund Quarterly,* vol. 35, No. 2 (April 1957), pp. 202-223.

8. Harold F. Dorn and Arthur J. McDowell, "The Relationship of Fertility and Longevity," *American Sociological Review,* vol. 4, No. 2 (April 1939), pp. 234-246.

9. Bettie C. Freeman, "Fertility and Longevity in Married Women Dying after the End of the Reproductive Period," *Human Biology,* vol. 7, No. 3 (September 1935), pp. 392-418.

10. World Health Organization, *Manual of the International Statistical Classification of Diseases, Injuries, and Causes of Death,* vol. 1 (Geneva, 1957), p. xxii.

11. A. T. Hertig and John Rock, "A Series of Potentially Abortive Ova Recovered from Fertile Women Prior to Their First Missed Menstrual Period," *American Journal of Obstetrics and Gynecology,* 58: 968-993 (1949).

12. Sam Shapiro, Ellen W. Jones, and Paul M. Densen, "A Life Table of Pregnancy Terminations and Correlates of Fetal Loss," *Milbank Memorial Fund Quarterly,* vol. 40, No. 1 (January 1962), pp. 7-45.

13. *Ibid.,* p. 13. The article cited in this quotation is Edith L. Potter, "The Abortion Problem," *GP* (April 1959).

14. Carl L. Erhardt, "Pregnancy Losses in New York City, 1960," *American Journal of Public Health,* vol. 53, No. 9 (September 1963), pp. 1337-1352.

15. Shapiro, Jones, and Densen, "Life Table of Pregnancy Terminations," p. 14.

16. Ronald Freedman, Pascal K. Whelpton, and Arthur A. Campbell, *Family Planning, Sterility, and Population Growth* (New York: McGraw-Hill, 1959), p. 34.

17. Calculated from unpublished data.

18. Pascal K. Whelpton and Clyde V. Kiser, eds., *Social and Psychological*

Factors Affecting Fertility (New York: Milbank Memorial Fund, 1950), II, 312.

19. C. F. Westoff et al., *Family Growth in Metropolitan America* (Princeton: Princeton University Press, 1961), p. 46.

20. Arkansas, Colorado, Georgia, Hawaii, Maine, Mississippi, New York City, Oregon, Vermont, and Virginia.

21. Freedman, Whelpton, and Campbell, *Family Planning,* pp. 32-34.

22. Shapiro, Jones, and Densen, "Life Table of Pregnancy Terminations," p. 14.

23. *Ibid.,* p. 15.

24. *Ibid.,* p. 16.

25. *Ibid.,* p. 18.

26. R. J. Plunkett and J. E. Gordon, *Epidemiology in Mental Illness* (New York: Basic Books, 1960).

27. Metropolitan Life Insurance Company, "Hospitalization for Mental Disorders," *Statistical Bulletin,* vol. 46 (March 1965), p. 1.

28. Lee L. Bean, "The Fertility of Former Mental Patients," *Eugenics Quarterly,* vol. 13, No. 1 (March 1966), pp. 34-39.

29. Charles Goldfarb and L. Erlenmeyer-Kimling, "Mating and Fertility Trends in Schizophrenia," in *Expanding Goals of Genetics in Psychiatry,* ed. Franz J. Kallman (New York: Grune and Stratton, 1962), pp. 42-51.

30. *Ibid.,* p. 48. Table 7 is particularly interesting, comparing the New York State data with the Current Population Survey data of August 1959.

31. Erik Essen-Moller, "Mating and Fertility Trends in Families with Schizophrenia," *Eugenics Quarterly,* vol. 6, No. 2 (June 1959), pp. 142-147.

32. National Center for Health Statistics, *Vital Statistics of the United States, 1960,* vol. II, *Mortality,* Part A, Table 1-K, and *1964,* vol. II, *Mortality,* Part A, Table 1-8.

33. National Center for Health Statistics, *Hearing Levels of Adults by Age and Sex: United States, 1960-1962,* Public Health Service Publ. No. 1000, Series 11, No. 11 (October 1965).

34. National Center for Health Statistics, *Selected Impairments by Etiology and Activity Limitation: United States, July 1959-June 1961,* Public Health Service Publ., Series B, No. 35 (June 1962).

35. National Center for Health Statistics, *Methodological Aspects of a Hearing Ability Interview Survey,* Public Health Service Publ. No. 1000, Series 2, No. 12 (October 1965).

36. Diane Sank and Franz J. Kallman, "The Role of Heredity in Early Total Deafness," *Volta Review,* vol. 65, No. 9 (November 1963), pp. 461-470.

37. Brian F. McCabe, "The Etiology of Deafness," *Volta Review,* vol. 65, No. 9 (November 1963), pp. 471-485.

38. Jerome D. Schein, Gallaudet College, Washington, D.C., kindly provided the figures used here from his records.

Chapter 3. The Control of Fertility

1. These studies were conducted by the Survey Research Center of the University of Michigan and the Scripps Foundation for Research in Population Problems, Miami University, Oxford, Ohio. The 1955 study is reported in Ronald Freedman, Pascal K. Whelpton, and Arthur A. Campbell, *Family Planning, Sterility, and Population Growth* (New York: McGraw-Hill, 1959). The 1960 study is reported in Pascal K. Whelpton, Arthur A. Campbell, and John E. Patterson, *Fertility and Family Planning in the United States* (Princeton: Princeton University Press, 1966). The present chapter is largely a summary of Chapters 4-7 of the latter book.

2. The words "Subfecund" and "Fecund" are capitalized to indicate that they are being used in a special sense in this study. They are derived from the word "fecundity," which refers to the *ability* to reproduce. This word is often confused with "fertility," which, according to definitions adopted by the Population Association of America, refers to the actual number of children couples have had.

3. See also Clyde V. Kiser, "Fertility Trends and Differentials among Nonwhites in the United States," *Milbank Memorial Fund Quarterly,* vol. 36, No. 2 (April 1958), pp. 149-197. See especially pp. 190-196 for evidence on the extent of involuntary childlessness among nonwhite groups.

4. These are among the most important findings of the Princeton Study. See Robert G. Potter, Philip C. Sagi, and Charles F. Westoff, "Improvement of Contraception during the Course of Marriage," *Population Studies,* vol. 16, No. 2 (November 1962), pp. 160-174.

5. I. C. Winter, "The Incidence of Thromboembolism in Enovid Users," *Metabolism: Clinical and Experimental,* 14: 422-428 (March 1965).

6. *Time,* March 31, 1964, p. 39: 3 million; *Chemical Week,* April 4, 1964, p. 22: more than 3 million by the end of 1964; *Newsweek,* July 6, 1964, p. 55: 3.5 million; *Chicago Tribune,* June 27, 1965, sec. 1-A, p. 1: nearly 4 million.

7. Norman B. Ryder and Charles F. Westoff, "Use of Oral Contraception in the United States," *Science,* vol. 153, No. 3741 (September 9, 1966), pp. 1199-1205.

8. The total fertility rate is the sum of age-specific birth rates for single years of age for all ages in the reproductive span, observed in a given calendar year. See the discussion of completed fertility and total fertility in Chapter 13 for more detail.

Chapter 4. Fertility Rates by Color and Ethnic Group

1. For data on trends in venereal disease by color, see the monograph on venereal diseases in this series, by William J. Brown et al., in preparation.

2. As used here, the general fertility rate is the average number of live births occurring during a year per 1,000 females 15-44 years of age.

3. The net reproduction rate is a hypothetical concept based on the assumption that the age-specific fertility and mortality rates of women during one calendar year represent the experience of a cohort passing through life. The gross reproduction rate omits the reduction for mortality and assumes that the women in the synthetic cohort will survive the reproductive period. It should be mentioned that the differences in color based upon registration data may be exaggerated because of less adequate population bases for the nonwhite group, arising from under-enumeration.

4. U.S. Bureau of the Census, 1960 Census of Population, *Women by Number of Children Ever Born,* PC(2)-3A, Table 1.

5. *Ibid.,* Tables 6 and 7.

6. Computed from fertility rates for white and nonwhite ever-married women of staggered ages in the censuses of 1940, 1950, and 1960.

7. The country of origin for persons of foreign parentage was determined by the birth place of the father if the two parents were born in different foreign countries. For persons of mixed parentage, it was determined by country of birth of the foreign-born parent.

8. Wilson H. Grabill, Clyde V. Kiser, and Pascal K. Whelpton, *The Fertility of American Women* (New York: John Wiley and Sons, 1958), pp. 103-112.

9. For evidence of increasing differentials by color in marriage stability, see Daniel O. Price, *Changing Characteristics of the Negro Population: Trends in Migration, Occupation, Education, and Marital Status,* to be published by the Government Printing Office for the Bureau of the Census.

Chapter 5. Residence

1. Regions comprise the following states and the District of Columbia: *Northeast,* Connecticut, Maine, Massachusetts, New Hampshire, New Jersey, New York, Pennsylvania, Rhode Island, and Vermont; *North Central,* Illinois, Indiana, Iowa, Kansas, Michigan, Minnesota, Missouri, Nebraska, North Dakota, Ohio, South Dakota, and Wisconsin; *South,* Alabama, Arkansas, Delaware, District of Columbia, Florida, Georgia, Kentucky, Louisiana, Maryland, Mississippi, North Carolina, Oklahoma, South Carolina, Tennessee, Texas, Virginia, and West Virginia; *West,* Alaska, Arizona, California, Colorado, Hawaii, Idaho, Montana, Nevada, New Mexico, Oregon, Utah, Washington, and Wyoming.

2. U.S. Bureau of the Census, 1960 Census of Population, vol. I, *Characteristics of the Population,* Part 1, *U.S. Summary,* p. xxxviii.

3. Procedures for standardization are given in most textbooks on techniques of demographic analysis. For example, A. J. Jaffe, ed., *Handbook of Statistical Methods for Demographers* (U.S. Bureau of the Census, 1960), Chapter III, "Selected Statistical Methods for the Standardization of Population."

4. This is discussed further in the section on ecological correlations, later in this chapter. Another example is Otis Dudley Duncan and Albert J. Reiss, Jr.,

Social Characteristics of Urban and Rural Communities, 1950, Census Monograph Series (New York: John Wiley and Sons, 1956), Table B-5.

5. J. Allan Beegle, Dale E. Hathaway, and W. Keith Bryant, *The People of Rural America, 1960,* Census Monograph Series, to be published by the Government Printing Office for the Bureau of the Census.

6. Michael Sadler, *Law of Population* (England, 1830).

7. *Memoirs of John Quincy Adams,* ed. Charles Francis Adams, 12 vols. (Philadelphia: J. B. Lippincott, 1874-77), entry for April 10, 1822.

8. Warren S. Thompson, *Ratio of Children to Women, 1920,* Census Monograph XI (U.S. Government Printing Office, 1931).

9. National Resources Committee, *The Problems of a Changing Population* (U.S. Government Printing Office, 1938).

10. *The People of Rural America, 1960.*

11. David Goldberg, "The Fertility of Two-Generation Urbanites," *Population Studies,* vol. 12, No. 3 (March 1959), pp. 214-222.

12. Otis Dudley Duncan, "Residential Areas and Differential Fertility," *Eugenics Quarterly,* vol. 2, No. 2 (June 1964), pp. 82-89.

Chapter 6. Migration in Relation to Fertility

1. U.S. Bureau of the Census, 1960 Census of Population, vol. I, *Characteristics of the Population,* Part 1, *U.S. Summary; Detailed Characteristics,* PC(1)-1D, Table 164.

2. Clyde V. Kiser, "Fertility Rates by Residence and Migration," *Proceedings, International Population Conference, Vienna, 1959* (Vienna: International Union for the Scientific Study of Population, 1959), pp. 273-286.

3. Clyde V. Kiser, "Residence and Migration," in *The Third Child,* by C. F. Westoff, R. G. Potter, Jr., and P. C. Sagi (Princeton: Princeton University Press, 1963), pp. 157-182.

4. Clyde V. Kiser, "Residence and Migration," in *Family Growth in Metropolitan America,* by C. F. Westoff, R. G. Potter, Jr., P. C. Sagi, and E. G. Mishler (Princeton: Princeton University Press, 1961), pp. 278-279.

5. Henry S. Shryock, Jr., *Population Mobility Within the United States* (Chicago: Community and Family Study Center, University of Chicago, 1964), p. 9.

6. "The 1960 instructions specified that place of birth was to be reported in terms of mother's usual State of residence at the time of birth rather than in terms of the location of the hospital if the birth occurred in a hospital." U.S. Bureau of the Census, 1960 Census of Population, *Women by Number of Children Ever Born,* PC(2)-3A, p. xii.

Chapter 7: Marital Characteristics

1. U.S. Bureau of the Census, *Current Population Reports,* Series P-20, No. 108, Table 5.

Chapter 8. Illegitimacy

1. Arthur A. Campbell, "Fertility and Family Planning among Nonwhite Married Couples in the United States," *Eugenics Quarterly,* vol. 12, No. 3 (September 1965), pp. 124-131.

2. *Ibid.*

3. William F. Pratt, "Premarital Pregnancy in a Metropolitan Community." Paper presented at the 1965 Annual Meeting of the Population Association of America.

4. Campbell, "Fertility and Family Planning among Nonwhite Married Couples in the United States."

5. For additional evidence on this point, see Clyde V. Kiser, "Fertility Trends and Differentials among Nonwhites in the United States," *Milbank Memorial Fund Quarterly,* vol. 36, No. 2 (April 1958), pp. 190-196. See also the monograph on venereal diseases in this series by William J. Brown et al., in preparation.

6. See Chapter 12, particularly the discussion of the Easterlin hypothesis.

Chapter 9. Education and Fertility

1. Wilson H. Grabill, Clyde V. Kiser, and Pascal K. Whelpton, *The Fertility of American Women* (New York: John Wiley and Sons, 1958), pp. 183-261.

2. *Ibid.,* pp. 191-192.

3. *Ibid.,* pp. 195-198.

4. "Fertility of the Population: June 1964 and March 1962," *Current Population Reports,* Series P-20, No. 147 (January 5, 1966), p. 17.

5. The "base rates" for women of given age, marital status, color, and type of community were standardized to the 1950 distribution of women or ever-married women. Operationally, for a given age, color, marital status, and type of residence group for 1940 and 1960, the fertility rates by educational attainment were weighted according to the percentage distribution of women or ever-married women by educational attainment in 1950. This was done to avoid possible bias accruing from temporal shifts in *composition* by educational attainment.

6. Attention is called to the fact that the data for 1940 relate to native white ever-married women whereas those for 1950 and 1960 relate to white women.

7. See monograph on marriage and divorce in this series by Hugh Carter and Paul C. Glick, in preparation.

8. Clyde V. Kiser and Myrna E. Frank, "Factors Associated With the Low Fertility of Nonwhite Women of College Attainment," *Milbank Memorial Fund Quarterly,* 45: 434-435 (October 1967).

Chapter 10. Occupation in Relation to Fertility

1. Wilson H. Grabill, Clyde V. Kiser, and Pascal K. Whelpton, *The Fertility of American Women* (New York: John Wiley and Sons, 1958), p. 115.

2. Joseph A. Hill, *Fecundity of Immigrant Women,* U.S. Immigration Commission Reports (Washington, D.C., 1911), XXVIII, 731-784.

3. Edgar Sydenstricker and Frank W. Notestein, "Differential Fertility According to Social Class," *Journal of the American Statistical Association,* 25: 9-32 (March 1930).

4. Census of England and Wales, 1911, vol. XIII, *Fertility of Marriage* (London: General Register Office, 1917).

5. U.S. Bureau of the Census, 1940 Census of Population, *Differential Fertility, 1940 and 1910–Fertility of States and Large Cities* (1943); *Standardized Fertility Rates and Reproduction Rates* (1944); *Women by Number of Children under 5 Years Old* (1945); *Women by Number of Children Ever Born* (1945); *Fertility by Duration of Marriage* (1947).

6. "Fertility of the Population: June 1964 and March 1962," *Current Population Reports,* Series P-20, No. 147 (January 5, 1966), p. 17.

7. Clyde V. Kiser and Myrna E. Frank, "Factors Associated With the Low Fertility of Nonwhite Women of College Attainment," *Milbank Memorial Fund Quarterly,* 45: 427-449 (October 1967).

8. Sydenstricker and Notestein, "Differential Fertility," p. 31.

9. See monograph on marriage and divorce in this series by Hugh Carter and Paul C. Glick, in preparation.

10. National Center for Health Statistics, *Fertility Measurement, A Report of the United States National Committee on Vital and Health Statistics,* Series 4, No. 1 (September 1965), pp. 15-18.

11. Grabill, Kiser, and Whelpton, *Fertility of American Women,* pp. 180-182.

Chapter 11. Income and Other Social and Economic Factors

1. Pascal K. Whelpton and Clyde V. Kiser, eds., *Social and Psychological Factors Affecting Fertility,* vol. II (New York: Milbank Memorial Fund, 1950), p. 395.

2. Charles F. Westoff, Robert G. Potter, Jr., and Paul C. Sagi, *The Third Child* (Princeton: Princeton University Press, 1963), p. 119.

3. Deborah Freedman, "The Relation of Economic Status to Fertility," *American Economic Review* (June 1953), p. 422.

4. "Fertility of the Population: June 1964 and March 1962," *Current Population Reports,* Series P-20, No. 147 (January 5, 1966), p. 17.

5. Frank W. Notestein, "The Relation of Social Status to the Fertility of Native-Born Married Women in the United States," in G. H. L. F. Pitt-Rivers, *Problems of Population* (London: Allen and Unwin, 1932), p. 158.

6. Gwendolyn Z. Johnson, "Differential Fertility in European Countries," in *Demographic and Economic Change in Developed Countries,* A Report of the National Bureau of Economic Research (Princeton: Princeton University Press, 1960), p. 61.

7. It is not possible to equate precisely the rental value of owned homes with the actual rental of rented homes. However, except at the lower rental and value levels, the categories used in the classifications by value and rent in the 1960

fertility data permit comparisons of approximately equated classes of owners and renters. For instance, a rental of $100-$149 is assumed to be approximately equivalent to a value of $10,000-$14,999. The "$150 or more" rental is assumed to be equivalent to the three top value categories combined.

8. U.S. Bureau of the Census, 1960 Census of Population, *Women by Number of Children Ever Born,* PC(2)-3A, Table 44.

9. Ronald Freedman, Pascal K. Whelpton, and Arthur A. Campbell, *Family Planning, Sterility, and Population Growth* (New York: McGraw-Hill, 1959), pp. 275-277.

10. Whelpton and Kiser, *Social and Psychological Factors,* vol. I (1946), p. 8.

11. Westoff, Potter, and Sagi, *The Third Child,* p. 238.

12. *Ibid.*

13. *Official Catholic Directory* (New York: P. J. Kenedy & Sons, 1910-).

14. Dudley Kirk, "Recent Trends of Catholic Fertility in the United States," in *Current Research in Human Fertility* (New York: Milbank Memorial Fund, 1955), p. 104.

15. Ronald Freedman, David Goldberg, and Dorothy Slesinger, "Current Fertility Expectations of Married Couples in the United States," *Population Index* (October 1963), p. 378.

16. C. Joseph Neusse, "Recent Catholic Fertility in Rural Wisconsin," *Rural Sociology* (December 1963), p. 391.

Chapter 12. The Relation Between Fertility and Economic Conditions

1. See Chapter 13 and Appendix A for definitions.

2. Richard A. Easterlin, *The American Baby Boom in Historical Perspective,* Occasional Paper No. 79 (New York: National Bureau of Economic Research, 1962); Virginia L. Galbraith and Dorothy S. Thomas, "Birth Rates and the Interwar Business Cycles," *Journal of the American Statistical Association,* vol. 36, No. 216 (December 1941), pp. 465-476; Dudley Kirk, "The Influence of Business Cycles on Marriage and Birth Rates," in *Demographic and Economic Change in Developed Countries* (Princeton: Princeton University Press, 1960), pp. 241-257.

3. Raymond W. Goldsmith, *A Study of Saving in the United States* (Princeton: Princeton University Press, 1955).

4. G. U. Yule, "Why Do We Sometimes Get Nonsense Correlations between Time-Series," *Journal of the Royal Statistical Society,* 89:2 (January 1926).

5. This relates to 1920-57, excluding 1942-46, for birth probabilities, and to 1919-56, excluding 1941-45 for economic indicators.

6. This is a rough estimate based on data from the Indianapolis Study. The median is about 2 months for the first pregnancy and 5 months for the second and third.

7. For example, the proportion of pregnancies that were planned by discontinuing contraception was 33 percent for the second pregnancy, 10 percent for

sixth and higher pregnancies. Ronald Freedman, Pascal K. Whelpton, and Arthur A. Campbell, *Family Planning, Sterility, and Population Growth* (New York: McGraw-Hill, 1959), p. 72.

8. Easterlin, *The American Baby Boom.*

9. *Ibid.,* p. 31.

10. Richard A. Easterlin, "On the Relation of Economic Factors to Recent and Projected Fertility Changes," *Demography,* vol. 3, No. 1 (1966), pp. 131-153.

11. *Ibid.,* p. 149.

Chapter 13.   Cohort Fertility

1. National Office of Vital Statistics, "Fertility Tables for Birth Cohorts of American Women, Part 1," *Vital Statistics–Special Reports,* vol. 51, No. 1 (January 29, 1960). See Methodological Appendix, pp. 105-129.

2. Wilson H. Grabill, Clyde V. Kiser, and Pascal K. Whelpton, *The Fertility of American Women* (New York: John Wiley and Sons, 1958), pp. 429-435.

3. Ronald Freedman, Pascal K. Whelpton, and Arthur A. Campbell, *Family Planning, Sterility, and Population Growth* (New York: McGraw-Hill, 1959). See "high assumptions" on p. 357.

4. Ronald Freedman, David Goldberg, and Larry Bumpass, "Current Fertility Expectations of Married Couples in the United States," *Population Index,* vol. 31, No. 1 (January 1965), p. 10.

5. See monograph on marriage and divorce in this series by Hugh Carter and Paul C. Glick, in preparation.

6. Grabill, Kiser, and Whelpton, *Fertility of American Women,* p. 5.

Bibliography

Since the 1950 census monograph *The Fertility of American Women* contained a fairly extensive bibliography for the years up to 1958, the following one is restricted largely to the period since that year and to publications not cited at the end of chapters of this volume.

Books

Chipman, Sidney S., Abraham M. Lilienfeld, Bernard G. Greenberg, and James F. Donnelly, eds. *Research Methodology and Needs in Perinatal Studies* (Springfield, Ill.: Charles C. Thomas, 1966).

Coale, Ansley J., and Melvin Zelnik. *New Estimates of Fertility and Population in the United States* (Princeton: Princeton University Press, 1963).

Driver, Edwin D. *Differential Fertility in Central India* (Princeton: Princeton University Press, 1963).

Folger, John K., and Charles B. Nam. *Education of the American Population* (Washington: U. S. Government Printing Office, 1967).

Gebhard, Paul H., Wardell B. Pomeroy, Clyde E. Martin, and Cornelia Christenson. *Pregnancy, Birth and Abortion* (New York: Harper, 1958).

Handel, Gerald, and Lee Rainwater. "Persistence and Change in Working-Class Life Style," in *Blue-Collar World,* ed. Arthur B. Shostak and William Gomberg (Englewood Cliffs, N.J.: Prentice-Hall, 1964).

Johnston, Denis Foster. *An Analysis of Sources of Information on the Population of the Navaho,* Smithsonian Institution, Bureau of American Ethnology (Washington: Government Printing Office, 1966).

Kiser, Clyde V., ed. *Research in Family Planning* (Princeton: Princeton University Press, 1962).

Lopez, Alvaro. *Problems in Stable Population Theory* (Princeton: Office of Population Research, 1961).

Miller, Herman P. *Income Distribution in the United States* (Washington: U.S. Government Printing Office, 1966).

Okun, Bernard. *Trends in Birth Rates in the United States since 1870* (Baltimore: Johns Hopkins University Press, 1958).

Rainwater, Lee. *And The Poor Get Children* (Chicago: Quadrangle Books, 1960).
——*Family Design: Marital Sexuality, Family Size and Contraception* (Chicago: Aldine Publishing Co., 1965).

Sauvy, Alfred. *Fertility and Survival: Population Problems from Malthus to Mao Tse-Tung* (New York: Criterion Books, 1961).

Spiegelman, Mortimer, *Introduction to Demography* (Chicago: Society of Actuaries, 1955); revised edition, Cambridge, Mass., Harvard University Press, 1968.

Thomlinson, Ralph. *Population Dynamics: Causes and Consequences of World Demographic Change* (New York: Random House, 1965). See especially

Chapter 9, "Fertility Trends and Differentials," pp. 159-185, and Chapter 10, "Family Planning," pp. 186-209.

Thompson, Warren S., and David T. Lewis. *Population Problems* (New York: McGraw-Hill Book Co., 1965).

Tien, H. Yuan. *Social Mobility and Controlled Fertility* (New Haven: College University Press, in collaboration with the Australian National University, Canberra, 1965).

Yaukey, David. *Fertility Differences in a Modernizing Country: A Survey of Lebanese Couples* (Princeton: Princeton University Press, 1961).

Articles and Pamphlets

Anderson, Ursula M., Rachel Jenss, William E. Mosher, and Virginia Richter. "The Medical, Social, and Educational Implications of the Increase in Out-of-Wedlock Births," *American Journal of Public Health,* vol. 56, No. 11 (November 1966), pp. 1866-1873.

Bachi, Roberto, and Judah Matras. "Family Size Preferences of Jewish Maternity Cases in Israel," *Milbank Memorial Fund Quarterly,* vol. 42, No. 2 (April 1964), pp. 38-56.

Bajema, Carl Jay. "Relation of Fertility to Educational Attainment," *Eugenics Quarterly,* vol. 13, No. 4 (December 1966), pp. 306-315.

Bakker, Cornelius B., and Cumeron R. Dightman. "Psychological Factors in Fertility Control," *Fertility and Sterility,* vol. 15, No. 5 (September-October 1964), pp. 559-567.

Bayer, Alan E. "Birth Order, Father's Education, and Achievement of the Doctorate." Paper presented at April 1966 Conference of the Population Association of America. For Abstract, see *Population Index,* vol. 32, No. 3 (July 1966), p. 326.

Beasley, Joseph D., Carl L. Harter, and Ann Fisher. "Attitudes and Knowledge Relevant to Family Planning among New Orleans Negro Women," *American Journal of Public Health,* vol. 56, No. 11 (November 1966), pp. 1847-1857.

Beegle, J. Allen. "Social Structure and Changing Fertility of the Farm Population," *Rural Sociology,* vol. 31, No. 4 (December 1966), pp. 415-427.

Berelson, Bernard, and Ronald Freedman. "A Study in Fertility Control," *Scientific American,* vol. 210, No. 5 (May 1964), pp. 29-37.

Bertrand, Alvin L. "The Emerging Rural South: Under Confrontation by Mass Society," *Rural Sociology,* vol. 31, No. 4 (December 1966), pp. 449-457.

Blake, Judith. "The Americanization of Catholic Reproductive Ideals," *Population Studies,* vol. 20, No. 1 (July 1966), pp. 27-43.

Burch, Thomas K. "The Fertility of North American Catholics: A Comparative Overview," *Demography,* vol. 3, No. 1 (1966), pp. 174-187. Spanish Summary.

Campbell, Arthur A. "Concepts and Techniques Used in Fertility Surveys," in *Emerging Techniques in Population Research* (New York: Milbank Memorial Fund, 1963), pp. 17-38.

——"Design and Scope of the 1960 Study of Growth of American Families," in *Research in Family Planning,* ed. Clyde V. Kiser (Princeton: Princeton University Press, 1962), pp. 167-183.

——"White-Nonwhite Differences in Family Planning in the United States," *Health, Education and Welfare Indicators,* February 1966, pp. 13-21.

Carlsson, Gösta. "The Decline of Fertility: Innovation or Adjustment Process," *Population Studies,* vol. 20, No. 2 (November 1966), pp. 149-174.

Day, Lincoln H. "Fertility Differentials among Catholics in Australia," *Milbank Memorial Fund Quarterly,* vol. 42, No. 2 (April 1964), pp. 57-83.

Dice, Lee R., Philip J. Clark, and Robert I. Gilbert. "Relation of Fertility to Education in Ann Arbor, Michigan, 1951-54" *Eugenics Quarterly,* vol. 11, No. 1 (March 1964) pp. 30-45.

——"Relation of Fertility to Occupation and to Income in the Male Population of Ann Arbor, Michigan, 1951-54," *Eugenics Quarterly,* vol. 11, No. 3 (September 1964), pp. 154-167.

——"Relation of Fertility to Religious Affiliation and to Church Attendance in Ann Arbor, Michigan, 1951-54," *Eugenics Quarterly,* vol. 12, No. 2 (June 1965), pp. 102-111.

Donnelly, J. F., C. E. Flowers, and R. N. Creadick. "Maternal, Fetal, and Environmental Factors in Prematurity," *American Journal of Obstetrics and Gynecology,* 88:918-931 (April 1, 1964).

Duncan, Otis Dudley. "Farm Background and Differential Fertility," *Demography,* vol. 2, (1965), pp. 240-249.

Duncan, Otis Dudley, Ronald Freedman, J. Mitchell Coble, and Doris P. Slesinger. "Marital Fertility and Size of Family Orientation," *Demography,* vol. 2, (1965), pp. 508-515.

Duncan, Otis Dudley, and Robert W. Hodge. "Cohort Analysis of Differential Fertility," in *International Population Conference, New York, 1961* (London: International Union for the Scientific Study of Population, 1963), I, 59-66.

Erhardt, Carl L., and Frieda G. Nelson. "Reported Congenital Malformations in New York City, 1958-59" *American Journal of Public Health and the Nation's Health,* vol. 54, No. 9 (September 1964), pp. 1489-1506.

Farley, Reynolds. "Recent Changes in Negro Fertility," *Demography,* vol. 3, No. 1 (1966), pp. 188-203.

Frank, Myrna E., and Clyde V. Kiser. "Changes in Social and Demographic Attributes of Women in Who's Who," *Milbank Memorial Fund Quarterly,* vol. 53, No. 1 (January 1965), pp. 56-75.

Frank, Richard, and Christopher Tietze. "Acceptance of an Oral Contraceptive Program in a Large Metropolitan Area," *American Journal of Obstetrics and Gynecology,* 93:122-127 (September 1, 1965).

Freedman, Deborah, Ronald Freedman, and P. K. Whelpton. "Size of Family and Preference for Children of Each Sex," *American Journal of Sociology,* vol. 66, No. 2 (September 1960), pp. 141-146.

Freedman, Ronald. "American Studies of Family Planning and Fertility: A Review of Major Trends and Issues," in *Research in Family Planning,* ed. Clyde V. Kiser (Princeton: Princeton University Press, 1962), pp. 211-227.

——and Larry Bumpass. "Fertility Expectations in the United States: 1962-1964," *Population Index,* vol. 32, No. 1 (April 1966), pp. 181-197.

Freedman, Ronald, and Lolagene C. Coombs. "Childspacing and Family Economic Position," *American Sociological Review,* vol. 31, No. 5 (October 1966), pp. 631-648.

——"Economic Considerations in Family Growth Decisions," *Population Studies,* vol. 20, No. 2 (November 1966), pp. 197-222.

Freedman, Ronald, Lolagene C. Coombs, and Larry Bumpass. "Stability and Change in Expectations about Family Size: A Longitudinal Study," *Demography,* vol. 2, (1965), pp. 250-275.

Gibson, J., and M. Young. "Social Mobility and Fertility," in *Biological Aspects of Social Problems,* ed. J. Meade and A. Parkes (New York: Plenum Press, 1965), pp. 69-80.

Goering, John M. "The Structure and Processes of Ethnicity: Catholic Family Size in Providence, Rhode Island," *Sociological Analysis,* vol. 26, No. 3 (Fall 1965), pp. 129-136.

Gold, Edwin M., Carl Erhardt, Harold Jacobziner, and Frieda G. Nelson. "Therapeutic Abortions in New York City: A 20-Year Review," *American Journal of Public Health and the Nation's Health,* vol. 55, No. 7 (July 1965), pp. 964-972.

Goldberg, David. "Another Look at the Indianapolis Fertility Data," *Milbank Memorial Fund Quarterly,* vol. 38, No. 1 (January 1960), pp. 23-36.

Goldscheider, Calvin. "Fertility of the Jews." Paper presented at the April 1966 Conference of the Population Association of America. Abstracted in *Population Index,* vol. 31, No. 3 (July 1966), p. 330.

—— "Nativity, Generation and Jewish Fertility," *Sociological Analysis,* vol. 26, No. 3 (Fall 1965), pp. 137-147.

——"Socio-economic Status and Jewish Fertility," *Jewish Journal of Sociology,* vol. 7, No. 2 (December 1965), pp. 221-237.

Goldstein, Sidney, and Kurt B. Mayer. "Residence and Status Differences in Fertility," *Milbank Memorial Fund Quarterly,* vol. 43, No. 3 (July 1965), pp. 291-310.

Goldzieher, J. W. "Future Approaches to Conception Control. Conclusion," *Pacific Medicine and Surgery,* 73:69-73 (February 1965).

Grabill, Wilson H., and Lee Jay Cho. "Methodology for the Measurement of Current Fertility from Population Data on Young Children," *Demography,* vol. 2, (1965), pp. 50-73.

Grabill, Wilson H., and Maria Davidson, "Recent Trends in Childspacing by American Women." Paper presented at the Meetings of the Population Association of America, Cincinnati, Ohio, April 28-29, 1967.

Hair, P. E. "Bridal Pregnancy in Rural England in Earlier Centuries," *Population Studies,* vol. 20, No. 2 (November 1966), pp. 233-243.

Hakanson, E. Y. "Family Planning in the City-County Hospital Setting: A Preliminary Report," *Minnesota Medicine,* 48:1557-1561 (November 1965).

Hall, R. E. "Therapeutic Abortion, Sterilization, and Contraception," *American Journal of Obstetrics and Gynecology,* 91:518-532 (February 15, 1965).

Hellman, Louis M. "One Galileo is Enough: Some Aspects of Current Population Problems," *Eugenics Review,* vol. 57, No. 4 (December 1965), pp. 161-166.

Jarrett, William H. "Family Size and Fertility Patterns of Participants in Family Planning Clinics," *Sociological Analysis,* vol. 25, No. 2 (Summer 1964), pp. 113-120.

Kiser, Clyde V. "Differential Fertility in the United States," in *Demographic and Economic Change in Developed Countries,* A Report of the National Bureau of Economic Research (Princeton: Princeton University Press, 1960), pp. 77-116.

——"Fertility Rates By Residence and Migration," *Proceedings, International Population Conference, Vienna, 1959* (Vienna: International Union for the Scientific Study of Population, 1959).

——"Types of Demographic Data of Possible Relevance to Population Genetics," *Eugenics Quarterly,* vol. 12, No. 2 (June 1965) pp. 72-84.

Kiser, Clyde V., and Myrna E. Frank. "Factors Associated with the Low Fertility of Nonwhite Women of College Attainment," *Milbank Memorial Fund Quarterly,* vol. 45, No. 4 (October 1967), pp. 427-449.

Kistner, R. W. "Medical Indications for Contraception: Changing Viewpoints," *Obstetrics and Gynecology,* 25:285-288 (February 1965).

Kunz, Phillip. "The Relation of Income and Fertility," *Journal of Marriage and the Family,* vol. 27, No. 4 (November 1965), pp. 509-513.

Leasure, J. William, and Nicholas W. Schrock. "White and Nonwhite Fertility by Census Tract for 1960," *Eugenics Quarterly,* vol. 11, No. 3 (September 1964), pp. 148-153.

Lehfeldt, H. "The First Five Years of Contraceptive Service in a Municipal Hospital," *American Journal of Obstetrics and Gynecology,* 93:727-733 (November 1, 1965).

Lunde, Anders S. "White-Nonwhite Fertility Differentials in the United States," *Health, Education and Welfare Indicators,* September 1965, pp. 23-38.

Marguilies, L. C. "Intrauterine Conception: A New Approach," *Obstetrics and Gynecology,* 24:515-520 (October 1964).

Matras, Judah. "The Social Strategy of Family Formation: Some Variations in Time and Space," *Demography,* vol. 2, (1965), pp. 349-362.

Nam, Charles B., and Mary G. Powers. "Variations in Socioeconomic Structure by Race, Residence, and the Life Cycle," *American Sociological Review,* vol. 30, No. 1 (February 1965), pp. 97-103.

New York Academy of Medicine [Group of Articles on Family Planning],

Bulletin of the New York Academy of Medicine, 42:46-64 (January 1966).

Pincus, Gregory, et al. "Effectiveness of an Oral Contraceptive," *Science,* vol. 130, No. 3367 (July 10, 1959), pp. 81-83.

Powers, Mary G. "Socioeconomic Status and the Fertility of Married Women," *Sociology and Social Research,* vol. 50, No. 4 (July 1966), pp. 472-482.

——"Progress in Family Planning," *Consumer Reports,* 29:400-403 (August 1964).

Rhodes, A. Lewis. "The Validity of 'Years of School Completed' as an Indicator of Educational Attainment." Paper presented at the April 1966 Conference of the Population Association of America. Abstracted in *Population Index,* vol. 32, No. 3 (July 1966), p. 327.

Ryder, Norman B. "The Cohort as a Concept in the Study of Social Change," *American Sociological Review,* vol. 30, No. 6 (December 1965), pp. 843-861.

Saunders, Lyle. *Family Planning Research and Evaluation: Needs for the Future* (New York: Ford Foundation, [1966]).

Spiegelman, Mortimer. "The Organization of the Vital and Health Statistics Monograph Program," in *Emerging Techniques for Population Research* (New York: Milbank Memorial Fund, 1963), pp. 230-249.

Sutton, Gordon F., and Gooloo S. Wunderlich. "Estimates of Marital Fertility Rates by Educational Attainment Using Survey of Mothers," Paper presented at the April 1966 Conference of the Population Association of America. Abstracted in *Population Index,* vol. 31, No. 3 (July 1966), pp. 330-331.

Westoff, Charles F., and Raymond H. Potvin. "Higher Education, Religion, and Women's Family Size Orientation," *American Sociological Review,* vol. 31, No. 4 (August 1966), pp. 489-491.

Westoff, Charles F., and Norman B. Ryder. "United States: Methods of Fertility Control, 1955, 1960, & 1965." *Studies in Family Planning,* A publication of The Population Council, No. 17 (February 1967), pp. 1-16.

——"The United States: The Pill and the Birth Rate, 1960-1965." *Studies in Family Planning,* A publication of The Population Council, No. 20 (June 1967), pp. 1-8.

Whelpton, Pascal K. "Cohort Analysis and Fertility Projection," in *Emerging Techniques in Population Research* (New York: Milbank Memorial Fund, 1963), pp. 39-64.

——"Why Did the United States' Crude Birth Rate Decline during 1957-1962?" *Population Index,* vol. 29, No. 2 (April 1963), pp. 120-125.

Woolf, C. M. "Stillbirths and Parental Age," *Obstetrics and Gynecology,* 26:1-8 (July 1965).

Public Documents

UNITED NATIONS.

Demographic Yearbook, 1965 (New York, 1966). Special topic: natality statistics; 1966 (New York, 1967).

Population Bulletin of the United Nations, No. 7 (1963). Special reference to conditions and trends of fertility in the world.

Proceedings of the World Population Conference, Belgrade, 1965. Vol. I, *Summary Report* (New York, 1966); Vol. II, *Selected Papers and Summaries: Fertility, Family Planning, Mortality* (New York, 1967); Vol. III, *Selected Papers and Summaries: Projections, Measurement of Population Trends* (New York, 1967); and Vol. IV, *Migration, Urbanization, Economic Development* (New York, 1967).

U.S. BUREAU OF THE CENSUS

U.S. Census of Population, 1960 (Washington: Government Printing Office, 1961—).

Vol. I, Parts 1 to 57. *Characteristics of the Population.* (The 57 parts are those for the United States as a whole, each of the 50 states and District of Columbia, Puerto Rico, Guam, Virgin Islands, American Samoa, and Canal Zone.)

PC(1)-1A. *Number of Inhabitants.*
PC(1)-1B. *General Population Characteristics.*
PC(1)-1C. *General Social and Economic Characteristics.*
PC(1)-1D. *Detailed Characteristics.*

Vol. II. Subject Reports.

PC(2)-1A. Nativity and Parentage.
PC(2)-1B. Persons of Spanish Surname.
PC(2)-1C. Nonwhite Population by Race.
PC(2)-1D. Puerto Ricans in the United States.
PC(2)-1E. Mother Tongue of the Foreign-Born.
PC(2)-2A. State of Birth.
PC(2)-2B. Mobility for States and State Economic Areas.
PC(2)-2C. Mobility for Metropolitan Areas.
PC(2)-2D. Lifetime and Recent Migration.
PC(2)-3A. Women by Number of Children Ever Born.
PC(2)-3B. Childspacing. (Report in preparation.)
PC(2)-3C. Women by Children Under 5 Years Old. (Report in preparation.)
PC(2)-4A. Families.
PC(2)-4B. Persons by Family Characteristics.
PC(2)-4C. Sources and Structure of Family Income.
PC(2)-4D. Age at First Marriage.
PC(2)-4E. Marital Status.
PC(2)-5A. School Enrollment.

PC(2)-5B. Educational Attainment.

PC(2)-5C. Socioeconomic Status. (Report in preparation.)

PC(2)-6A. Employment Status and Work Experience.

PC(2)-6B. Journey to Work.

PC(2)-6C. Labor Reserve.

PC(2)-7A. Occupational Characteristics.

PC(2)-7B. Occupation by Earnings and Education.

PC(2)-7C. Occupation by Industry.

PC(2)-7D. Characteristics of Teachers.

PC(2)-7E. Characteristics of Professional Workers.

PC(2)-8A. Inmates of Institutions.

PC(2)-8B. Income of the Elderly Population.

PC(2)-8C. Veterans.

Vol. III. Selected Area Reports.

PC(3)-1A. State Economic Areas.

PC(3)-1B. Size of Place.

PC(3)-1C. Americans Overseas.

PC(3)-1D. Standard Metropolitan Statistical Areas.

PC(3)-1E. Type of Place.

CURRENT POPULATION REPORTS.

"Marriage, Fertility, and Childspacing, August, 1959," Series P-20, No. 108 (July 12, 1961).

"Continuing Increase in the Average Number of Children Ever Born: 1940 to 1964," Series P-20, No. 136 (April 16, 1965).

"Fertility of the Population, June 1964 and March 1962," Series P-20, No. 147 (June 5, 1966).

Siegel, Jacob S., Meyer Zitter, and Donald S. Akers. "Projections of the Population of the United States, By Age and Sex: 1964 to 1985," Series P-25, No. 286 (July 1964).

OTHER

National Center for Health Statistics, *Natality Statistics Analysis,* United States– 1963, Public Health Service Publ. No. 1000, Series 21, No. 8 (March 1966).

National Center for Health Statistics, *Natality Statistics Analysis, United States– 1964,* Public Health Service Publ. No. 1000, Series 21, No. 11 (February 1967).

Schachter, Joseph, "Child Spacing as Measured from Data Enumerated in the Current Population Survey: United States, April 1950 to April 1954," *Vital Statistics–Special Reports,* vol. 47, No. 3 (October 9, 1958), pp. 81-127.

INDEX

Abortion, 2, 9, 13, 14, 18, 145
Abstinence, as contraception, 51
Adams, John Quincy, 97
Africa, 1, 3
Age, differential by: and maternal mortality, 9; and fetal mortality, 17, 18; and fecundity, 31; and contraception, 40, 42-45 *passim;* and residence, 61, 62, 67, 68-69, 74, 78, 79, 83, 107, 205; and socioeconomic factors, 148-149, 181-182, 208, 224-227 *passim;* in regions, 74, 75, 108, 109, 110; in counties, 99; and migration, 104, 107, 108-110; and foreign-born, 106; and region of birth, 108, 110; and ever-married women, 114; and proportion women married, 115; in birth cohorts, 115-116, 259-260, 263; in marriage cohorts, 117, 265-269 *passim;* of husband and wife jointly, 119, 120, 121; of husband, 120, 121; and illegitimacy, 137; and postwar baby boom, 150, 173; and education, women *(1940-60),* 168-170 *passim,* 173, 174, 176, 216; and occupation, 182, 184, 185, 190, 196-200 *passim,* 204, 205; and parity progression ratio, 200-203; and children ever born, 208, 209; and husband's income, 208, 210, 212, 216; and labor force status of women, 220-221; and employment of women, 223-225; and housing, 226-230 *passim;* and economic conditions, 250, 251. *See also* Marriage, age at
Age cohorts of completed fertility, 11
Age-parity-specific birth probabilities, 240-246, 250-252, 295-296
Alaska, 75, 76, 82
American Indians, 56, 67, 72
Arizona, 69
Asia, 1
Asian Indians, 56
Asiatic Barred Zone, 56
Australia, 10
Austrian birth, Americans of, 72, 73
Averages, moving, 243-244

Baby boom, *see* World War II, fertility after
Bean, Lee L., on mental illness and fertility, 21
Beegle, J. Allan, 96, 101
Bethesda, Md., 95
Birth cohort, *see* Cohorts, birth
Birth control, *see* Contraception
Birth-death ratio in SMSA's, 87
Birth injuries, 9

Birth probabilities, age-parity-specific, 240-246, 250-252, 295-296
Birth rates: after World War II, 1, 2, 57, 74, 238; outside U.S., 2, 3, 5; U.N. prediction for *1965-2000,* 3; crude, 5, 57, 81-84 *passim,* 237; *1915-47,* 57; *1950-65,* 59; intrinsic, 59; District of Columbia, *1960,* 82; Catholic, 234; age-order-specific, defined, 240; central, cumulative, 294, 295
Births: live, *1963,* 8; attendance at and place of delivery, *1963, 1964,* 9, 18, 19, 28; and excess fertility, 47; region of, 108, 110; order of, and birth probabilities, 251; timing of, 260-264; order of, and color differential, 276, 277-278, 280; order of, and cohort analysis, 276-282; records of, and data on children ever born, 305-310
Bogue, Donald J., 97
Boston SMSA, 89
Bryant, W. Keith, 96, 101

California, 69, 134
Campbell, A.C., 231
Canada, 2, 3
Canadian birth, Americans of, 70
Catholic Church, 2, 33, 51
Catholics: and contraception, 40, 42, 51; and fecundity impairments, 42; fertility rates of, 231, 233, 234; and family planning, 234
Census: of England and Wales, *1911,* 180, 217; of British family, *1946,* 265
Census, U.S.: *1890,* 114; *1910,* 180, 217, 265, 272; *1920, 1930,* 180; *1940,* 11, 27, 147, 180, 196, 265, 269; *1950,* 11, 13, 27, 147, 180, 181, 182, 219, 265, 269; *1960,* 11, 13, 27-28, 56, 60, 68, 84, 106, 108, 147, 180, 182, 184, 208, 212, 219, 220-221, 230, 265, 269, 272, 297-301, 307-310; Current Evaluation Study of, 302-303, 305-307
Census, U.S. Bureau of the, 3, 180, 292, 302
Censuses, U.S.: factors affecting reliability, 11; questions on education in, 147; questions in on children ever born, 180, 297-299; questions on occupation in, since *1820,* 180; question on religion in, 229-231; quality of data of, 297-303, 305-310; comparisons between, 299-300
Central birth rate, 294, 296
Central cities, 63, 85-87, 89, 90, 92; defined, 85
CES, *see* Current Evaluation Study